TRADITIONAL HEALTH PRACTICES OF KUMAONI WOMEN

CONTINUITY AND CHANGE

Concept's Discovering Himalayas Series

- People's Participation in Himalayan Eco-System Development: A Plan for Action/ **M.L. Dewan**
- Nut Fruits for the Himalayas (CDHS)/ **M.L. Dewan, M.C. Nautiyal** and **V.K. Sah**
- Vedic Philosophy and Himalayan Eco-System Development/ **M.L. Dewan** and **B.D. Joshi (Eds)**
- People's Movement for Himalayan Rejuvenation : 2nd Revised and enlarged edition/ **M.L. Dewan**
- Water User's Associations In Andhra Pradesh: A Quick Assessment from the field / **Jasveen Jairath**
- Images of Women in the Folksongs of Garhwal Himalayas / **Anjali Capila**
- Himalayan Snow and Glaciers : Associated Environmental Problems, Progress and Prospects/ **Jagdish Bahadur**

About the Author

Anjali Capila is presently Associate Professor in the Department of Community Resource Management and Extension at the Lady Irwin College, New Delhi. She teaches Development Communication and has worked extensively with women at the grassroots level in North India, especially Haryana and Uttaranchal in the past two decades. She is the Deputy Coordinator for the Development Support Assistance (DSA) Unit funded by the University Grants Commission, and Coordinator of the Michigan State University Study Abroad Programme, at the Lady Irwin College.

Based on her Ph.D. research her first book *'Images of Women in the Folk Songs of Garhwal Himalayas'* is a pioneering research on cultural communication and understanding the lives of women in hill communities as reflected in their songs.

She serves on several technical advisory committees like the 'Environmental Restoration Project through Watershed Management' funded by the Indo-Canadian Environment Facility (ICEF) for the NGO, INHERE in the Kumaon Hills. She has also been a consultant to CHIRAG – Central Himalayan Rural Action Group for setting up a learning centre for adolescent girls in the hills.

Her deep personal interests include areas associated with women's development, particularly in fields like Panchayati Raj, information on health issues including reproductive health and HIV/AIDS. A consultant for the United Nations, she has worked with UNIFEM on 'Mapping HIV/AIDS education programmes for student youth in India – a gender sensitive approach'; UNICEF on developing IEC materials for training field functionaries in the ICDS programmes.

Her publications are self-illustrated and despite the busy travelling and teaching schedule, she has time to devote to her family and close friends and music.

Address : 4, Doctor's Lane, New Delhi - 110 001 (India) Tel. : 23364529.
E-mail : dr_capila@rediffmail.com.

Concept's Discovering Himalayas Series-8

TRADITIONAL HEALTH PRACTICES OF KUMAONI WOMEN

CONTINUITY AND CHANGE

ANJALI CAPILA, *Ph.D.*
Reader, Lady Irwin College,
University of Delhi
Delhi

CONCEPT PUBLISHING COMPANY, NEW DELHI-110059

ISBN 81-8069-146-2

First Published 2004

Published and Printed by
Ashok Kumar Mittal
Concept Publishing Company
A/15-16, Commercial Block, Mohan Garden,
NEW DELHI-110059 (India)

Phones : 25351460, 25351794
Fax : 091-11-25357103
E-mail : publishing@conceptpub.com

FOR

- The tiny lights on the hill side
  That merge into the stars . . . . .

- The little paths
  That hug the mountain slopes . . . . .

- The layers and layers of mountains
  That rise into the majestic Himalayas . . . . .

- The 'Home' away from home
  That provided space, care and support . . . . .

- All the Kumaoni Women.
  The Community Health Workers,
  And the Dais,
  Whose wisdom enriched this journey. . . . .

PREFACE

The present book examines the traditional health practices of women in the Kumaon Hills, Uttaranchal, with special reference to Reproductive and Child Health. Modern Health-Care systems are primarily concerned with the 'medicalization of life' which has taken away the power of people to heal and take care of themselves. This fragmented approach to health as a sector of development has ignored the holistic knowledge system of traditional societies where health is seen as a 'way of life'.

To reiterate the interconnectedness of culture, health and development, a study was conducted in the Nainital district of the Kumaon Hills where the NGO CHIRAG (Central Himalayan Rural Action Group) has been working in the area of health-care for the past fifteen years. The methodology, combines the quantitative data from a questionnaire and integrates the 'unheard voices' of the women of Kumaon who are the holders and practitioners of the traditional wisdom and knowledge. Community Health Workers, Dais, and women and adolescent girls from various villages participated in this research. Their 'dialogue' has enriched this journey, building towards an alternate paradigm for understanding women and their health.

Chapter 1 introduces the conceptual framework and builds on Ivan Illich's concept of medicalization and commercialization of life. It introduces the major health concerns of women in India as outlined by various authors.

Chapter 2 establishes the context, *i.e.* the geographical, historical, cultural and demographic profile of Kumaon. This background provides the canvas against which the traditional health practices, myths and rituals related to health have been studied.

In Chapter 3 in order to understand the health-care delivery system the detailed primary health-care system of the government in Nainital district has been outlined. Also the health-care infrastructure of the NGO CHIRAG has been presented in detail to understand how a community health programme is put into action at the grassroots, what services are provided and what is the role of health-care providers.

Chapter 4 examines the reproductive and child health management practices of Kumaoni women with special reference to menstruation, pregnancy, delivery, antenatal and postnatal care, immunization and child health. Voices of women, Dais and CHWs (Community Health Workers) are integrated with the findings, in order to bring authenticity to the research. Interviews with various resource persons have also been added to bring in a wider perspective on the issue. The major health concerns of women, their traditional knowledge and wisdom related to each phase of their reproductive life and the common foods eaten and avoided by them for the preventive, promotive and curative aspects of health care have also been included.

Chapter 5 focuses on the emerging trends of this study. What emerges is that women's health is linked to community participation, traditional and sustainable agriculture, natural resource management practices, water resources, the habitat, her self-esteem, her position in the family and society, her education status, food habits, access to information and male participation. Some salient findings have been presented as highlights of the first part of the book.

Chapter 6 is based on the insights from the first phase of the book and addresses the health needs of adolescent girls in Uttaranchal. A module on Reproductive and Child Health was developed keeping culture-specifics of this region in mind and building on the traditional knowledge and wisdom of women. As a follow up, an action plan was devised for training adolescent girls in collaboration with the NGO, CHIRAG. This training intervention was a much-needed initiative that was appreciated by the girls and the community at large.

16th March, 2004 ANJALI CAPILA

ACKNOWLEDGEMENTS

There are many people who walked with me on this journey to the Kumaon Hills. I gratefully acknowledge the following:

- Dr. Satinder Bajaj, Director, Lady Irwin College and members of the Governing Body for enabling me to pursue this research.
- The entire CHIRAG family, especially Kanai Lall, Chairman, and his wife Lakshmidi, Rajesh Thadani, Executive Director and his wife Ritika; Bipin Kabedwal, Sunder Nial, Anil Bajpai, Pratima Singh, Laksmi Kumari and Adil Rizvi for their support both in terms of inviting me as a consultant for the adolescent learning centre and for providing the logistics for the extensive field work.
- The Health team at the Sargakhet clinic of CHIRAG: Ram Singh, Gangu, Neomi, Kunti and Zarina for sharing their experiences in the area of maternal and child health. Lata Harbola, in-charge of the women's programme for accompanying me on my visits to several villages, and Basanti, Durga Bisht and Kamla Bisht.
- The KSK team headed by Pratima Singh, Lalita, Ganga Aneria, Radha Bisht, Rekha Kumari; all of whom made the dream of a Kishori Shikshan Kendra a reality.
- The Community Health Workers and Dais whom I interacted with over a period of one year. Their warmth and enthusiasm in participating in my journey of understanding the traditional health practices of women in the Kumaon Hills was indeed special.
- All the women in the villages I visited with the health team of Central Himalayan Rural Action Group (CHIRAG), for sharing their wisdom and health concerns with me, especially Kishni Devi whose knowledge and 'common sense' regarding health issues facing women in the Kumaon Hills always stumped me.
- The Deputy Chief Medical Officer, Nainital district; the staff and doctors at the Primary Health Centre, Padampuri; and the ANMs who shared their work roles and other concerns with me.
- Bharat and Sonali Bisht from INHERE, located at Masi, Almora district; Dr. Sushil Sharma from AAROHI, for sharing their experiences about the issues facing the new hill state of Uttaranchal and providing the contextual background for my work. Yashodhara Das, Abhijit Das from SAHYOG, Almora for sharing relevant materials.

- Reetu Sogani from AADHAR, Almora district, who spent several days sharing the traditional knowledge and wisdom of women and their food consumption patterns.
- Bhagwati Pande who has worked with the health team of SAHYOG at the grassroots level for providing useful insights into the rituals and practices of women in the Kumaon Hills.
- Vinita Nathani, Executive Director, PRERNA, New Delhi, and her training team Bimla Raj and Pushpa for agreeing to train adolescent girls in Reproductive and Child Health Issues in Kumaon.
- Prof. S.C. Malik for valuable theoretical and editorial inputs that went into several drafts.
- Discussions with Prof. M.M. Agrawal, Sharat Kumar, Janet Chawla (MATRIKA), Mary and Harry Andrews (Michigan State University, (USA), Kusum and Prem Budhwar; all of which added different and rich dimensions to the work.
- Shri Pritam Singh Mehra and his family, Bimal, Manoj and others for providing insights into the changing scenario in Kumaon.
- All my colleagues in the department of Community Resource Management and Extension, Lady Irwin College especially Mrs. H.K. Sawhney and Dr. Archna Kumar for their interest in my work. Also Ms. Sushma Zutshi, Assistant Librarian, Shri K.N. Jha, and Mr. Ajit Kumar at the India International Centre Library for their support.
- Elizabeth Huff and Beth Taylor students from Michigan State University who were working in CHIRAG as part of the Lady Irwin College 'study abroad programme', for all the photographs in the book. Elizabeth also assisted me in the analysis of the Mother and Child Health management practices in Kumaon Hills.
- The support of my family, especially 'Appanji', my mother-in-law, Vinay Capila, my husband, Pranav Capila, my younger son who designed the cover and my elder son Ishan and his wife Priya.
- My parents, siblings, friends and other family members for their support and interest in my work.
- Dr. M. L. Dewan for his constant encouragement and support, and Shri Ashok Mittal for undertaking this publication.

And, finally, no work can be accomplished without the grace of 'Thakur' Shri Ramakrishna and Sharada 'Ma'.

CONTENTS

LIST OF PLATES

PROLOGUE

The songs of the women of Garhwal Himalayas have become a part of my being. My previous book *Images of Women in the Folk Songs of Garhwal Himalayas – A Participatory Research* (2002) had focused on the song as a source material for understanding culture and the lives of women in the hill communities. While the songs had revealed many aspects of the life of the women, one issue that I had not looked at was the Health Care Practices of women, their access to Health Services and their traditional knowledge and wisdom related to health.

On a visit to the Kumaon Hills (Sargakhet, Mukteshwar) in the summer of 2001, I saw a small white building with a sloping roof and an orange logo representing the 'Diva' (oil lamp), light. I walked in and introduced myself to the resident doctor, Dr. Sivaraman, his Clinic supervisor Shri Ram Singh and to the three women whose warm smiling faces disarmed me totally; they were Neomi, Kunti and Zarina (all Health Extension Workers) with the clinic, I had supposedly walked into.

We talked about their work in Health Care, the area they covered, the services they provided and the conversation meandered to 'who they were' and how they were there. "The logo outside the clinic building represents the acronym of the NGO we work for CHIRAG (Central Himalayan Rural Action Group), Kanai Lall is the chairperson and founding member of this NGO", they continued. In a few moments, I was on the phone introducing myself to him, and had got myself an invitation to have 'brunch' with him and his wife Laxmi the next day at Sitla.

The walk to Sitla (6,800ft. above m.s.l.) from the P.W.D. Rest House at Mukteshwar, takes about thirty minutes. The path goes through a forest of Oak, Rhododendron and rich undergrowth. A dried up natural spring with a small temple on the side, under a tree had me transfixed, as I moved along the stony path thinking about my meeting with Kanai Lall.

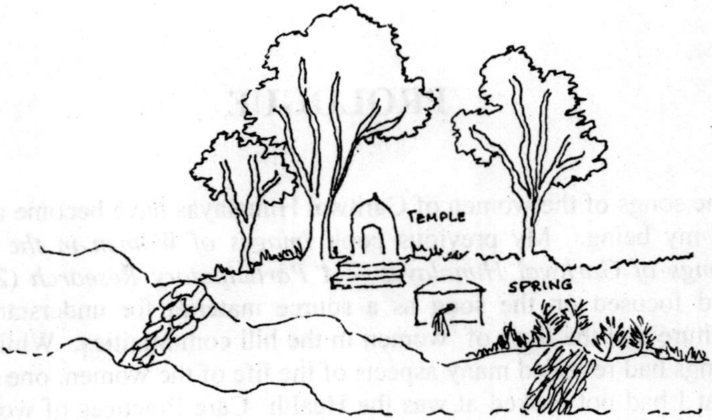

Diagram 1 : On the way to Sitla

The Sitla estate, home for Kanai and Laxmi for over two decades envelopes one in its wilderness. A stony path leads one to the house; and the garden so exquisitely kept by Laxmi Lall overawes one with the variety of flowers, bushes and trees. Fortunately for me it was a clear day. It had rained the previous night, and across the house rising above, to touch the sky were the majestic Himalayas – Nanda Devi, Trishul, Chaukhamba, Neelkanth, Nandagunthi, Nandakot and the Panchchuli peaks. Where does one look I thought, the eyes moving quickly to absorb everything?

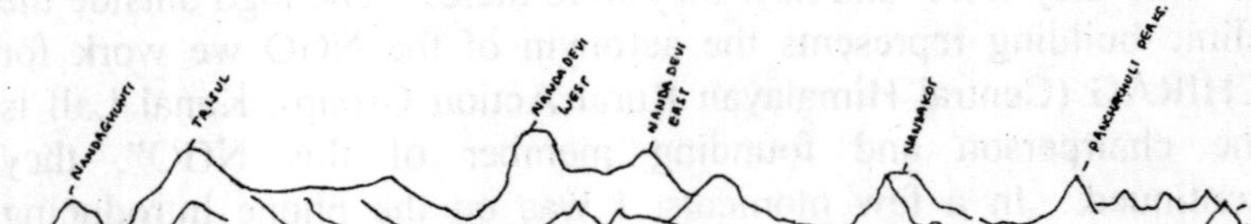

Diagram 2 : The Kumaon Himalayas as I saw them from Sitla

The silence was broken by Kanai Lall's warm welcome and we soon got down to an animated conversation about my work in the Garhwal Himalayas, some common friends (the Late Joseph Allen Stein and Margaret) and my job at the Lady Irwin College.

Kanai-Da, as I had now started referring to him said, " I have a dream for the adolescent girls of Uttaranchal who are the future mothers of this society, if they are given training in skills or issues related to their lives in the hill communities one would be making a great contribution to their well being". In fact after saying this he produced a concept note on this issue, and asked me for my comments.

We were soon joined by Rajesh Thadani, the Executive Director of CHIRAG who also felt that perhaps this programme should start with the Reproductive and Child health component, as Health was a major area of focus with CHIRAG. My research work with post-graduate students at the Department of Community Resource Management, Lady Irwin College, had recently been focusing on assessing the Information needs of Adolescent Girls with special reference to Reproductive Health Issues in the urban slums of Delhi. I thought, this work in Kumaon would provide me with an opportunity to expand the horizons of our 'learning' in a different socio-cultural environment. I was completely enrolled into this dream.

On returning to the college, with motivation and support from the people who had seen me interact with the women in the Kumaon Hills, I presented an application for a one year sabbatical to conduct research on "Existing Health Systems in the Kumaon Hills", leading to the education of adolescent girls. I was delighted that the leave was sanctioned for a period of one year, October 2001 to October 2002. Another year of working in the mountains with women filled me with joy, as I had already spent three years in the Garhwal Himalayas listening to the women's songs.

I joined the CHIRAG family as an Honorary Consultant for the 'Yuvati Shikshan Kendra", as it was then called to develop training modules on reproductive and child health for the adolescent girls in the CHIRAG outreach villages. Since it was a new project there was a lot of flexibility and freedom to build this 'brick by brick'. Ms. Pratima Singh who had joined CHIRAG in July 2001, with a Master's degree in Social Work, was in-charge of this programme.

I had several meetings in Delhi with professionals who had been working in this area, Ms. Abha Bhaiya who founded Jagori, Ms. Malini Sharma from Nirantar, Ms. Mridula Seth from UNFPA, Ms. Vinita Nathani from PRERANA, and they all were of the opinion that we should not reinvent the wheel, since there was so much material already prepared in training on RCH. They suggested that I do a desk review of available modules and build the regional-cultural specifics into that.

THE PROCESS

While I visited various libraries and institutions to collect material, Pratima Singh designed a questionnaire for adolescent girls in the CHIRAG target area (32 villages) to find out the perceptions of the adolescent girls to the 'Yuvati Shikshan Kendra' and also identify areas of their interest (presented in Chapter 6).

Based on the desk review the next step was to develop a five day training module on Reproductive and Child Health for adolescent girls. However, at this juncture I felt that it was absolutely imperative to study the existing health care practices of women especially during the reproductive phase, to identify their major health concerns, their health-seeking behaviour, access to health care, the rituals and ceremonies associated with the important life-cycle events like menstruation, pregnancy, delivery, post-delivery and child rearing. Also, it would be important to understand their food consumption patterns, changes if any, and how they address their major health problems, i.e. their traditional knowledge and wisdom. This background I felt would be important as adolescent girls also live in the same socio-cultural environment and this knowledge would help to contextualise their learning.

Keeping the above in mind, Pratima Singh, Ms. Laxmi Kumari (who has extensive field experience of working with CHIRAG on the Swajal project) and I developed a questionnaire, which went through several changes before it was finalized for administration in the field (The details are presented in Chapter 4).

Since I had a two-fold task, one of writing my book and the other of assisting with the Yuvati Shikshan Kendra, while the quantitative data was being collected by the Health Extension Workers of CHIRAG, I interacted with at least 200 women at the village level in order to understand from their lived experience all the aspects related to Health-Care Practices mentioned above. Their voices are presented as verbatim reports interwoven in the text in Chapter 4. On daily field visits with the health team to a village, I had conversations with Community Health Workers and Dais to understand in detail the delivery practices and document in their knowledge and wisdom.

In order to get a holistic picture I interacted with women in villages even where CHIRAG did not have its health outreach programme, but was working in other sectors. I accompanied Lata Harbola, in-charge of the women's programmes, especially the Self-

Help Groups (SHGs) and income generation, on her field visits to villages Sunderkhal, Gunialekh, Sarna and Kanarkha in Dhari block, Nainital district. The women who had gathered for the SHG meeting, became an important entry point for interactions on Health Practices. (Diagram 3)

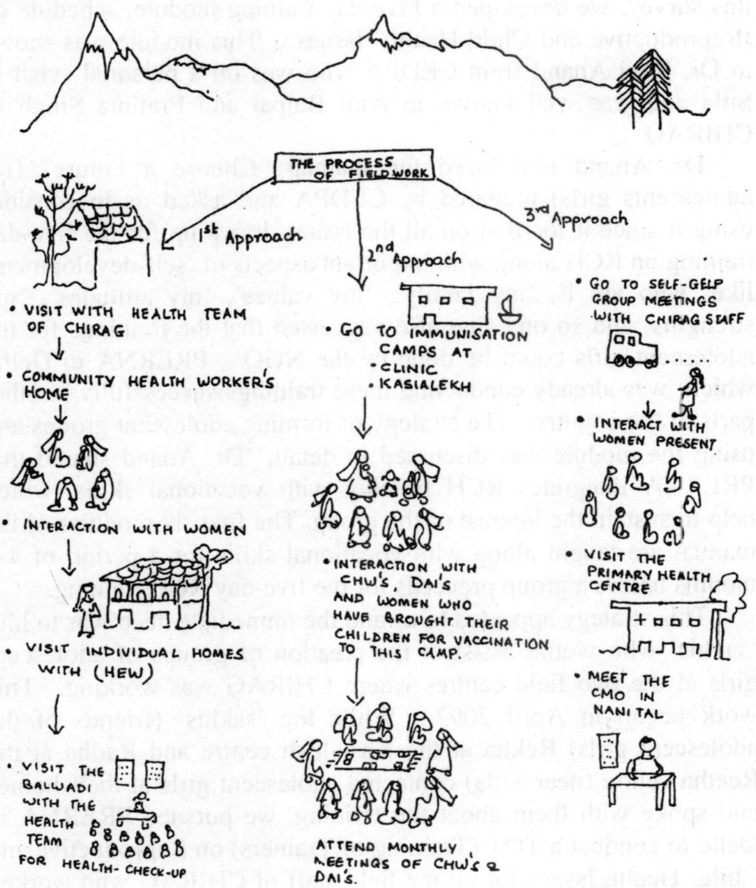

Diagram 3 : The process of Field Work

Since women identify closely with all aspects of their reproductive life there was always a great amount of sharing. There was so much that I was 'listening' to, that in a way reproducing that energy in words is not easy. In my earlier work also I have referred to listening to the 'hum' behind the words, the 'in-dwelling' and articulating the lived experience of women into constructs of knowledge, which indeed is a challenge to all field workers (Capila : 2002). The interviews with the community health workers and Dais are also presented in Chapter 4.

Based on the quantitative and qualitative aspects emerging from this survey, we developed a Five-day training module, schedule on 'Reproductive and Child Health Issues'. This module was shown to Dr. Ravi Anand from CEDPA who was on a personal visit to Sitla and was well known to Anil Bajpai and Pratima Singh of CHIRAG.

Dr. Anand introduced the manual "Choose a Future" (for adolescents girls) prepared by CEDPA and asked us to consider using it since it focused on all the issues drawn up for the five-day training on RCH along with important aspects of 'self-development' like 'who am I', 'my family', 'my values', 'my attitudes', 'my strengths' and so on. She also suggested that the trainings for the adolescent girls could be done by the NGO – PRERNA in Delhi, which was already conducting these trainings successfully in other parts of the country. The strategy of forming adolescent groups and using the module was discussed in detail, Dr. Anand shared that PRERNA integrates RCH training with vocational skills, which help to sustain the interest of the group. The first six modules of the manual are taught along with vocational skills for a period of 4-6 months before a group proceeds for the five-day RCH training.

This strategy appealed to us and the immediate need was to hire 'sakhis' who would assist in the creation of groups of adolescent girls at the two field centres where CHIRAG was working. This work began in April 2002. While the 'sakhis' (friends of the adolescent girls) Rekha at the Kasialekh centre and Radha at the Reetha centre (near Sitla) contacted adolescent girls at their homes and spoke with them about the training, we pursued PRERNA in Delhi to conduct a TOT (Training of Trainers) on Reproductive and Child Health Issues for all the field staff of CHIRAG who worked in the health and social sector.

By the end of April the group at the Reetha centre was formed and on three days a week they were given two hours of vocational training in stitching and tailoring, and two hours of life-skill education. The second group was formed in June 2002. The socio-economic and cultural environment of these adolescent girls as well as their educational status was different from the girls at the first centre, and more efforts were needed to sustain this group.

The training of trainees for CHIRAG staff was conducted by the PRERNA team in early June 2002 and this was followed by a more detailed RCH training in August 2002. Since it was the health team and the field staff working in the social sector that were indirect contact with the families of the adolescent girls, it was crucial to educate them about the salient features of the manual "Choose a Future" and orient them to its innovative methodology, so that they could answer any queries that the parents had.

The integrated sessions of vocational training and life-skill education continued at both the centers (Monday, Tuesday, Wednesday at Reetha and Thursday, Friday, Saturday at Kasialekh). Several approaches were used to strengthen the group at Kasialekh, follow up home visits, parents meetings and what was really unique was that members of the CHIRAG health and social sector team adopted a girl from the community and became *'abhivavaks'* (parents) to her, in terms of support and convincing her parents about the value of her participation and presence.

The big achievement came when the first batch of adolescent girls of twenty from the Reetha centre were trained at a Residential Camp for five days at Dhokane Training Centre (Almora district) in September 2002. Since the second batch was created later their training was held in November 2002. The details of the training and their impact are presented in Chapter 6.

The above is a brief description of the process and the issues addressed in this book. It is not often that research translates into action, all in the period of one year. For me that was a new and rich experience and perhaps the 'learning' on this journey can give insights to other such initiatives.

PART – I

TRADITIONAL HEALTH PRACTICES OF KUMAONI WOMEN

1

INTRODUCTION

1.1 What is Health Care for Women? Conceptual Framework – Traditional and Modern

Modernity has brought about fragmentation in every sphere of human society because one of the underlying premises was to make separate categories and treat them as if these are independent of each other. It was only at the end of the late twentieth century the realization came that this perception was totally flawed since it had created havoc at every level of human society, not only in terms of wars but disease, epidemics and ill-health especially for those living in the underdeveloped or developing nations. Modern thought, it is obvious, distinguishes, culture, politics, religion, ethics, etc. as separate and independent units without giving any due consideration to their intimate interconnectedness. From various researches carried out, we know now that in earlier traditional societies, generally speaking, these subparts or segments were integrated into a holistic whole; culture touched every aspect of life, as did religion. These were interchangeable concepts in terms of interconnectedness at the day-to-day level of living.

In pre-modern societies, in all probability and especially in India, health was a part of culture, defined as a total way of life by the people themselves. Thinking about health was integrated into the way of living as a whole. Here, the important notion was to focus on creating a "healthy living", meaning thereby that the physical, social, mental and religious aspects were intertwined with each other. In contrast, today's focus generally is on curing diseases as such, within a simple one-to-one model:

cause ⟷ effect ⟷ cure.

On the other hand, earlier, life-style and living in general was a holistic way of being. It appears that both at the conceptual and practical level, because health practices were encompassed within the many shared aspects of traditional knowledge, these were also connected with one or the other aspects of culture. In this sense these health practices and health care in general was 'life-giving'. This is why today it is very imperative that development models take the following linkages into account:

Culture ⟷ Health ⟷ Development

In other words, health cannot be divorced from culture, or a way of life as a whole. To illustrate, this traditional wisdom, in one of the interviews, Kishni Devi from village Sargakhet, said ".... health and life are not two separate things, for example, trees are connected to life, they are deified, plants such as tulsi, neem are sacred. This kind of knowledge is inherent in the culture of Kumaon, it is integral to our way of life."

The present work focuses on the health practices of women in Kumaon hills and the knowledge-related to these practices. The sectoral approach to health has been fragmented so far. On the other hand, in a holistic approach health is integrated with the way of life.

Health ⟷ Culture

How it is so, is shown by the fact that behind traditional practices governing women in Kumaon hills, especially during the important events of their lifecycle like menstruation, childbirth, and the rearing of children, there is knowledge of how these practices contribute to 'health'. In short, there is a conceptual connection between culture, considered as a way of life and the social practices, which embody them. Health through the traditional knowledge of life is inherent in all its aspects.

Culture ⟷ social practices ⟷ traditional knowledge ⟷ health

However, it is equally true that when the traditional knowledge behind a practice is lost, the practice becomes a superstition, and therefore, it becomes in many cases counterproductive.

Because our living conditions are sufficiently changed in the modern times, and we are using many new food items and other consumer products, changes in our social environment make these practices either redundant or very difficult to engage in. Only when we retrieve the knowledge behind these practices may one see whether they still serve a useful purpose.

In the context of health, thus, giving value to traditional practices is not just for the sake of giving value but also for the positive benefit that we may derive from them. The usefulness lies here because of their rootedness in the culture, i.e. these are easily understood because of having a moral backing to them, in the sense of being known through a familiar worldview rather than an alien one. Alternatively, if the same benefits can be derived by more efficient means then one may modify these practices without the loss of value that is attached to them. The idea is sound because it is suited to the cultural resources of the practitioners in that society.

Revealed knowledge is most likely the source of traditional knowledge, and is often sheer common sense logic, backed by a worldview that reflects an aura of sacredness, i.e. it is sanctified in the sense that it gives meaning to the people who practice it. Thus, calling it or perceiving that knowledge as revealed is to establish and justify its authority for posterity.

1.2 Medicalization – Technologization of Traditional Health Care Systems

The above brief statement implies that today a reassessment is required of what one defines as a good health care system. This implicitly means that a study of health, within the terms of a pragmatic conceptual framework must equally re-examine the taken for granted notions of 'progress' and its publicized benefits. A model of social assessment of technological progress is what Illich (1976) uses to look at health as a sector of development. The paradigm he uses in terms of optimal limited health care, is what he calls as the recovery from society in terms of iatrogenetic disease which will be explained later on. This he says is a political task, not a professional one, which for him must be based on a consensus of grassroots voices between the civil rights to an equitable health care. In this way, rightly, the social commitment to provide citizens with unlimited outputs of the medical system threatens to destroy the environmental and cultural conditions. It has led to a life, which has become so fragmented that it is far removed from our inner harmony. In this disjointed world is it possible to live a life of autonomous healing?

Illich continues to say that it is only a political ideology aimed at the limitation of professional health management that will enable people to rediscover their powers for healthcare. He continues in this strain to say that a professional physician based health care system has grown beyond critical bounds, and it is sickening for three major reasons as follows:

1. It produces clinical damage that outweighs its potential benefits.
2. It enhances even as it obscures the political conditions that render society unhealthy.
3. It tends to mystify and to expropriate the power of the individual to heal himself and to shape his or her environment maintenance.

For more than a century analysis of disease trends has shown that the environment is the primary determinant of the state of general health of any populations. The social history of attitudes towards illness, for instance, have shown that food, water, and air in correlation with the level of socio-political equality and the cultural mechanisms that make it possible to keep the population stable, play the decisive role in determining how healthy grownups feel and at what age adults tend to die. Today, a new kind of malnutrition is becoming the most rapid modern epidemic. One-third to one-half of humanity go hungry every night, perhaps the percentage was less in the stone age, so that at a time of the greatest technical power, starvation is an institution which no one seems to be willing to admit. Thus, while on the one hand, one-third of humanity survives on a level of undernourishment, on the other more and more rich people absorb even greater amounts of poisons and mutagens in their food. (Illich, *ibid*)

It is equally true that some modern medical techniques indeed have been optimally effective when they have become part of the culture and environment, and in this manner have affected changes in general health. Among these are contraception devices, small-pox vaccination of infants, and such non-medical health measures as the treatment of water and sewage, the use of soap and scissors and some antibacterial and insecticidal procedures. It has been found out that the new techniques for recognizing and treating such conditions as pernicious anemia and hypertension, etc. redefines but has not reduced morbidity. This is most likely because often doctors tend to gather where the climate is healthy, where the water is clean, and where people are employed and can pay for their services. It is well known that hardly any doctors, especially the younger ones seldom want to work in rural, village areas, and very hard to get any doctor to work in the clinics in the mountains. Awe-inspiring medical technology has combined with egalitarian rhetoric to create the impression that contemporary medicine is highly effective. Illich clearly shows that this is very doubtful, because there are skyrocketing medical expenditures destined for the kind of diagnosis and treatment

At another level the so-called health professionals have an even deeper culturally health denying effect in so far as they destroy the potential of people to deal with their human weakness, vulnerability, and uniqueness in a personal and autonomous way. The patient in the grip of contemporary medicine is but one instance of mankind in the grip of its pernicious techniques. This cultural iatrogenesis (Illich, 1976, p.34) is the ultimate backlash of hygienic progress in the paralysis of healthy responses to suffering, impairment and death. It occurs when people accept health management designed on the engineering model, as if to produce a commodity which is called "better health". Iatrogenesis has become medically irreversible at all levels: a feature built right into the medical profession. This inevitably results in the managed maintenance of life on high levels of sub-lethal illness. This is the ultimate evil of "medical progress".

The reversal of this dangerous trend can only come from within man and not from yet another managed source depending once again on presumptuous expertise and subsequent mystification, the interaction of culture and health care, just as culture and development should go hand in hand, in fact culture being kept as the dominant parameter for an all around healthy growth of society. Until recently, before the modern era, medicine attempted to enhance what occurs in nature. It fostered the tendency of wounds to heal, of blood to clot, and of bacteria to overcome by natural immunity.

Today, the net contribution of medicine to society's burden of disease comes from outside the profession. Illich uses the word "social iatrogenesis" to mean that medicine undermines health not only through direct aggression against individuals but also through the impact of its social organization on the total milieu, i.e. when medical damage to individual health is produced by a socio-political mode of transmission. This is when people are rendered impotent to cope with their milieu, when health care is turned into a standardized item, a staple; when all suffering is "hospitalized" and homes become inhospitable to birth, sickness, and death; when the language in which people could experience their bodies is turned into bureaucratic jargon; or when suffering, mourning, and healing outside the patient role are labelled a form of deviance. In this way when professional autonomy degenerates into a radical monopoly and people are rendered impotent to cope with their milieu, social iatrogenesis becomes the main product of the medical organization. This can only be reversed by political action that retrenches professional dominance. This remedy would shake the foundations of medical power much more profoundly than any catalogue of medicine's technical faults!

Each culture has its own characteristic perception of disease and thus its unique hygienic mask. Disease takes its features from the physician who casts the actors into one of the available roles. Medicine is a moral enterprise and therefore built into it. In traditional societies it is obvious that in the exercise of medical skill, the recognition of moral power is implied. But for modern man, medicine is exercised by full-timed specialists who control large populations by means of bureaucratic institutions, exercising a unique kind of control over their own work. The divorce between medicine and morality has been defined on the ground that medical categories unlike those of law and religion, rest on scientific foundations exempt from moral evaluation. "This is narcissistic scientism, to claim to be value-free cure and care which obviously is nonsense, and the phenomenal rise in cost of health service is a clear example." (Illich, *ibid.*)

In the same manner there is a pharmaceutical invasion, and cultures have become a prey to this, and it usually causes more damage than profit to health. Ultimately it establishes a new attitude in which the body is perceived as a machine run by mechanical and manipulating switches. Today drugs are more plentiful, more powerful, and more dangerous; they are sold by television and radio. Self-control by the profession on such matters has never worked, or self-regulation. This invasion fits industrialized man who has learnt to purchase whatever he fancies. To take a drug no matter which and for what ever reason, is a last chance to assert control over him, to interfere on his own with his body rather let others interfere. This invasion of medication, by himself and by others, reduces his ability to cope with his body for which he can still care.

The fact that modern medicine has become very effective in the treatment of specific symptoms does not mean that it has become more beneficial for the health of the patient especially in the villages and rural areas. Like genetic selection, those who fit into that machine are the logical next step of medico-social control.

All traditional cultures, on the other hand, derive their hygienic function from their ability to equip the individual with the means for making pain tolerable, sickness or impairment understandable, and the shadow of death meaningful. Health in such cultures is a traditional way of consoling, caring, and comforting people while they heal, and most sick-care is a form of tolerance extended to the afflicted. Only those cultures survive that provide a viable code that is adapted to a group's genetic makeup, to its history, to its environment, and to the peculiar challenges represented by competing groups of neighbours. The ideology promoted by contemporary cosmopolitan medical enterprise runs counter to these functions. It radically undermines the continuation of old cultural programmes and prevents the emergence of new ones that would provide a pattern of self-care and suffering. Medicalization constitutes a prolific bureaucratic programme based on the denial of each man's need to deal with pain, sickness and death. The goals of metropolitan medical civilization are thus in opposition to every single cultural health programme they encounter in the process of progressive colonization.

This is what Illich calls the third level of cultural iatrogenesis, a dimension of medical health-denial. Professionally organized medicine has come to function as domineering moral enterprise that advertises industrial expansion as a war against all suffering. It has thereby undermined the ability of individuals to face their reality, to express their own values, and to accept inevitable and often irremediable pain and impairment, decline, and death. It is easily forgotten that culture and health coincide, i.e. there is a unique gestalt of health. For instance, medical civilization tends to turn pain into a technical matter and thereby deprives suffering of its inherent personal meaning.

If traditional cultures confront pain, impairment, and death by interpreting them as challenges soliciting a response from the individual under stress; then, medical civilization turns them into demands made by individuals on the economy, into problems that can be managed or produced out of existence. If cultures are systems of meanings, cosmopolitan civilization is a system of techniques. Traditional cultures made everyone responsible for his own performance under the impact of bodily harm or grief. Thus, technological and traditional civilization start from opposite assumptions, and as culture is medicalized the social determinants of pain are distorted.

1.3 Women and Health in India

In the context of the preamble stated above, in India, women are very vulnerable to health risks at every stage of their lives — from conception to old age – such as maternal deaths, anaemia, tuberculosis, work-related health risks and violence on them. All this is clearly linked to poverty, economic dependence, lack of decision-making opportunities, appropriate health services, limited access to information and so on. This is why the entire issue requires a multi-pronged approach, clear policy directions where there is a collaboration of various sectors so that a holistic viewpoint is possible for resolving these complex health challenges.

In discussing women's health it is seldom realized that women are exposed in the same way as men when the discussion is about prevalent common diseases in India. However they get attention much later than men, if at all they do, and they are likely to be treated at home rather than by a doctor or at a medical centre, women are more likely to face serious consequences including death. Moreover, for example, because women are different as a result of their biological and physiological make-up anaemia is more prevalent in women, and blood depleting diseases like malaria, affect women's health more. Furthermore, health needs are influenced by socio-political and economic conditions within specific cultural settings. This is why any discussion on the health of women has to take into consideration the hierarchical and patriarchal nature of the society. Until recently, women's health needs in official policies has only taken into account mainly their role as producers of children, such as maternal and child health is included in the health services.

Then again, segregated and asymmetrical gender relations are present not only in discriminatory treatment meted out to daughters in the family but they are strengthened by the marriage practices. Marriage as a social institution is seen as an alliance of patrilineal kin groups, so that early marriage to a man senior in age, practice of village exogamy and patrilineal residence upon marriage ensure that women submit to fulfilling traditional gender roles. Under such situations, women's problems are defined in terms of family needs rather than their own unequal access to health resources.

The neglect of women's health needs has continued in spite of the fact that time and again, several committees have looked into the health conditions in India and have recommended policies for modifications and improvements in the health care system. These reports have pointed out that health services are inadequate to cater to the needs of the large sections of the rural and urban poor as the biases are in favour of the rich and the geographic and cultural needs of the people are not taken into account, especially the requirements of the women. It is also pointed out that medical professionals are largely concerned with profits for themselves rather than the improvement in the health of the people. The way the family planning programme has been functioning; it has not helped improving the health of women. It does not focus on the regulation of fertility since women bear a heavy burden due to their role in reproduction. There is an urgent need to reduce medicalization of the women's bodies and to empower them to get control over bodies and their sexuality, as against the fact that the programme is more interested in promoting the interests of the pharmaceutical industry by introducing newer methods even when they are harmful to the health of the women. (Karkal, 1995)

Population control programmes talk of environmental degradation and poverty. Women are rarely causes of environmental degradation, but they are certainly their victims. Shortages of water, fuel, and fodder are known to increase women's workload. Being protectors of health of the family as well as being health workers, women face additional burdens of these problems. It is also clear that poverty cannot be abolished by the capitalist system since it is actually produced and perpetuated by the very logic of its functioning. It is for this reason that DAWN's (Development Alternatives for Women) New Era says:

> "While traditional gender based systems of subordination have been considerably transformed by the forces of economic growth, commercialization, and market expansion, subordination itself persists, although in some case more impersonal forces in the labour market replace the direct control

of women within the patriarchal rural households. We must understand the impact of these processes on women's relative access to recourses, income and employment, as well as sexual division of labour. The almost uniform conclusion of the research is that, with a few exceptions, women's relative access to economic resources, incomes and employment has worsened, their burdens of work have increased, and their relative and even absolute health, nutritional and educational status has declined."

At the root of the population problem – both qualitative as well as quantitative – is the status of women in the society. Thus, improving the health of women requires not only looking at the health conditions, generally discussed by the health professionals but also involves in large part, reexamining sexuality with social and cultural mores and therefore, hierarchical and patriarchal nature of the society. It entails improving male, as well as adolescent sexual health and more importantly, involving men in the health programmes. In short, securing women's health is the crucial means for bringing about social transformation.

Health conditions of women are closely linked with the conditions of poverty, their family structure that restrains them from availing of the health services, as well as accepting healthier life-styles and the political power that empowers them for equal share in the social resources. It is clear that the importance of the social context has to be taken into account. To illustrate, in 1974, at the International Population Conference the key to improving women's health was advocated to be increasing CPR (Couple Protection Rate – through contraception), in 1994 at their conference 20 years later, the key was ensuring women's health and their economic well-being through their empowerment and their rights over their bodies and their sexuality. (Karkal, *ibid.*)

It may be noted critically that traditional and folk systems of health care which are the mainstay of medical support to thousands of poor people in remote rural areas, have not been seriously promoted and much structural support has not been given by the government to traditional mainstreams of medical care.

In recent times, globalization is affecting lives of millions of women and children adversely, because medicalization issues are becoming very expensive. It is causing economic dependency and thereby creating unsustainable health problems. Thus, the roots of all this lies in the worldwide socio-economic inequities, and environmental degradation that we see all around us everywhere.

Furthermore, while knowledge on diseases is available, the gaps that exist between knowledge and information with regard to health awareness of the public are very wide indeed. Most likely, low literacy levels within a multi-lingual society requires the task of health requirements to be culture sensitive and gender sensitive in the process of health education. Therefore, the interventions of education are necessary. This is a problem of communication that requires the capacity to listen to the voiceless. In the absence of such an approach, medical solutions are becoming as a consequence increasingly costlier, dependency creating unsustainable medical solutions that are being promoted by multi-nationals and others, for health problems of women whereby there is an imposition of alien models on many indigenous cultures.

It is clear that in order to deal with the magnitude of diverse health problems, all reductionist approaches have to be avoided, since these are based on a mechanical and fragmentary approach that is a hangover of outdated paradigms. Health is not a mere bio-medical treatment of the individual. In a holistic approach it needs to be addressed comprehensively at multiple levels. This means that the existing wisdom experience of the non-literate and the systems of medicine in use since thousands of years has to be kept in mind when approaching health problems. This requires a multi-pronged strategy in terms of planning, designing programmes for the elimination of disease, (the etymological roots of which means 'not at ease'), i.e. making it imperative to correct cultural, psychological and mental problems beyond the mere diagnosis of the bio-physical symptoms of the specific disease.

In other words, the gender specific health problems need to be understood in their total context and not merely as a problem of reproductive health. The health worker him/herself and those at the top need to approach their own lives from this viewpoint if results are to be produced at a deeper level that is lasting. The vulnerability of women to various diseases even during their reproductive needs requires a critical notice, and not merely to be confined to addressing contraception, safe childbirth and safe abortion. All this is connected to the larger concerns of women in this context, namely, infertility, childlessness, and a high incidence of low birth weight babies, high neo-natal mortality and high maternal mortality. This is the only way to counteract such health care practices that have become unethical and exploitative because of the increasing commercialization of health services as a commodity of trade – an area in this sense being socially unhealthy. It, therefore, urgently requiring social control, regulation, and accountability.

The marginalization of women and their health concerns has been a major focus of the women's movement in India that includes activists and NGO's who are intensively agitated by the neglect of women's health, specifically as a gender issue. They have independently addressed this issue in the course of their work. However, until now the attention has largely been on their reproductive role, contraceptive responsibilities of women; all this mainly for population control. But this approach ignores other dimensions of women's health, as mentioned above, the gender perspective that is conspicuously absent in the formulation of specific policies and programmes that have hitherto not shown the links between women's education, social and economic status on the one side and their nutritional and health status associated with their morbidity and mortality on the other. (Gopalan and Shiva, 2000)

However, it may be mentioned here that the Women Health Development Cell of WHO has taken the initiative to highlight women's health concerns in their global agenda. Their goal is to prepare regional and national profiles of women's health and development in order to identify the current status of women's health and specific areas requiring focus. In this way it is hoped that this exercise highlights the linkages between investment decisions of governments and the repercussions of these decisions on different strata of men and women in different socio-cultural situations. The basic idea is to develop parameters to monitor health status of women within countries and between countries.

At this point it may be useful to briefly summarize the national health policy to give a background for the work that follows in the context of women and health.

1.4 National Health Policy : Organization of Health Care System

Policy and Planning, Approach and Objectives for Health

Around Independence, it may be mentioned, that a national health care in policy and planning was started after a Health Survey and a Development Committee known as the Bhore Committee in 1940 submitted its comprehensive proposal in 1946. Its mandate was to "survey" health conditions and organizations and make recommendations for their development. Among its more important suggestions were :

1. That no individual should lack access to medical care because of inability to pay for it;
2. That medical relief and preventive health care should be urgently provided to rural people;
3. That special emphasis should be placed on preventive methods;
4. That health services should be as "close to the people as possible in order to ensure the maximum benefit to the community to be swerved";
5. That the active cooperation of people in the health programme should sought;
6. That health units should be established according to a set pattern;
7. That physicians should receive three months training in social and preventive medicine, and
8. That all facilities for diagnosis and treatment should be available in the health service system when it is fully developed.

As these recommendations had hardly been achieved, they were all reiterated in the National Health Policy Statement!

The enunciation of a National Policy by the Government of India in 1982 raised hopes among those concerned with India's poor health that the government is serious about its commitment to provide "health for all". It states many ambitious possibilities in its goals, calling the redress of the many mistakes made in the past, embodying many concepts of social justice and democratization that have been eclipsed in the process of health development. (Chatterjee, 1988)

However, the shortcomings of the past are reflected in the rapid population growth; high morality among women, infants and children; extensive malnutrition; a high incidence of blindness, leprosy, tuberculosis and other infectious disease; a lack of a lack of access of rural people to potable water and basic sanitation; and inadequate trained birth attendance. This poor health situation is based on the adoption of a "hospital based, curative approach to health services and manpower which has been at the cost of providing comprehensive primary enhancing dependency and weakening the community's capacity to cope with its problems health care to all". This has lead to the neglect of preventive, promotive, rehabilitative and public health measures. The curative approach is deemed "inappropriate" and "irrelevant" to the country's needs, and is blamed for "instead of improving awareness and building up self-reliance". It is also held responsible for creating a cultural gap between the people and personnel providing care. Further, it is suggested that achieving satisfactory health status calls for "involving the community in the identification of their health needs and priorities as well as in the implementation and management" of programmes.

The overall goal of the Policy was the "universal provision of comprehensive primary health care services" which are "relevant", "affordable by the people" and "participatory" of communal and voluntary organizations. On the subject of medical education and training personnel, the major recommendation is that manpower development should concentrate on imparting a greater orientation to community health and an integrated "health team" approach.

The public sector provides many services through various bodies of the Centre and the States, which are, integrated in the sense that curative, preventive and promotional health care are combined. The service rendered by the private sector is also mainly curative. However, the NGOs, Charitable Trusts and Societies have a strong presence in institutional health care. While most of these are non-profit and non-commercial organizations, they charge fees to recover the costs for their services except some that are run purely on philanthropic basis. Some funding also comes from external support. All this is also curative except for those NGOs that are involved in community health care and other such development and welfare activities.

Health Care System in India

Thus, health care system in India is very complex and diverse with, further, co-existence of different systems of medicine such as Allopathic, Ayurvedic, Unani, Homoeopathy, Naturopathy, Yoga, etc. The Chopra Committee established in 1940 drew up a plan for health services comprising a primary level health care system based mostly on the indigenous system of medicine and secondary and tertiary levels integrated with the modern system, and this has not quite happened, except recently when the traditional medicine systems have been incorporated into the healthcare system to offer a "synthesized" medicine. (Chatterjee, *ibid*)

***National Health Proramme*s**

Several National Health Programmes were developed on the recommendations of the Bhore Committee through the various five-year plans.

The Bhore Committee, in fact, laid down norms for a rural health infrastructure with short (10 years) and long term (20-40 years) goals.

The construction of Primary Health Centres (PHCs) was begun in the early 1950s in accordance with the Bhore Committee's recommendations, although some of the norms were changed. The pattern adopted envisioned one PHC for every Community Development Block which at that time had a population of 60,000 on an average. By the 1970s, this ratio (one PHC per block) had been achieved but, significantly, the average population of a block had increased by then to 1,00,000. It currently stands at over 120,000. While there were to be three sub-health centres per block initially, this ration was later increased to one sub-centre per 10,000 people. The pattern proposed now is one sub-centre per 5,000 people. There is still a long way to go to achieve this ration, leave alone the Bhore Committee's recommendations for this level.

1.5 Structure of Health Care Services

This service now provides a network of Sub-centres and Primary Health Centres (PHCs) of the Government in rural areas, hospitals and dispensaries in government as well as private health sectors. The table shows the figures, which is below the recommendation of the Bhore Committee, i.e., PHCs is 30,000 rural population against 20,000 recommended except in hilly areas (20,000 for tribal and hilly areas) sub-centres for 5,000 population.

Rural Health Centres—Average Population Served, 1996

Item	Population Norm	Average Population Served
Sub-Centre	3,000 to 5,000	4,737 (4-7 villages)
PHC	20,000 to 30,000	28,375 (25-27 villages)
HC	100,000+	260,000

The PHCs are functioning sub-optimally because of one or more the following factors:

1. Inappropriate location, poor access, lack of maintenance;
2. Lack of professional staff at the critical posts;
3. Mismatch between the requirement and availability of health professionals especially physicians;
4. Lack of funds for essential drugs;
5. Lack of first referral units (FRUs) for linkage of referral services.

These problems need urgent solution at the local level, for which strengthening of Panchyati Raj institutions with funds is necessary.

Human Resource for Health Care

Medical Professionals

One doctor for a population of 1500 and one nurse for a population of 500 was recommended by the Bhore Committee in 1946. The Bajaj Committee in 1987 recommended that population ratio, inter-professional ratio and manpower mix must be considered in assessing health manpower requirement. The present status for this purpose is very low, which is required for the Rural PHC. The posts sanctioned are far below what is required. The personnel in position are even less than the posts sanctioned. This is indeed a sad situation.

In rural areas, the non-allopathic doctors provide the first contact for medical care for a majority of people, and that too many are unqualified and unlicensed practitioners, who again have information gathered from other people! There are now provisions for the modernization of traditional systems under separate laws for the registration of those doctors qualified in those systems. Many of these also practice modern medicine, it is estimated that one-third of those in the PHCs come from this stream. However, at village micro-level studies show that a majority of the population use non-modern system facilities that are not even captured in the household level health surveys. For instance, a recent survey, 1998 by the Centre for Social Studies in Surat (Gujarat) that traditional healers were practicing it with herbal medicine and faith healing in 27 villages, and this does not include Ayurvedic medicine.

Nurses

The doctor-nurse ratio recommended is 1:3 generally, but in India it is 2.1:1. Nursing is almost a female profession, except 4.2 per cent are males, in the General Midwife category. It is a policy of the Government to not to train male nurses as ANMs, even though the job-description for both is the same, except that the female nurse has to be responsible to undertake deliveries.

Traditional birth attendants, it may be noted, known as Dais are not part of the public health care delivery system. However the Government had initiated systematic programme for Dais in 1970s, in basic hygiene practices since they attend to a large number of deliveries in the rural areas. Trained Dais are supplied with a delivery kit. By March 1993, the Government had trained 6,09,506 dais in the rural areas. Dais receive a token payment for each delivery and this depends on the efficient functioning of the PHC. The contribution of Dais continues to be great and is reflected on the decreasing maternal morbidity rate and child mortality. Their services and contribution to health care has not been recognized nor studies properly. They will continue to be needed in local health for many years to come. (Gopalan and Shiva, *ibid.*)

1.6 Health Status and Socio-economic Development

The health of a population is dependent on the socio-economic development of any given region/state/country, namely, standard of living, sanitation, housing, water supply, education, employment, health consciousness, personal hygiene, health services, etc. The lack of such services and factors is clearly reflected in many states of India, where all these facilities are not available. This is so despite the tremendous amount of scientific advancement in the field of curative medicine in the world. The WHO defines Health "as a state of complete physical, mental and social well being, and not merely the absence of diseases or infirmity". Such a holistic definition, until recently has not been reflected in most states of India. There is yet to evolve an accurate set of yardstick to measure the health status of a community. While traditional methods for measuring the health status exist in the form of vital rates and morbidity studies, it is debatable whether these are appropriate and sensitive in the present context. (VHAI Report, 1995).

Preventive Public Health

In general it is clear that in India despite 40 or more years of developmental planning there has been no change in the pattern of occurrence of the high incidence of disease and death. Data and observations both clearly show that the largest chunk of morbidity and mortality is due to preventable and communicable diseases. Clearly there has been a lack of emphasis on preventive health programmes. For instance, medical expenditure has been very high in comparison with public health expenditure, i.e. the concern is with expensive and advanced technology in urban areas. All this deprives peripheral health institutions of inexpensive but essential tools and techniques. Consequently, instead of evolving a health system resting on paramedical staff to strengthen the periphery, a centralized system dependent on doctors has evolved. Catering to the minority, economic reforms have increased the chasm between these two systems of health, and there is no commitment for providing free and comprehensive health services to the entire population. The health of impoverished India as a whole assumes importance only when there is an outbreak of an epidemic. Not surprisingly as soon as the epidemic is over, the emphasis on public health disappears once again. It goes to show that solutions to problems of ill-health and diseases does not lie with medical technology alone.

Compared to this, in the West the improvement was due to a public health revolution in the nineteenth century, i.e., due to the improvement in nutrition, water supply, sanitation and levels of living. In India public health is not on the political agenda. If health for all is to be made a reality, the need for high priority in the domain of poverty eradication and investment in public health has to be addressed.

Underdevelopment, regional imbalances and social inequalities and nutritional deficiencies and communicable diseases, along with eradication of child labour, burdening of women because of male migration to urban areas, etc. has to be urgently looked into and deserves an urgent need for a multi-pronged action by all concerned. In short, problems of public health care are a political matter.

Maternal Health and Child Health

This area of maternal health and child health has to be given top priority in every region of India because not only do they form the largest chunk of the population, they are the most vulnerable segment of our population. The following areas are most important:

- Women's role in health development,
- Maternal nutrition,
- Iron deficiency anemia,
- Safe motherhood,
- Maternal morbidity and mortality,
- Infant mortality and morbidity,
- Diarrhea disease,
- Breast feeding and weaning, and
- Acute respiratory tract infection.

Maternal Health

It is a truism to state that the role of women in the economy of India and their status in society as principal providers of care and support for the family is crucial for development. They are responsible for almost all physical and mental development of the next generation. They have, therefore, to be trained in the technology of nutrition, hygiene, surrounding sanitation and family its healthcare in sanitation, and education in these areas. The current indicators show that there is a fundamental bias and discrimination against women, i.e. figures of mortality rates, life expectancy, women work force participation, maternal mortality, etc. clearly indicates. For instance, the nutrition of girls is placed second to that of boys on the whole in north India.

Iron Deficiency Anaemia

Women are a recognized vulnerable group for iron deficiency anaemia. It is associated with protein energy malnutrition and further aggravated by high levels of hook worms infestation. It constitutes the most serious hazard to maternal survival, and contributes significantly to pre-term births, low birth weight babies and therefore to peri-natal mortality. It can be prevented by an adequate intake of green leafy vegetables in the diet, with additional supplements.

Safe Motherhood

There are many women in India who die in the process of giving life, which can be prevented if enough knowledge and information is made available then the risks of pregnancy can be drastically reduced. Safe motherhood can be promoted through :

- Periodic check up during pregnancy,
- Ensuring immunization again tetanus,
- Ensuring that a trained person is available at birth,
- Ensuring that the pregnant women gets adequate nutrition and rest,
- Avoiding pregnancies under the age of 18 and over the age of 35 could reduce maternal death by 25 per cent,
- Spacing births at least 2 years apart,
- Ensuring that female children and adolescent girls are well nourished, and
- Detecting the danger signs during pregnancy such as intra-uterine growth retardation toxemia, bleeding, fever, etc.

Maternal Mortality and Morbidity

The risk of dying of causes related to pregnancy and child birth is 40-100 times higher than the developed world in India. A large percentage of these women die in the desperate attempt to terminate unwanted pregnancies, other maternal deaths are due to abortion and sepsis, and due to toxemia's and anemia, and when referral services are not available. All these cases are preventable.

Infant Mortality and Morbidity

Several studies in Uttranchal and elsewhere in India have shown that there is high rate of IMR. The main cause of child deaths in the first of life have been assessed as tetanus, acute respiratory tract infection and diarrhoeal disease, in addition to the most common the infection of the umbilical cords.

Infant Breast Feeding

Infant feeding practices studied show that gastro-intestinal disorders amongst breast-fed infants is low as compared to bottle-fed infants. It is clear that the conditions under which bottle feeding is practiced favour infections especially among poorer communities where environmental sanitation and safe water supply is not available. It is well-known that breast milk particularly the colostrums secreted during the first five days after delivery contains a wide range of anti infective substances including lymphocytes, secretary immunoglobulins, zinc and vitamin A. The antibodies protect the absorbing surfaces of the intestinal lining against infections of E.coli, Shigella, Salmonella and Rota which cause diarrhoeas. The importance of this, starting breast feeding soon after birth and its advantage needs to be stressed.

Acute Respiratory Tract Infections

Acute respiratory tract infections (ARI) is the number two killer of infants. As the National ARI envisages the reduction of such morbidity can be reduced by the management of the following components :

1. Early discrimination of cases at the community level on, rapid breathing and chest in drawing.
2. Appropriate anti-microbial therapy by the frontline worker in moderately severe cases.
3. Referral of severe cases to the health centre.
4. Strengthening of immunization programme against measles, pertusis, diphtheria, childhood TB and Vit. A prophylaxis.

Maternal and Health Services

Maternal health services were started as early as 1866 by Church missions, and later by Chelmsford League, the Indian Red Cross, and still later by the Maternity and Child Welfare centres which were set up for preventive services. It was later merged with Family Planning and the into Family Welfare Services.

Reproductive Health and Family Welfare Programme

Women's groups and NGOs have attempted to focus attention on the use of women as guinea pigs in various experiments. Family planning methods have concentrated wholly on women and not included men at all. In this way the control that women have over their fertility has been taken away from them without any active participation from them. (VHAI, *ibid.*)

Health and family planning services are provided through a network of sub-centres, primary health centres, community health centres, post partem centres, voluntary organizations and other facilities. The family welfare programme is voluntary everywhere, leaving the choice to the individual couple. Mass media and interpersonal communication are used to explain the various methods of contraception and to remove socio-cultural barriers among the people. Even after expensive infrastructure and programme hardware expenses, the outcome is still questionable. Another way of assessing the impact is to see whether the decline in crude birth rate shows greater association with literacy or with Family Welfare expenditure. The impact of literacy in terms of cost effectiveness of this massive national programme seems to be meagre.

Women's Participation and Perspectives

The present trend shows that there is something inherently wrong with the family welfare programme. The question is, are women supposed to be a mere object of this programme? Nowhere is this technological determinism more evident than in the family planning,

Programme, through which poor women is said to be the cause of the country's poverty have come victims of whatever contraceptive technology is in fashion. If anything, fashionable medical intervention has added to the morbidity burden borne by the poor women.

Need for a Holistic Approach

The success of population education and family planning programmes in a variety of settings demonstrates that informed individuals everywhere can and will act responsibly in the light of their own needs and those of their families and communities. Any form of coercion has no part to play. Thus, the family planning and welfare programmes should aim at :

1. To help couples and individuals meet their reproductive goals in a framework that promotes optimum health, responsibility and family well being,
2. To prevent unwanted pregnancies and reduce the incidence of high-risk pregnancies and morbidity and mortality,
3. To make quality family-planning services affordable, acceptable and accessible to all who need and want them,
4. To improve the quality of family planning advice, information, education, communication, counseling and services,
5. To increase the participation and sharing of responsibility of men in the actual practice of family planning, and
6. To promote breast-feeding to enhance birth spacing.

Health Priority Areas and Challenges for NGOs

In general the focus in this chapter has been on issues of community health and its detrimental factors. There are however certain challenges which both the government and NGOs have to face. These include regional imbalances at the micro and macro levels. These often generate a lot of socio-political anger and dissatisfaction that shapes the nature of political situation of a region. The hill regions, for instance, are characterized by low productivity, high or low density population, difficult terrain and topography, inadequate infrastructure, unfavourable demographic and recurrence of natural of calamities like floods and droughts. However, in spite of the lack of agro-industrial indicators of development, the hill regions despite poverty are well ahead of other regions in the demographic and socio-economic realms. Even in respect of infrastructural facilities of health and education the hill region comes first. Nevertheless despite these indicators, the status of women in the hills is not better, even though woman work participation is higher yet it does not improve her status in the family. They are more anaemic and have to work harder than those in the plains.

There is an urgent need to work for creating awareness among poor and working class to sensitize them on issues related to the following :

- Gender sensitivity and reproductive health,
- Iodine deficiency disorders,
- Prevention of other communicable diseases,
- Safe Drinking water,
- STD/HIV/AIDS,
- Mother and Child care,
- Elimination of child labour.

Thus NGOs can and have played a role in developing alternative models as well as providing low cost and effective health services in many parts of the country. They have been able to develop village based health cadres, educational material and appropriate technology. They also have helped in filling the critical gaps that exist in government health services. However there can be no prototype and a system should evolve out of the people themselves. Moreover, these NGOs, health groups are also divided on ideological grounds, i.e. those following traditional or modern medicine, etc. Most of them are dominated by a group of elites, for whom even paramedics and village health workers are mere functionaries and not agents of change.

It is recognized, of course, that the NGOs are indispensable allies in the delivery of Primary Health Care. Their advantage is that they have personalized approach, motivation, necessary zeal, sympathy for the deprived/weaker sections, responsiveness to the people's needs, creativity and above all flexibility to experiment with innovative and alternative approaches in solving health problems. They also provide people with information, technical support and decision making possibilities. The following areas can be considered most significant to the community health movement:

1. Links with the socio-political process;
2. Commitment to individual and community awareness building;
3. Process of "community building" including increasing the participation of those who do not/cannot participate at present;
4. Quest for medical pluralism (including promoting traditional/indigenous systems of medicine);
5. Acceptance of conflicts of interest within the community;

6. Confrontation of various factors in the medical model of health care including over-medicalization of health, over professionalization of skill and knowledge, and over-emphasis on the physical dimension of health; and
7. Increasing commitment, accountability and medical audit.

Protection of Girls and Women

Finally, one of the most potent weapons to protect women against their degraded position is to empower them in order to avoid unwanted pregnancies and births at whatever age. The most effective way to do this is to provide women with the means of social and economic self-determination. This means giving them full rights in the family and society, i.e. access to income and career development, education and health care, and an equal say in the decisions that affect their live, including family size, and motivate adolescent girls to avail of learning opportunities for the development of their self-image and prepare them for better motherhood. In this respect the NGOs have a vital role to play, in organizing and sustaining women's groups, centred around economic activities needs to be visualized. There being a need to assist them through a communication and training process, consisting of discussion and debate leading to decision and action, and especially to reduce exclusive reliance on bureaucracy as a problem solving agency, in fact to keep check on the working of the bureaucracy (VHAI : 1995.)

Keeping the above focus in mind this research looks at the traditional health practices of women (especially during their reproductive phase) in the Nainital district (Ramgarh and Dhari Blocks) of Kumaon Hills. The Government Health infrastructure at the district and block level and the role of the NGOs has been looked at in detail in Chapter 3. The following chapter gives a geographical, socio-historical and cultural profile of the Kumaon region in order to contextualise the background of this research.

KUMAON – A PROFILE

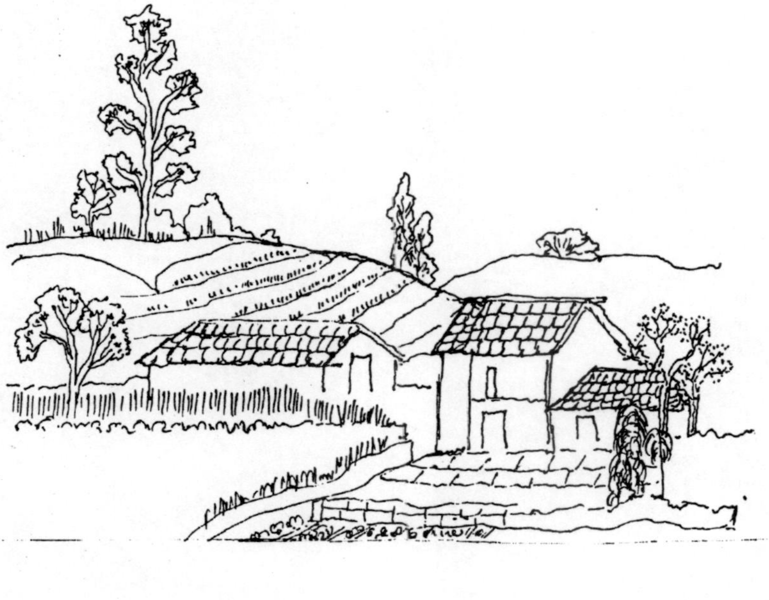

2

KUMAON
Geographical, Historical and Cultural Outline

2.1 Geography

Lying between the latitudes 28°44′ N and 30°49′ and longitudes 78°45′ and 81°1′ E, Kumaon is situated at the tri-junction of Nepal, Tibet and Himachal Pradesh. A natural water-divide separates it from Tibet, the Kali River defines its eastern border with Nepal, high transverse mountain spurs separate it from the Chamoli and Pauri districts of Garhwal, and the southern limit of the Terai belt demarcates its southern boundary. Kumaon comprises all the four longitudinal physiographic subdivisions, namely, the Outer Himalayas with the Terai and Bhabar belt and Siwalik Range, the Lesser Himalayas (Himanchal), the Great Himalayas (Himadri) and the Trans-Himalayan Tethys domain of Bhotland. (Valdiya: 1988)

It thus constitutes a distinct geographical entity that is spread over 21,035 square km area. The Kumaon Division earlier comprised three districts – Nainital, Almora and Pithoragraph, which were divided into 14 tehsils and 41 development blocks. After the creation of the new hill-state of Uttaranchal, Kumaon comprises six districts, namely, Nainital, Almora, Pithoragarh, Champawat, Bageshwar and Udhamsingh Nagar.

The region is mountainous with altitudes ranging mostly between 600 to above 3500 metres above m.s.l. In this region, the lifestyle is heavily dependent on local natural resources, and although agriculture is the main occupation, poor yields force men to migrate out for jobs. As in other regions all over India, women do a lot of physical work. The women of this region shoulder most of the burden for collecting fuelwood, fodder, water, and other forest produce, do all the back-breaking work in the field, take care of all aspects of animals husbandry, as well as handle household work. Along with this, they are mostly non-literate and marginalized from most social decision making processes. Even where the husband is away, women do not dare to make any independent decision on their own. More about all this elsewhere in this chapter and in other chapters throughout the book. (Jalal, 1988.)

Climate

The altitudinal variations and the slope aspects have given rise to varying climates in the different eco-zones of Kumaon. It is hot and moist (tropical) in the sub-montane zone and in the river valley below 600 m in elevation. At higher elevations the climate becomes subtropical up to the altitudes 1,200m, cool–temperate up to 1,800m and cold-temperate 1,800 and 2,400m. At still higher altitudes the climate is extreme cold.

The mean temperature in the month of January ranges around 21°C in the submontane belts of Terai and Bhabar (Kichha, Ramnagar and Tanakapur) and the river valleys lying below 600m in elevation, 8°C in the in the valley and spurs (Hawalbagh, Dharchula, Pithoragarh, Almora and Ranikhet) and 6°C on higher mountain range lying between 1,800 and 2,400m (Nainital and Mukteshwar). The corresponding temperature records for the month of June are around 40°C for the Terai and Bhabar belts, 24°C for inner valley and spurs with a few exceptions, and 20°C for the higher ranges. (Jalal, *ibid.*)

Settlements

Of the total estimated population of around 2.4 million of Kumaon, the people live in 7000 villages including the uninhabited forest localities of various sizes. The population size of the rural settlements varies from one person in Kabhara village in the Ramgarh Block to 9,218 per person at Nagla in the Rudrapur Block in the Terai area. The density of population, excluding the forest area, varies from 14 persons per two km in the Dharchula Block to 412 persons per two km in the Haldwani Block.

According to the size of population, the rural settlements fall into six groups. Out of the total number of 6,999 inhabited villages, 55 per cent, 30.8 per cent, 10.5 per cent, 3.1 per cent and 0.6 per cent settlements fall in the population size group of below 200, 200-499, 500-999, 1000-1999 and 2000-4999 persons, respectively.

The percentages for the small-sized settlements, are in general in increasing order from the Outer, the Lesser and the Great and Trans-Himalayan blocks.

> "Two types of rural settlements can be generally seen, viz. agglomerated or nucleated, and dispersed settlements. The agglomeration is on account of the clusters of community groups. A village may have one or more clusters of houses. Dispersion is caused by isolation of farmsteads due to ruggedness of the terrain or due to intervening forests. Under such conditions, landholdings are dispersed and fragmented.
>
> In some localities 'twin villages' are also common, that is, a person may own two houses, one at the lower altitude in the valley and the other at a higher altitude or ridge. The former is used during winters and the latter in the summers. The winter habitations form compact settlements, whereas the summer habitations are temporary abodes in scattered state. Earlier, groups of people in large numbers practiced seasonal migration and occupied the dwelling by turn.
>
> However, this practice is decreasing on account of the induction of modern technology, which ensures higher agricultural yields. Conse-quently, many of the high altitude settlements are now deserted.
>
> The number of urban settlements was 26 in 1981 and rose to 31 in 1986. They had the population of about 0.4 million person in 1981. The population size of these settlements varies from 1,702 persons at Champawat to 77,300 at Haldwani-Kathgodam. Out of the total 31 towns, respectively 15, 9, 5 and 2 centres fall in the population size groups of below 5000, 5000-20,000, 20,000-50,000 and 50,000-1,00,000 persons." (Jalal: *ibid.*)

Land Utilization

Out of the total 21,035 square km. area of Kumaon, 6,794 square km. land is in the Nainital district, 5,385 square km. in the Almora district and 8,856 square km. in the Pithoragrh district. Reserved civil, panchayati forests, including the forests belonging to local bodies, comprise 53.4 per cent area of Kumaon. The forest land is 57.4 per cent in Nainital, 52.2 per cent in Almora and 50.4 per cent in Pithoragrah. It may be emphasized that the percentages of the area shown as forests do not refer to the extent of the actual tree-covered area but also include non-forest land use such as settlements, agricultural farms, roads, etc. falling within the limit of the forest blocks. The actual forest cover is thus considerably less than indicated.

Village pastures (*gauchar*) and high altitude pasture (*dhura* and *bugyal*) comprise 6.3 per cent of the land – 0.2 per cent in Nainital, 6.9 per cent in Almora, and 12.3 per cent in Pithoragrh. More than 3.1 per cent of the land is barren – 0.9 per cent in Nainital, 4.6 per cent in Almora and 3.8 per cent in Pithoragarh. The high-altitude areas are generally included in the category described as wasteland.

Over 2.9 per cent of the land is under built-up areas (settlements, roads, canals, etc.) within the revenue-areas – 4.3 per cent in Nainital, 2.9 per cent in Almora and 2.2 per cent in Pithoragarh. The area which can effectively be used for other purposes but at present are left unused (waste and fallow), accounts for 8.9 per cent in Kumaon, 5.7 per cent in Nainital, 10.3 per cent in Almora and 10.9 per cent in Pithoragarh.

Orchards constitute 4.7 per cent of the land in Kumaon, 4.7 per cent in Nainital, 5.2 per cent in Almora and 6.9 per cent in Pithoragrah. More than 20.7 per cent of the land in Kumaon is utilized for agriculture – 29.3 per cent in Nainital, 18.9 per cent in Almora and 13.5 per cent in Pithoragarh. (Jalal, *ibid.*) **(Plate 1)**

2.2 History

In ancient times Kumaon together with Garhwal, formed one single politico-cultural unit linguistically termed as Central Pahari Region. The ancient history of Kumaon, therefore, cannot be separated from that of Garhwal. However, with the passage of the time socio-political horizons have progressively narrowed until it has become confined to the present-day Kumaon. (Joshi:1988)

The present setup of the Kumaoni society is a result of immigration of different peoples during the Medieval period. The immigrants from the plains, in the course of time, probably because of socio-economic and political exigencies mixed with the local cultural traditions to form a new social order. It was a combination of orthodox and liberal views. However, at all social levels most of the household and agricultural work was and continues to be carried out by the women; this is the indispensability of women in the agricultural communities of all caste levels. Most likely, the reason being that tilling of the land with one's own hand using the plough by a high caste man (Brahman and Kshatriya) was looked down upon by the orthodox section of the society. While the resourceful and economically well off Brahmans employed agricultural labourers, the poorer and weaker Brahmans were obliged to work hard in their fields in order to earn their livelihood and were relegated to a lower social status. (Joshi, *ibid*).

Yet another curious feature of the Kumaoni society was its behaviour towards the 'Shudras' who enjoyed certain privileges, recognized even by the state. With this background, it is possible to explain different vertical and horizontal sections of the Kumaoni society in its historical perspective –

(a) Descendants of prehistoric and proto-historic communities.
(b) Descendants of early migrants other than the tribal groups, such as the Shaukas, the Tharus, the Rajis, etc.
(c) Descendants of later migrants who maintained strict social distance with the earlier communities.
(d) Descendants of the joint stock of liberal later migrants and 'a' and 'b'.
(e) The Sah or Shah community considered to be a merchant class, but some claiming to be high-class Kshatriyas. Significantly, the Sahs and the Chaudharis do have matrimonial alliance with the high-class local Kshatriyas.
(f) Artisans – the Shudras – whether or not descendants of the indigenous groups, form an intergral part of the Kumaoni society. (Joshi:1988)

Uttrakhand is an oft mentioned region in Indian mythology and scriptures, and has always been a centre of activities at different times. This on-going process of struggle and assimilation has a time span of at least five thousand years. Today the oldest Shilpkars, Banrajis, Shaukas, Tharus, Boksas, Gujars, the Khasas and the people who came in medieval and modern times, are all living together, even though at different stages of development. The most probable reasons being the geographical conditions and inaccessibility of terrain which have been the prime drawbacks for the variations in social development.

The ancient history of Uttrakhand is intertwined with myths, so much so that even some historians are have forgotten to mention important historical facts. For instance, it is evident that the initial society was that of hunter-gatherers which in the course of time became nomadic-pastoral, and later pastoral-agrarian, pastoral-trader and finally, agrarian-pastoral or agrarian communities. (Pathak, 1988).

"These stages can be observed in the process of movements going from the valleys to the mountains and settling there, in later times the opposite flow from the innermost valleys back to the foothills. Owing to their weaknesses generated by the instability, many societies failed to stop the arrival of rival societies and were compelled to desert the habitat or get destroyed. The stability possessed over the centuries was diluted owing to the dynamism and mobility of every new society. The elements of struggle, compromise and assimilation played their role differently." (Pathak, *ibid.*)

Language and Dialects

Kumaoni is one of the two constituent languages of the Central Pahari group. In the context of linguistics, the word *'Pahari'* denotes all the Indo-Aryan languages spoken in the southern slopes of the Himalaya extending from Bhadarwah in Jammu and Kashmir to Nepal. However, from the point of their structural peculiarities, these have been classified into three main groups, namely Western Pahari, Central Pahari and Eastern Pahari. The natural dividing line between the Western and Central Pahari is the River Yamuna, and between the Central and Eastren Pahari is the River Kali (Sharada). Roughly speaking, the term Central Pahari stands for all the Indo-Aryan languages spoken in the region to the east of the Kinnaur, Sirmaur and Mahasu districts of Himachal Pradesh upto the western border of Nepal, embracing the region known in ancient times as 'Sapadalaksa' or 'Khasamandala'. (Sharma, 1988)

Origin of the term 'Kumaoni'

Formerly, the region around Champawat in District Pithoragarth was known as *'kumu'* and the language spoken in that region as *'Kumaiyya'*. With the expansion of the domain of the rulers of *'Kumu'*, the whole territory under their control came to be known as Kumaon; hence all the varieties of the language spoken in this region are designated as Kumaoni. Writing about the language of this area, Grierson says: 'In the south-east of the Almora District, there is a peak over 7000 ft high named Kanadeo, the old name of which was Kurmachala, 'the mountain of Kurma' related to the legendary 'Kurma' incarnation of Lord Vishnu. However, some authors on the ground of phonetic changes derive the word from Kurmaangaka or Kurmaangaka > Kurmaanngaka> Kummao > Kumaun > Kumu/Kumaon. (Sharma: *ibid*).

Kumaoni language, its possible origins

It is commonly believed by scholars, true or not, that the Uttrakhand region was inhabited by many Aryan and non-Aryan races in historical past, but there is a complete lack of inscriptional records. Hence, varied hypotheses have been propounded to explain its origin. Some authorities believe that its source is the same Sauraseni Prakrit from which Rajasthani and Brij Bhasha originated. Undeniably, the outside settlers did add some vocabulary items of common use. However, there are a number of linguistic peculiarities of Kumaoni which do not indicate in any way the linguistic tendencies attested in Hindi or its dialects. Moreover, diachronically too the various rules prescribed by the Prakrit grammarians regarding sound changes are not applicable to Kumaoni. (Sharma: *ibid.*)

Kumaon has a very rich tradition of art and literature. One view is that the people of this region were well-versed in Sanskrit, while others feel that it would not be correct to link the Kumaoni language with Sanskrit. In this way, there are two views regarding the origin of the Kumaoni – it is possibly linked to Dardokhas Prakrit. Alternatively, it is a corruption of Sourseni. However, one view again is that as the Khasas were actually the Yakshas, who lived in Kumaon before the advent of the Aryans, that Kumaoni is a synthesis of the languages of the Aryans and the Yakshas-Gandharvas-Nagas-Kiraats. Nevertheless, it is true that in this language there are subtle differentiations on the basis of caste and social status. This fact implies that Kumaoni was influenced from time to time by other languages of the immigrants. (Sharma: *ibid.*)

2.3 Culture

Folk Songs

(a) Kumaon folk literature embraces primarily folk songs and folk epics and tales, especially it has a rich store of folk songs. These songs, also known as 'Muktaks', are usually placed in two categories. The first deals with customs and traditions and the second with seasons and their festivals. The songs of the first category are the *"Shakunaakhar"* or auspicious words, through which all the gods and goddesses are extended invitation for taking part in the ceremony being held. While asking for the blessings of Ganesh, Shiva, Brahma, etc. invitations are also extended to all the relatives. These songs are sung during child birth-*'Nawaan'* (the christening ceremony), *'Yagyopaveet'* (sacred-thread ceremony) and *'Bya'* (weddings). The following is an example of *'Shakunaakhar'* :-

From the aesthetic point of view the 'Muktak' songs are the most attractive of all the Kumaoni songs. In them emotions pre-dominate; there are imaginative flights of fancy concerning love and beauty, as well as deep expressions of sorrows, disappointment and pity. This is but an indication of the contradictory aspects of the lives of the people of this region. There are various categories of *'Muktak'* songs.(Bisht:1988)

(b) Kumaon has a rich store of folk epics, which depict the entire gamut of the experiences in the mountains. The epics narrate the valorous deeds of those who laid down their lives in combats and difficult situations. The epics are such an amalgam of facts and fiction, that they can neither be described as being purely imaginative, nor wholly historical.

Malu Sahi is the most popular folk epic of Kumaon. It has a very wide geographic canvas encompassing the whole region extending from the Tibetan border to the Bhabar belt. There are five versions of this tale. It depicts the love story of Rainju, the daughter of Sunpati Shauka and Malu Sahi the King of Bairath. Rajuli is sometimes called Rainju, Raijula. Malu Sahi was probably a Katyuri King whose capital Bairath, is said to have been somewhere near the present-day Chaukhutia-Gewar. This place is now called Rangili Bairath.

'Naatak' and 'Sutak'

Kumaonis observe *'Naatak'* and *'Sutak'* when there are, respectively, births and deaths in the family. *'Naatak'* is related to the birth of a child. The mother and newly born are considered unclean until formally purified through *pujas*. The worship of the family goddess and purification ceremony starts on the sixth day with the accompaniment of merriment and feasting. On the eleventh day, following the final purification of the mother the child is given a name along with a horoscope by the priest. The christening ceremony is known as *'Nawaan'*.

In the event of death a unique aspect is that all persons participation in the funeral ceremony – *'Malaami'* – are given sweets and fried potatoes after the cremation, presumably as a token of expression of obligation for having participated in the cremation ceremony. The close relatives of the deceased observe *'Sutak'* or mourning for ten days. The person performing the last rites, with his head shaven, sits in mourning. He cooks his own food in a secluded corner, and observes absolute abstinence. Relatives, friends and mourners call on him only on Tuesdays and Saturdays, bringing as they do dry fruits presumably to supplement his nutrition. The purification ceremony is done on the twelveth day when *'pujas'* and *'havan'* are performed. (Shah: 1988)

Ceremonial 'Aipan'

For the *'Namkaran Sanskar'*, a ceremony when the child is given a name, the *'Aipan'* on the wooden *'Chauki'* comprises motifs of sun, moon, bell, conch shell and the utensils used in *'Puja'*.

In the *'Janyo'* (sacred-thread) ceremony initiating a boy to the social rituals, the *'Aipan'* shows the zodiacal sign of polar stars (Sapta Rishis) arranged in hexagons. This is to invoke the blessings of the very learned and sagacious Sapta Rishis. In the *'Bya'* (*Vivaah* or marriage) ceremony the *'Dhuligarh Chauki'* (wooden seat for the bridegroom) bears a design of big water-jar, symbolising primordial water from which the universe emerged. The upper portion has a crown and at the centre is a motif drawn by four horizontal and bisecting lines making nine squares. This motif is encircled by lotus petals. The *'Kanyadaan Chauki'* bears marks of *'Shakti'* and *'Swastic Peeth'* surrounded by lotus and footprints representing Vishnu and Lakshmi, respectively.

The womenfolk of Kumaon have played quite a role in perpetuating the traditions of folk art. The style of painting is locally known as *'Aipan'*, as noted above. Using their nimble fingers and palms, the Kumaoni women have not only preserved the memories of past events, and the styles, designs, etc., but also have given expressions to their own ideas and conceptions on aesthetic values. During ceremonies and festivals the women set themselves to decorating the floor and walls of their houses with designs and patterns. The floor paintings are usually associated with some ritualistic figures. The floor of the worship room and specially the seat of god and goddess, is decorated with specific tantric motifs called *'Peeth'*. The kitchen walls are painted with animalistic motifs. The entrance doors are done with symbols boding good omens. The material used is the paste of rice mixed with ochres. (Shah: *ibid*). (Fig. 2.1 and 2.2)

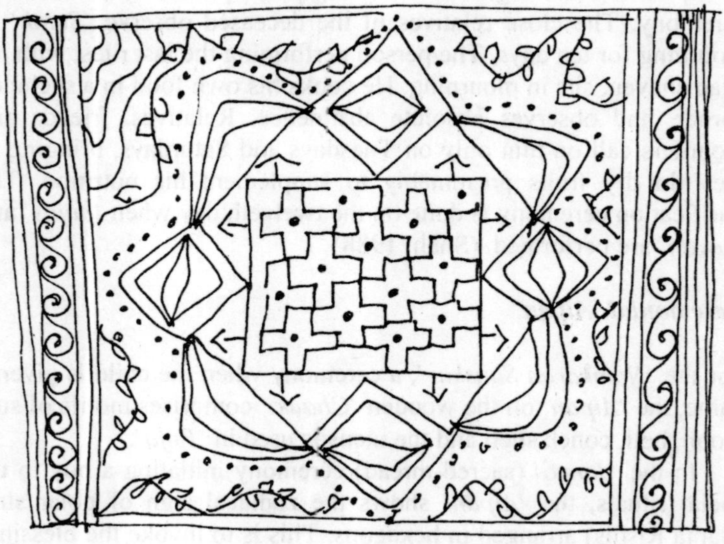

Fig. 2.1 : "NAV SWASTIK" Peeth used for all dieties

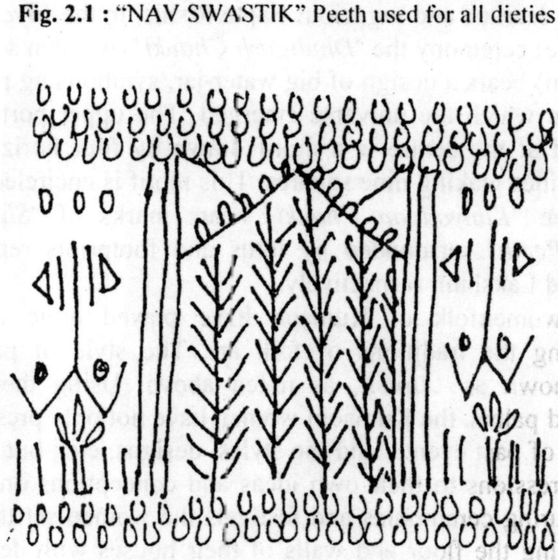

Fig. 2.2 : "NATA" Kitchen Wall Painting

Rangwali : A Unique Cloth Design

The tradition of colourful ornamentation on 'Anchal' cloth is unique Kumaoni tradition rooted deep in its long history. In all ritual ceremonies women wear colourful 'Pichhora' known as 'Rangwali' or 'Kusumia'. A piece of muslin cloth, 3 by 1-1/2 metre, is dyed yellow and dried under shade. It is then spread on the floor and printed with designs. This is done with a padded wooden stick, using red colours. At the centre is the sign of Swastik, and the motifs of sun, moon, bell and conch shell. Around this motif, red concentric circles are stamped with the help of padded small coins. The outermost ring ends up in zig-zag ornaments.

In the Brahman tradition the lemon yellow background bears pink or rose red patterns, whereas in the 'Kusumia' tradition of Shahs on the yellow base crimson red pattern are embossed. The red coloured is the symbol of abiding conjugal life (*Suhaag*), the warmth of fire and sun, health and wealth, the joy of spring; and the golden colour means attachment for the material world. The combination of the two colours is symbolic of the focal theme of a functional life.

Some Customs of Kumaon

Kumaoni art heritage, according scholars, is a combination of many aesthetic traditions that have been based and labelled as Animistic, Tantric, Buddhist, Shivaite, Shakta and Vaishnavaite philosophies. In other words, Kumaoni customs represent the many socio-cultural influences on the Kumaonis. These customs have exercised great influence on the society and kept it a closely knit unit. The customs are quite distinct from the rest of the country.

Religious Fairs and Festivals

It is most likely that the awe-inspiring and in some places forbidding natural environment of the Himalayas has had its deep impression on the various customs of Kumaon and profoundly shaped the outlook of its people. This is why, perhaps, every season has its own appropriate festival, and the ceremonies associated with them give expression to the needs of the people during that particular season. Thus the arrival of winter is heralded by 'Khataruwa' or the 'Festival of Bonfire', and the coming of spring is celebrated with 'Phool Deyi' or the 'Festival of Flowers'. A sort of correlation exists between the seasonal changes and the rituals of the Kumaoni festivals. Some of the festivals, which are distinctive in characters and are unique to Kumaon are described below.

In Kumaon a number of fairs are held throughout the year, but are concentrated during the winter. About a hundred fairs are held in the district of Almora alone, out of which nearly forty are held from October to February. The reason why most of the fairs are held in winter is that during this period villagers are relatively free from their agricultural chores. These fairs, generally centred round shrines, have three aspects :

1. Business, entailing buying and selling of food, clothing and articles of daily needs. The fairs provide a good opportunity for marketing of products of the farmers, horticulturists and artisans and craftsmen;
2. Religious, consisting of a ritual of a dip in the river, if the fair is held on the river bank and worship of the presiding deity of the region; and
3. Socio-cultural, meeting friends and relatives with attendant merry-making and enjoyment. In their best and colourful costumes, men and women in groups sing and dance to the accompaniment of drum beats (*Hurka*). Kumaoni folk dancers from far and near assemble in these fairs and participate with gay abandon. (Shah : *ibid.*)

'Bya' or Marriage

1. The custom of marriage or *"Bya"* is somewhat different among the Kumaonis while the high-caste and well to do people give away their daughters in gift (*Kanyadan*) to worthy grooms with all the customary social fanfare, the very poor and helpless fathers accept bride-price and literally sell their daughters without ceremony. Between these two extreme types of marriage ceremonies of varied forms are known, the main being the 'Anchal', 'Dola' and 'Mandir' marriages. In all these marriages, the bride is decked with typically Kumaoni ornaments and garments. (Fig 2.3).

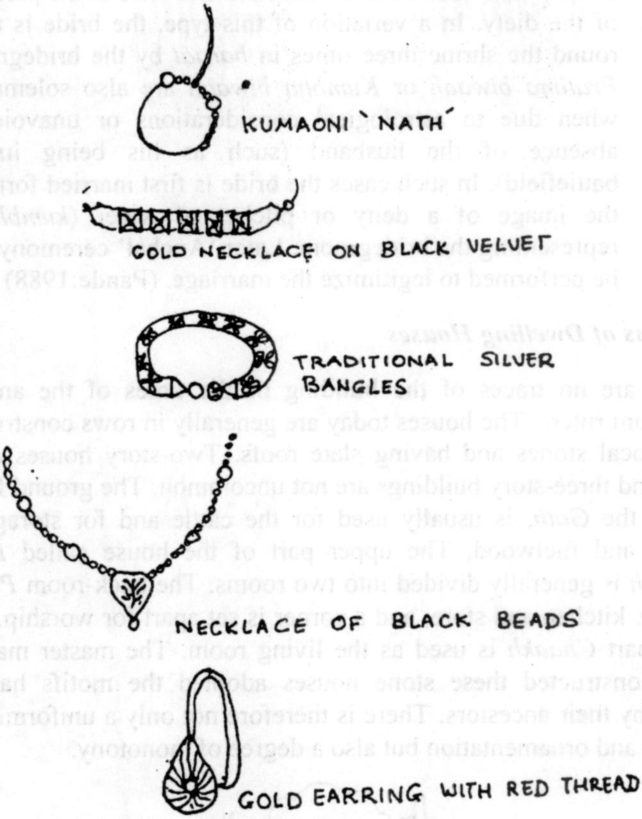

Fig. 2.3 : Traditional Jewellery of Kumaon

These consist of

i. *Natth* or nose-ring,
ii. *Charau* or necklace of black beads,
iii. *Ghaghra* or skirt tied at the waist,
iv. *Pichhaura* or colourful shawl, and
v. Bangles of glass, silver or gold.

2. In the 'Anchal' marriage tying together of the *Anchal* (shawls) of the couple is the principal and essential ceremony. In the *Dola* marriage (also known as 'Sarol' or 'Barkha') it is not necessary for the bridegroom to be present in the marriage ceremony. The groom may be represented by the sword he would have worn or such like things. A marriage can be performed in a temple where the

couple take each other as husband and wife in the presence of the diety. In a variation of this type, the bride is taken round the shrine three times in *baraat* by the bridegroom. *Pratima biwaah* or *Kumbha biwaah* are also solemnized when due to astrological considerations or unavoidable absence of the husband (such as his being in the battlefield). In such cases the bride is first married formally the image of a deity or pitcher of water (*kumbh*) as representing the bridegroom. Later 'Anchal' ceremony may be performed to legitimize the marriage. (Pande:1988)

Designs of Dwelling Houses

There are no traces of the building of the times of the ancient Kumaoni rulers. The houses today are generally in rows constructed with local stones and having slate roofs. Two-story houses are a rule, and three-story buildings are not uncommon. The ground floor, called the *Goth*, is usually used for the cattle and for storage of folder and fuelwood. The upper part of the house called *Paeri Chaakh* is generally divided into two rooms. The back-room *Pan* is used as kitchen and store, and a corner is set apart for worship. The front part *Chaakh* is used as the living room. The master masons who constructed these stone houses adopted the motifs handed down by their ancestors. There is therefore not only a uniformity of design and ornamentation but also a degree of monotony.

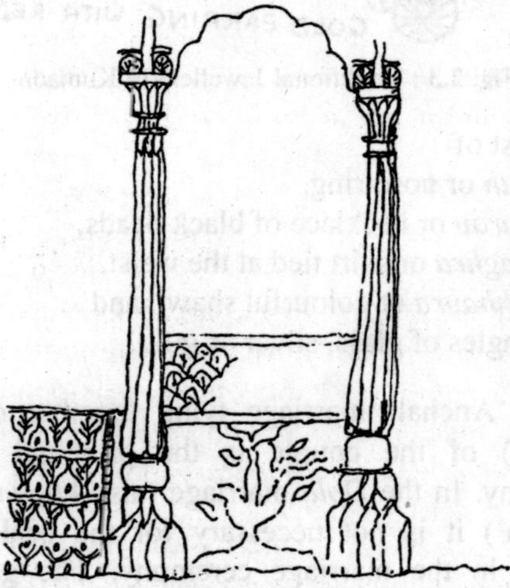

Fig. 2.4 : Carved Wooden Pillars in a Typical Kumaoni House

The façade of the upper storey are usually made of wood, and often artistically carved. The traditional small window-aperture resembles pigeon-holes, cut in wooden panels. Designs of creepers and floral forms based on lotus, pomegranates and grapes, images of human, birds, animals and other sacred signs and emblems find expression in the wood carvings on door panels, window and ceilings. The motifs, ordinarily of the gods or goddesses, add to the richness of the carvings. The Kumaoni craft man also does specific lattice-work to fill in the open space of the windows in order to give a screen like effect.

The open courtyard, which is locally known as 'Pataangan' or 'Khala', is the most significant ordering element in the hill habitation. They are kept private by low parapet walls, serving as benches for the family members and guests. The courtyard serves as a multipurpose space, extending the working area of the householders' activities and is used for such activities as cloth washing, fodder-preparation, dish-washing, drying of seeds, repairing of agricultural tools, etc. (Pande: *ibid.*) **(Plate 2)**

2.4 Role and Status of Women in Kumaon

Social Inequalities

It is not uncommon to see men talk loudly and passionately day in and day out about international, inter-regional and inter-state inequalities, but not a whisper is heard on the neglect of the women in the Indian society. This is especially true about the backwardness of women in general and rural women in particular. It is a truism to state that the growing ills of the exploding population are the direct consequence of the miseries of the women. For example, labelling the work-participation of women and their contributions as economically unimportant and looking down on them as unpaid domestic servants, instead of treating them as co-workers is indeed underestimating the significance and magnitude of the contribution of the women in the development and well-being of the Kumaoni society. It goes without saying that this component of society is restlessly toiling day in and out without demur and protest. However, they have no say even in the matter of bearing their children and are forcibly burdened with the agonies of unwanted births. Over-occupied with breeding and nursing, the rural mothers have no time even to think about their own comforts, status, recognition and independent career .(Pande: 1988)

The life of the Kumaoni women is unbearably difficult in the absence or scarcity of basic amenities of life. Their main responsibilities are fetching water, fuel, fodder, routine unavoidable chores of household, besides looking after and nursing old ones and children. There are 11,58,887 such females in Kumaon (1981 Census).

Constraints of Living

Living in the mountains is not very easy. Basic requisites of even a moderate living, such as potable water, fuelwood, fodder, hospitals and maternity centres, veterinary services, schools, postal and telegraph services, roads and vehicular transport, marketing and banking centres are not easily available. The far-flung habitations in the mountains remain largely secluded. The villages are of very small-sized and scattered far and wide. Electricity is unknown in a large part of Kumaon and even kerosene oil is not available in the remote villages. In the last two decades there has been a tremendous change in respect of the availability or access to certain services including road transport, while the emphasis on programme of basic needs has ensured betterment in essential supplies. The deteriorating ecological conditions are said to be the root cause of the depletion of underground water reserve and the resultant drying up of springs.

Scarcity of Potable Water

Water has to be fetched from deeper ravines or streams or distant springs. Furthermore, water gets scarce in summers when these springs dry up. It may be inferred from this that the availability of potable water in the mountains is in the Almora district, 1.5 per cent in the Pithoragarh district and less than one percent villages in the Nainital district get water from a distance of 1 to 3 kilometres in years of normal rainfall. During summers when many springs go dry, the accessibility becomes very difficult. From a door to door survey of the Okhalkanda block, it has been reported that 66.7 per cent villages where potable water was obtained from remote distances outside the village area. It was further noted that the availability of drinking water in about 33 per cent of the villages of Kumaon is totally insufficient, while 12 per cent villages suffer from this deficiency practically throughout the year. During rains the running water in mountains becomes dirty and unusable for drinking without adequate filtering.

Nearly 90 villages in Almora have to carry water from a distance of 3 kilometres and similarly in Pithoragrah nearly 30 villages have to cross this distance to fetch potable water. Those villages where water is obtained from places within one kilometre are only 9 per cent – about 200 villages in Pithoragarh district. Such habitations are nearly 150 in Almora district. The inconvenience of potable water supply is the primary reason for population deserting the 19 revenue villages which have now been declared uninhabited villages. The process of migration continues.

Now the details are available for only 6889 inhabited villages. The Seventh Five Year Plan of Hill Region (1985) mentions that in 7889 inhabited villages of the area, 4505 were the notified problem – villages in the year 1972 regarding potable water. The Fifth Plan covered 2157 villages and the Sixth covered 4112. The problem facing villages were expected to be around 392 by the end of the Sixth Plan. In 1980, there were 1184 villages having acute problem of potable water. (Pande: *ibid.*).

Far-flung Hospitals and Schools

Service of allopathic Hospitals, to illustrate, can be obtained in rural area of the Almora district after crossing mountainous tract of above 5 kilometres in more than 77 per cent villages. A similar distance has to be covered for reaching a maternity centre. Even in the Nainital district, which includes the plain areas of the Terai and Bhabar, nearly 47 per cent villages are at a distance more than 5 kilometres from the hospital or dispensary. In District Pithoragarh the condition is more difficult where nearly 79 per cent villages are more than 5 kilometres away from a public dispensary.

The Primary Health Centres (PHCs) in the mountains are so remotely located that the village can hardly make use of their amenities. In nearly 54 percent villages of the Almora district, 61 per cent villages in the Naintal district and 43 per cent villages in the Pithoragarh district, the Health Centres at a distance of more than 10 kilometres. The veterinary service centres are also very far from the villages.

Schools for girls are few and far between the rural area of Kumaon. Nearly 81 per cent villages in the Almora district, 63 per cent villages in the Nainital district, and 91 per cent villages in the Pithoragarh district have schools for girls at a distance of more than 5 kilometres. This means long treks in rugged terrain and difficult slopes. High schools or co-educational school up to the high school standard are beyond 5 kilometres in 97 per cent villages of the Almora district, 81 per cent are formidable barriers in the district Nainital and 86 per cent villages in the Pithoragarh district. These distances specially act as barriers in the pursuits of girls' education. There is no systematic governance of the schools and not very often, teachers do not attend the schools regularly. Remoteness and fragmented habitations involve exorbitant administrative costs while the schools lack in even the basic facilities like black-boards and floor matting.

Other Remotely Available Facilities

More than 92 per cent villages of the Pithoragarh distict, 73 per cent in the Nainital district and 42 percent villages in the Almora district have their closest telegraph office at more than 5 km distance. Similarly the villages, which have their nearest bus-station at more than 5km distance are 60 per cent in the Almora district, 36 per cent in the Nainital and more than 99 per cent villages of Pithoragarh.

These accounts of inaccessibilities speak of the constraints of living in the mountainous area of Kumaon. It is an irony that while electricity has reached quite a large number of villages, many of the households are not yet in a position to obtain electric connections. Thus the villages remain deprived of the benefits of electrification. (Pande: *ibid.*)

Fetching Water, Fuelwood and Fodder

Kumaoni women of the mountains suffer a great deal on account of fetching fodder, foliage and fuelwood and water, among the other things. The distances they have to trek barefoot to fetch them are excruciatingly tiring, specially because the slopes are steep, heights are great and negotiable paths are lacking.

It may be noted that for nearly 74 per cent rural households their daily supplies if fuelwood and fodder from very long distances ranging between 1 to 8 kilometres one way. As much as 15.5 per cent households have to go 8 to 10km, one way, to fetch them, and about 8 per cent have to go still further everyday. This fact illustrates the difficult life of the women in the mountainous terrain of Kumaon.

Table 2.1 : Distances Women Have to Trek to Fetch Fodder and Fuelwood

Distance of Sources of Fuelwood and Fodder (one way) (km)	Number of Households	Percentage
With 1 km	12	2.67
1 to 3	151	33.56
3 to 8	180	39.99
8 to 10	70	15.56
More than 10	37	8.22

Source : Pande, G.C., 1986.

Low Priority of Girls' Education

Girls' education is given lesser importance in so far as the parents are concerned. While the male children are sent to schools even if located in remote places, and they are not supposed to do domestic work. The girls on the other hand are compelled to dropout from schools at initial stages in order to help mothers in their domestic work including baby-care.

Adult education programme of the State Government have modestly attempted to open avenues of part-time education for rural women, but the overall achievement is not quiet assuring due to prohibitive distances and poor organization. Lack of proper education and information forces the girls to live within their traditional existence.

Dowry system in the marriage of girls is rather a newly emerging tradition in Kumaon and is prevailing particularly among the educated ones. The cost of marriage is rising steeply in view of the prices of gold ornaments and custom of giving gifts such as furniture and household effects to the brides. The girls are constrained to live under strain when income of the parents does not permit this scale of marriage expense. Among very low-income group, dowry system is still not that important. (Pande: *ibid.*)

Reproduction and Social Status

It is clearly established that there is an obvious link between the socio-economic backwardness of women and their reproduction behaviour in the hill area. The level of exposure to information and knowledge is closely interlinked with the adopted practices of contraception. Even in the case of girls who were admitted to schools, the dropout rate is more than 30 per cent in the first four years of education. One of the causes of dropping out of girls and high incidence of absenteeism is that they stayed at home to help their mother. The level of education among the women is closely related with their overall consciousness regarding health and sanitation in the context of the hill areas, and this has an impact on the level of fertility and mortality .

Drudgery and Deprivation

Kumaoni women are overburdened with work-load. Table 2.2 gives an idea of the working days on the farm, off-farm and domestic activities. The farm activities comprise cultivation, levelling, sowing, hoeing-weeding, harvesting, threshing, winnowing, drying and striate of grains and their bye-products. The off-farm activities include work relating to upkeep of the household – cleaning, washing cooking, handicraft, processing fruits, drying vegetables and grains, etc.

The social intercourses are intricately inter-woven with the domestic activities and form an integral part of their social life. It is customary among the villagers of Kumaon to work on an exchange basis in the fields. Small landholders share the field-work of large landholders on an exchange basis and get payment in kind, traditionally at the rate of 5 kg per day of corn. The work-days, as recorded from the household survey tend to vary with different size-groups of the land-holdings.

Besides the drudgery and monotony of life, Kumaoni women are compelled to contend with worries, and frustrations borne out to of their deep sense of helplessness against an extremely harsh nature and rigours of weather, the anxieties for their emigrant bread-winners, ailing old people, the under-nourished and uncared children, in the back-drop of natural hazards and living in isolated and secluded places where timely medical facilities are unavailable.

Table 2.2 : Working Days of Rural Women in Farm and Domestic and Other Activities

Size of Land–holding (hectares)	Economic Activities of Women		Domestic and other Activities	Total Working-days in a year
	Farm	Off-farm		
0.25 or less	079.76	55.69	195	330.45
0.25 – 0.50	108.77	49.53	177	335.29
0.50 – 1.0	156.19	47.01	139	242.20
1.0 – 2.0	187.09	42.56	126	355.65
More than 2.0	212.70	39.73	105	357.43
Total	128.86	49.09	154	344.21

Source : Nirmala Khetwal, 1980, p. 483.

Leafy foliage gets scarce after the month of March and the women folk have to trek long distances to collect it. Women are quite experienced in the art of climbing trees for fodder, but the risk of fall and resulting mortality or disablement is obviously enormous. They maintain a large number of cattle, but their productivity is disconcertingly low. The land-cattle ratio is about 1:0.7 (Annon, 1980). This adds to the workload of the womenfolk. Commodities like clothing, soap, kerosene, salt, medicines, matchbox, etc. are scarce and have to be procured from distant places. (Pande *ibid.*)

Marriage and Motherhood

The status and role of women is closely linked with the pattern of marriage. The mean age at the time of marriage in the Hill areas is different from that in the Bhabar and Terai belts. It is 15.53 years in the Hills. In the case of the Paharis settled in Terai, the mean age is 17.19, for the Boksas 14.31 years, and for Muslims with no educational background 15.27 years. There has been a noticeably fast change in the mean age at marriage in Kumaon in the last two decades between 1961 and 1971 (Tables 2.4 and Fig.2.5). However, the system of early marriage prevails, for some obvious gains in the labour classes. Marriage provides the benefit of an utterly loyal female worker without wage for all kinds of chores in the field and at home and that too unregulated by time and hours of work. Thus, marriage results in frequency of deliveries and the narrow average spacing between consecutive deliveries.

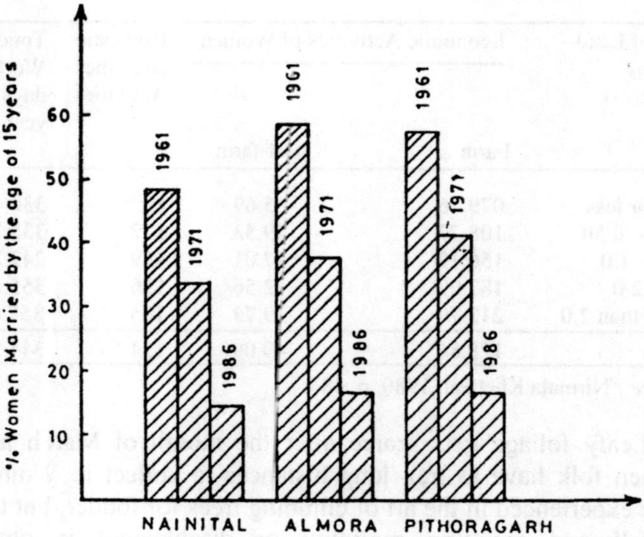

Fig. 2.5 : Girls Married by 15 years in Kumaon

The average spacing between the consecutive deliveries is around 2.64 years for the Paharis of Kumaon at the second birth and tends to fall till the fifth and then rises suddenly. The average live birth per mother is 3.8, which is less than that in other parts of Uttar Pradesh. The incident of still births, miscarriages and un-induced abortions is greater primarily due to early marriage of women and partly due to the extremely arduous life and difficult conditions of work, coupled with nutrition deficiency.

Table 2.3 : Kumaoni Girls Married by the Age of 15 years

District	Percentage of Married Women		
	1961	1971	Change
Nainital	48.36	33.88	(–) 14.48
Almora	58.61	37.93	(–) 20.68
Pithoragarh	57.15	41.02	(–)16.13
Kumaon average	54.71	37.70	(–) 17.09
U.P. average	61.75	51.38	(–) 10.29

Source : J.N. Srivastava, 1979 p. 12-17.

The customary early marriage of the female is very common among the socially backward and uneducated communities. Moreover, the marriage of immature girls with aged men, widowers and retired/pensioners is not uncommon.

The women of farming group followed by business group have the lowest mean age at marriage. The husband serving in armed forces had a higher age at effective marriage. (Pande: *ibid.*)

Table 2.4 : Age at Effective Marriage of Female in Different Occupational Categories of Husband. *(Percentages)*

Occupation of Husband	Age at : Effective Marriage (years)				Total Household	Mean Age
	Less than 14	14-16	16-19	20 and more		
Service	4.1	44.2	41.5	10.2	147	17.0
Sales & Business	13.3	38.6	33.7	14.4	83	16.7
Crafts	6.6	39.6	44.3	9.5	106	16.9
Farming	13.4	44.3	28.8	13.5	469	16.1
Armed forces	–	37.5	50.0	12.5	16	17.2
No occupation	13.0	26.2	30.4	30.4	23	17.1

Source : D.N.Saxena, 1976, p.73.

Literacy status of girls has a bearing on their age at effective marriage in rural Kumaon – only 11.7 per cent of the illiterate female entered into effective life at age about 19 years, as compared to 18.4 per cent with some level of education. Nearly 55 per cent of illiterate females consummated their marriage at the age below 17 years, against about 45 per cent with some education (Fig. 2.1).

Table 2.5 : Age at Effective Marriage of Literate and Illiterate Women in Kumaon Region

(Figures show percentage)

Age at Effective	Categories of Women		Total No. of
	Illiterate	Literate	Women
<14 years	11.8	5.7	92
14-16	42.8	39.0	360
16-19	33.7	36.9	292
20+	11.7	18.4	109
Total Women	712	141	853

Source : D.N. Saxena, 1976. p.73.

Srivastava (1974) noted that education had a positive role in promoting family planning in Kumaon, and has been an important determinant in deciding the marriage age. Female education is seen to exercise relatively greater influence on age at marriage than the male education. In respect of males, their literacy was not seen to exercise significant influence on the age of marriage. It is obvious emphasis needs to be given to female education (Srivastava, 1982).

Demographic Feature of Scheduled Castes Females

The age at marriage of girls of the Scheduled Castes is lower than that of the other castes primarily because these girls have exposure to education. In a study on the changing condition of Scheduled Caste population by Poorna Chandra Pandey it was found that the mean age at marriage was 13.03 years in the Hills and 12.93 years in the Bhabar and Terai areas.

Table 2.6 : Demographic Feature of Scheduled Castes Community in Kumaon

Feature	Kumaon Hills	Kumaon Plains	Average
1. Mean Age at Marriage (year)	13.01	12.93	12.97
2. Age at the birth of the first child (year)	17.85	17.13	17.49
3. Average spacing (year)		3.8	
4. Total conceptions (No.) per married female	8.84	7.22	7.93
5. Losses in abortions, miscarriages and still-borns per women	0.78	1.28	1.03
6. Normal births per mother of completed fertility	6.45	7.36	6.84

Source : Poorna Chandra Pandey, 1978, p.248.

Scheduled Caste community being at the lowermost rung of the social ladder, has a uniformity in hills and plains, but if we see the inter-occupational figures, the difference becomes evident (Table 2.6). The married female having attained menopause in active married career are treated mothers of completed fertility. The number of normal births per mother seems to be greater for the whole Scheduled Caste group in general and still greater in the Bhabar and Terai areas as compared to that in the Hill areas. The high incidence of losses shows the agony and miseries of the women

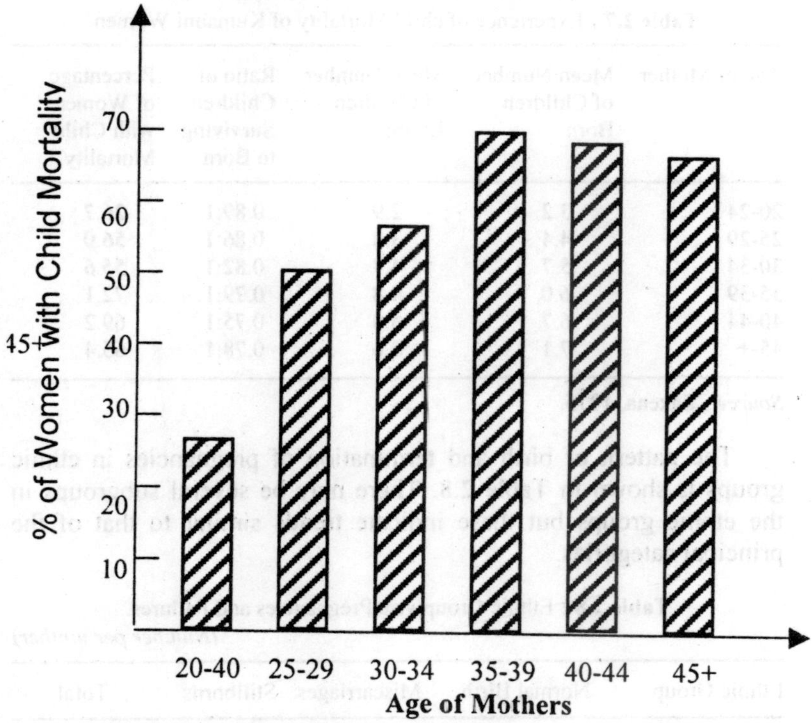

Fig. 2.6 : Child Mortality in Kumaon

of the Scheduled Castes. Illiteracy, poverty and lack of adequate health-care explain this miserable state. If child mortality is controlled and health of the women is looked after well, the success in the planned parenthood will be greater. Saxena (1975) remarks "Should the prospects of child survivorship undergo further improvement in rural areas, more and more couples are likely to come forward to accept even terminal methods with fewer living children and much earlier in their reproductive lives". The experience of child mortality has been quite traumatic in Kumaon as may be seen from Table 2.7 and Fig. 2.6.

Fertility Among Ethnic Groups

The fertility pattern of various ethnic groups in Kumaon was examined by Beena Tripathi (1980).

Table 2.7 : Experience of child Mortality of Kumaoni Women

Age of Mother	Mean Number of Children Born	Mean Number of Children Living	Ratio of Children Surviving to Born	Percentage of Women with Child Mortality
20-24	3.2	2.9	0.89:1	26.7
25-29	4.4	3.8	0.86:1	56.0
30-34	5.7	4.7	0.82:1	55.6
35-39	6.0	4.8	0.79:1	72.1
40-44	6.7	5.0	0.75:1	69.2
45-+	7.1	5.6	0.78:1	65.4

Source : Saxena, 1975.

The pattern of birth and termination of pregnancies in ethnic groups is shown in Table 2.8. There may be several subgroups in the ethnic groups but these indicate trends similar to that of the principal categories.

Table 2.8 : Ethnic Groupwise Pregnancies and Failures.

(Number per mother)

Ethnic Group	Normal Birth	Miscarriages	Stillborns	Total
Pahari	6.52	0.71	0.43	7.67
Tribals	6.84	0.72	0.56	8.13
Bengali immigrants	6.43	0.75	0.63	7.75
Sikh immigrants	6.67	0.73	0.45	7.82
Muslims	6.77	0.74	0.56	8.11
Average	6.68	0.73	0.52	7.92

Source : Beena Tripathi, 1980.

It is interesting to note that the intergroup variations in miscarriages are not very wide although it is slightly higher for the Bengali immigrants and Muslims. The number of stillborns seems to vary quite widely over a range of 0.43–0.63 per mother. It is highest among the Bengali immigrants and the lowest among the Paharis. Fertility seems to be greater among the illiterate females as compared to their educated counterparts. The study (Tripathi, 1980) showed that 81 mothers with completed fertility had 642 conceptions until menopause. 9.2 per cent among these conceptions resulted in miscarriages, 6.5 per cent had still-borns and 84.3 per cent had normal births.

Table 2.9 : Number of Surviving Children by Current Age of the Married Women in Kumaon Region

Age Group of Married Females	Number of Surviving Children									Total Females Studied	Total Mean
	0	1	2	3	4	5	6	7	8+		
15-19	78.1	18.8	2.1	-	-	-	-	-	-	64	0.3
20-24	30.0	41.5	21.5	5.2	0.6	-	-	-	-	130	1.1
25-29	11.9	19.7	23.2	26.7	12.7	4.2	1.6	-	-	142	2.3
30-34	5.2	9.7	23.1	26.1	17.2	11.9	6.8	-	-	34	3.0
35-39	2.7	5.4	15.3	18.9	21.6	18.0	9.9	5.4	2.8	111	3.9
40-44	5.5	3.3	13.2	17.6	19.8	13.2	14.3	4.4	8.7	91	4.2
45+	6.6	5.5	7.7	13.2	18.2	18.2	15.5	6.1	8.3	181	4.4
Total No. of Cases	133	126	137	142	111	8 87	63	21	26	853	2.9
Percentages	15.6	14.8	16.1	16.6	13.8	10.2	7.4	2.5	3.0	100	-

Source : D.N. Saxena, 1975, p.96.

Early marriage has been at the root of all ills the women suffer. Wherever the girls are educated up to High School or higher standards, their fertility was low. The incidence of fertility is greater in early age groups as compared to the later ones. Illness and deterioration of health of mothers is greater among those who have poor nutrition and overwork, the incidence of miscarriages was high. The fertility behaviour is charaterised by increasing pregnancies at short intervals till the age 24 years of the mother in active fertile union and then gradual decline tili the age of 34 years, after which the fertility falls steeply till the menopause.

The burden of motherhood falls on the immature girls when they are married between 14 and 18 years of age. Saxena (1975) reported that in rural Kumaon (Khatima, Ramgarh, Dwarahat, Bhikiasen, Berinag and Kanalichhina areas) nearly 18.8 per cent married women of 15-19 age-group had one surviving child and 3.1 per cent of them had two surviving children. In a duration of 4 years of marriage, 30.8 per cent mothers had a child and 5.6 per cent of them had two surviving children. By the age of 45 years or more, the married women had 8 children in 15.5 per cent cases and 4 to 5 children in 37 per cent cases. Those who had 1 to 3 children were 26.4 per cent only.

It is evident from Table 2.10 that the highest fertility among the Scheduled Caste mother is in the 16-24 age group, wherein nearly half of the total babies are born. Thereafter the fertility marks a noticeable decline. In order to bring down the growth rate of population the age of marriage needs to be raised to 20 years or above so that the fertility is reduced.

Table 2.10 : Pregnancies in Various Age Groups of Scheduled Castes Mother in Rural Kumaon

Age-Groups of Mothers (years)	Per cent Births Kumaon Hills	Per cent Births Kumaon Plains	Total (Year)
Less than 16	1.37	2.60	1.90
16-19	18.09	22.80	20.12
20-24	29.33	27.60	28.58
25-29	21.11	20.40	20.81
30-34	17.63	15.80	16.84
35-39	8.21	7.20	7.77
40-44	3.65	2.60	3.20
More than 45	0.61	1.00	0.78

Source : P.C.Pandey, 1978, pp. 351-451.

Impact on Women of Alcoholism Among Men

Alcoholism as a social evil that has existed in this region for a long time, received tremendous boost by induction of men in the armed forces. The men in armed forces got free alcoholic drinks at their places of posting; and when they retired they brought home this addiction. Until the advent of Independence this habit was discernible but rarely. With greater prosperity generated by developmental activities and due to closer contacts with outside world, the alcoholism has become ingrained in the social habit of the men in Kumaon. The liberal grants of licences for sale of liquor and granting of credits and subsidies for developmental excuses have greatly increased the sale of alcoholic drinks of all kinds. These habits of the Kumaoni males have led to atrocities on women and children in their families. (Pande: *ibid.*)

Gambling is intimately associated with alcoholism which leads to the loss of household assets of the addicts. The women folk in such households lead a miserable existence, a life of deprivation and penury.

2.5 Highlights

It is important to understand the lives of the Kumaoni women in a holistic perspective. The socio-economic environment, geography, physical features, cultural perspectives and rituals discussed above provide the background against which the Health Care practices of Kumaoni women were studied. As their voices and experiences unfold in the forthcoming chapters the linkages of the above canvas and their Health Practices become clear creating the total picture like the warp and weft of a piece of fabric.

This in a way is a step forward in establishing the interconnectedness of the

Environment ↔ Culture ↔ Health ↔ Development

paradigm which is the thread running throughout this book.

3

HEALTH SCENARIO OF UTTARANCHAL

In November 2000 the new state of Uttranchal was created out of the northern part of erstwhile Uttar Pradesh in the Himalayan region. It comprises thirteen districts, namely, (1) Uttarkashi, (2) Chamoli, (3) Rudraprayag, (4) Tehri Garhwal, (5) Dehradun, (6) Garhwal, (7) Pithoragarh, (8) Bageshwar, (9) Almora, (10) Champawat, (11) Nainital, (12) Udhamsingh Nagar, and (13) Hardwar. All of these districts, barring Hardwar of the foothill region and Udhamsingh Nagar of Terai region are hilly tracts. Uttranchal has 49 tehsils, 95 CD blocks and 16414 villages.

3.1 POPULATION AND ITS DISTRIBUTIONS

The provisional population of the new state as per 2001 census is 8,479,562; comprising 4,316,401 males and 4,163,161 females. While the state contributes 0.82 to the population of the country, with a total area of 53,483 sq. kms, its share of the land area is 1.69 per cent of the country.

The density of population per sq.km. is 159, with a wide variation between different districts. For instance, while Hardwar and Udhamsingh Nagar are densely populated (612 and 424 per sq.km. respectively), districts in the Northern part of the state have a low density, viz., Uttarkashi is 37, Chamoli is 48 and Pithoragarh is 65 per sq. km. respectively. (Sethi, *et. al.* : 2001)

Given the above statement, in this context the primary health care infrastructure has been developed as a three-tier system and is based on norms, which in comparison with the plain areas, are lower for the hilly areas. That is why applying a uniform norm for all the areas is not appropriate. These issues have been discussed in detail elsewhere in the book.

Growth Rate

There has been a decline (5.03 per cent) in the decadal growth rate from 24.23 per cent during 1981-91 to 19.20 per cent during 1991-2001. Barring Nainital, decadal growth has declined in all districts of the State. In Nainital, it has gone from 30.01 per cent in the previous decade to 32.88 per cent in the current decade. All this is likely to put an extra pressure on the amenities, thereby adversely affecting the health of the population in these districts.

Migration

Big population changes are usually attributed to migration flows. While Almora and Pithoragarh lose a sizeable proportion of their population due to outmigration, in the Nainital district the large-scale immigration augments its population much beyond what the difference between the birth and death rates would account for.

> "There are several reasons for the big upsurge in population in the Terai-Bhabar region of the Nainital district. The highly fertile land of Terai attracted people from the mountainous regions, big farms and forests drew labourers in large numbers from the eastern districts of Uttar Pradesh. The establishment in 1962 of Govind Ballabh Pant University of Agriculture and Technology at Pantnagar also opened new vistas of human settlement in the contiguous areas. Added to this, the eradication of malaria, which used to take a heavy toll of human life, and the provision for extensive medical facilities reduced not only the death rate, but also facilitated larger immigration. As a combined effect of these factors, the population increased by 71 per cent during 1951-61 in the Nainital district as a whole, by 137 per cent in the Kichha tehsil, 73 per cent in the Kashipur tehsil and 49 per cent in the Haldwani tehsil. In the hilly tehsil of the Nainital district, the population grew by only 20 per cent.
>
> A higher rate of growth of population of the Nainital tehsil in the hills, compared to that of Almora and Pithoragarh has been due to the fact that the Nainital township is a famous hill resort and tourist centre, the administrative headquarters of the Kumaon Division, and a seat of education with many schools, colleges and regional University. Nainital town also has had its share of general expansion of administrative and development activities in the form of opening of a number of new offices and

branches of varied organization. This has, obviously, led to a fast rise in its population." (Khanka: 1988)

Sex Ratio

This has been quite high in the hill districts as compared to the districts in the plains of erstwhile UP. The lowest is in Hardwar (868) followed by Dehradun (893), although the sex-ratio in 0-6 years has declined from 948 to 906, (i.e., 42 points) and this has adversely affected the females. It is possible that like in the neighbouring States, the greater availability of prenatal diagnostic facilities, the male child syndrome, may have started affecting Uttaranchal as well.

Sex ratio (defined as the number of females per 1,000 males) has consistently been adverse to females, owing to a number of social and cultural factors. Nonetheless, this negative aspect of the sex ratio is significantly less in Kumaon than in other parts of India.

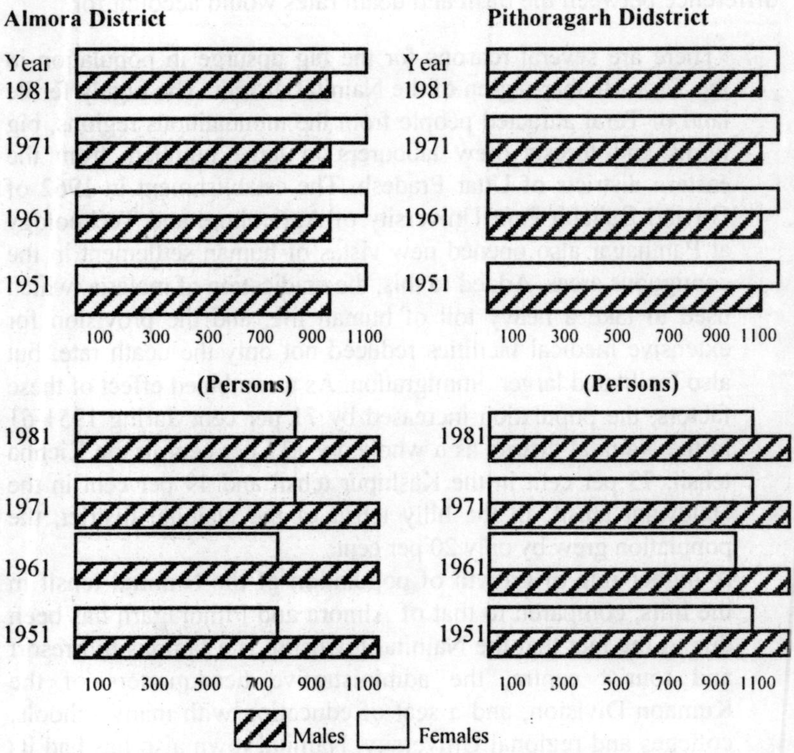

Fig.3.1 : The male and female population in the three districts of Kumaon in the last four decades.

Within Kumaon, the pronounced inconsistency in the sex ratio in the three districts is significant. An abnormally high sex ratio, even exceeding 1,000 in the Almora and Pithoragarh districts, and a negatives sex ratio in the Nainital district are primarily due to male outmigration from the former two districts and in-migration in the latter districts. A steady rise in the sex ratio of the Nainital district during the period is again due to special maternal and child-health measures taken during the period. Similarly, difference in the sex ratio between rural and urban areas are again due to the phenomenon of male migration from the rural to urban areas leaving back women-folk in the villages.

Age Structure

The structure of the population of Kumaon is characteristically pyramidal. The broad base of the pyramid consists of a large number of people in the age-group below 15-38 is 31 per cent in 1951 and 41.12 per cent in 1981. A relatively high birth rate combined with a low and declining rate of infant mortality account for this phenomenon. Notwithstanding, a declining proportion of children in 1981 over 1971 everywhere in the division is suggestive of declining birth rate resulting from family planning programmes during the period.

The population in the working age-group of 15-59 has gone down from 56.18 per cent in 1951 to 52.38 per cent in 1981 in the division as a whole. All the three districts reveal this trend. This relative decline is a result of the increase in the proportions of population in the age-groups below 15 and 16 and above.

The percentage of the population in the age-group 60 and above has increased from 5.51 to 6.50 per cent during 1951-81, which is suggestive of some improvement in life expectancy over the period. However, the overall situation in Kumaon is in contrast with the general position of females surviving more than males after crossing their reproductive age. Possibly, the out-migration of males affects their female counterparts, as the females have to bear excessive load of multifarious agricultural and household activities, in a condition of malnutrition and dearth of health facilities during their working age. This adversely tells on their health, resulting in early death of the women. (Khanka: *ibid.*)

Literacy

The State with 72.28 per cent literates is ahead of average literacy in the country (65.38 %), and the female literacy is also high (60.26 %), with Dehradun at the top (71.22%), followed by Nainital (70.98%) and in the other districts. With regard to state of literacy, in Kumaon there was a general improvement in the state of literacy in Kumaon from 18.8 per cent in 1951 to 38.1 per cent in 1981. However, the fact remains that about 62% of the population remained illiterate in 1981, nearly half of the population of males and three-fourth population of the females are still illiterate. An interesting feature is that in the last three decades (1951-1981) the female literacy registered a markedly higher increase compared to that of the male literacy everywhere in Kumaon. It is also interesting to observe that Nainital is the district which has the highest female literacy and the lowest male literacy throughout the period under reference, while Pithoragarh witnessed the highest increase in both male and female literacy followed by Almora, the lowest increase in both male and female literacy is noticed in the Nainital district.

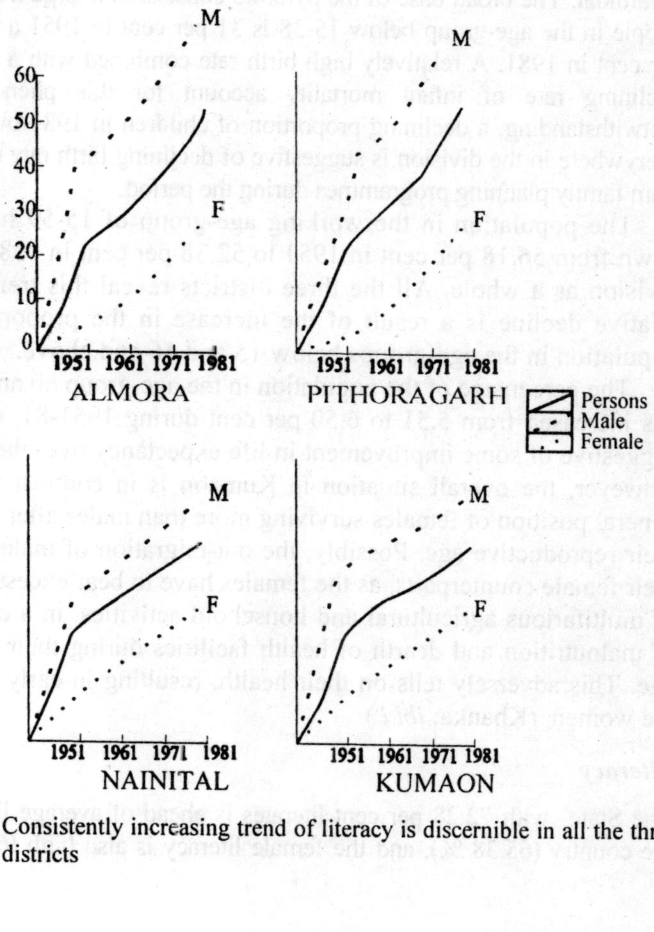

Fig. 3.2 : Consistently increasing trend of literacy is discernible in all the three districts

The lack of diversification of economies of Almora and Pithoragarh and over-concentration of female population in agriculture are the two basic reasons for the low female literacy in these districts. On the contrary, these constraints operate to a lesser extent in the Nainital district, particularly in its plain portion and, as a result female literacy is high.

Literacy was expectedly very high (55.33%) in the urban areas than in the rural areas (34.89%) in 1981. In respect of urban literacy, the Almora district stands on top and the Nainital district at the bottom throughout the period 1951-1981. As noted earlier, this difference is a reflection of the composition of the population of towns in these two districts. Most of the towns of Almora are administrative and educational centres, while a large number of towns in the Nainital plains are centres of trade and commerce and, thus, have a sizeable proportion of labour classes. (Khanka: *ibid.*)

Occupational Structure

The occupational structure of Kumaon is heavily loaded in favour of primary sector, with nearly three-fourth of its population engaged in agriculture and allied activities. The decline in the percentage of cultivators and the increase in the number of agricultural labourers which caused an overall decline of about 10 per cent in workforce in the primary sector during 1961-81 imply dispossession of tenurial rights; that is, downgrading of the tenancy of sharecroppers and agricultural labourers.

Particularly noticeable is the much lower proportion of the secondary sector in Kumaon, i.e., a low level of industrial development. In Kumaon the workforce engaged in the secondary sector has witnessed an increase from 6.53 per cent to 8.24 per cent during 1961-81.

A distinguishing feature of the occupational structure of Kumaon is the high proportion of the workforce in the tertiary sector-trade, commerce, transportation, communication and other services, and to note a significant increase in its proportion from 10.23 per cent to 18.89 per cent during 1961-81.

After agriculture, the biggest purveyor of employment in Kumaon is the ‘ other services’. In the case of Almora and Pithoragarh districts the service class is an euphemism for government and semi-government jobs and constitutes the bulk of the territory sector. In the Nainital district, existence of a considerable network of private enterprises in the service sector lends to sizeable contribution of the other components of the territory sector as well. In the districts of Almora and Pithoragarh, due to a low production base, and also the problem of inaccessibility in the rugged terrains, the trade and commerce as an economic activity are marginal. Industrial activity exists only nationally within its plains tract. In the Nainital district, trade and commerce alone provide above 6.57 per cent of the total employment, and another 3.11 per cent employment is generated by transportation and communication sectors.

Poverty

Health and living conditions go together, quite obviously, rather than depending upon mere health care services. This is where poverty conditions need to be taken into account as the root cause of most of the health problems in this State. A large proportion of the population live in conditions of poverty and social deprivation, and this is what remains the stumbling block to development. All this is often obscured by the spectacular mountain landscape which a casual observer sees, and often poverty conditions are under-estimated. While correlation between income levels and health status at the district and sub-district levels is not available, the poor nutritional status is not in doubt and hence people are very susceptible to disease; while those in the valleys are better off than those on the slopes/ridges, whereas those living in remote areas being usually the poorest.

Ecological Conditions

Ecological destruction during the last fifty years in the Himalayan belt has led to unprecedented poverty, as soil erosion has hastened a scenario of unproductive agriculture (particularly due to terrace cultivation these regions are not self-sufficient in the first place, and food consumption pattern therefore being too low), and deforestation making the collection of fodder, fuel, water etc. on a daily basis an impossibility. This particularly effects women, and weakening their health considerably.

All this bears adversely on the nutritional status of the population and health-status. Hence, there is the urgent need to address crucial issues related to food absorption and utilization, namely, food intake, clean drinking water, environmental sanitation, health education especially of women, etc.

Money Order Economy

It is well known that most of the men-folk from the hilly regions migrate in search of different jobs in the plains. They send their earning through Money Order to their families, especially as one person from every family is in the armed forces quite proudly.

Accessibility for health care centres is in proportion to small settlements which are seen more pronounced in Uttaranchal as these are also remotely located within geographical barriers. This is the rule rather than the exception, so that physical access to health care centres is a critical issue here in view of the difficult hill terrain, because of the non-availability of road communication and the distances involved. All this adversely affects supplies, cost of services, movement of trained manpower, frequency of supervision and access to health care. People walk for several hours to the nearest PHC, which often lacks both staff and supplies. For example, while 98 per cent of villages in Haryana are connected by *pucca* roads, the figure for the same is 61.5 per cent for Uttaranchal.

Household Amenities, Hygiene and Communicable Diseases

They are also poor, in terms of drinking water, toilet facilities, electricity and all this itself is a constraint that contributes to the various health problems. To top it all, there are poor household hygiene practices that contribute to a high incidence of diarrhoea. Water scarcity, housing problems limit the scope of personal and domestic hygiene that spreads disease.

Communicable diseases are deep rooted in this State, and morbidity status is high in say, TB, worm infestation and water-borne and water-related diseases. Prevalance of leprosy is also high in Uttarkashi, though malaria is much less compared to what it is in the foothill districts of the State.

Nutritional Disorder

Most of the districts especially the hill ones, lie in the endemic belt for Goiter, indicating iodine deficiency disorders. Since food insecurity is high in the State, it would not be wrong, in the absence of data, to assume that the poorest of the poor are the worst sufferers.

Reproductive and Child Health

About 50 per cent of the births here are of order three and above. The percentage of pregnant women receiving any kind of ante-natal care is around 40 per cent and those receiving full care remains absymally low, at 17.6 per cent. The extent of safe deliveries above 80 per cent exists only in Dehradun district. Only about two-third children receive their immunization, and one-fifth do not get covered at all.

All these issues have to be appropriately addressed by all concerned organizations. It must be said that despite difficult circumstances the people here have inculcated in them a great love of life and an abiding reverence for nature. Their tremendous potential and natural resources need to be harnessed in right earnest.

Existing Health Status of District Nainital

Since the research was conducted in the Nainital district in the blocks of Dhari and Ramgarh, health facilities infrastructure of this area were studied in greater detail.

The total population of the state of Uttaranchal is 84,79,562, according to the population survey of 2001, and that of district Nainital is 7,62,912 (9% of the state population). The data reflecting the Health Status of the mother and child in the district Nainital is as follows –

- Infant mortality rate is 52.4 per 1000 live births in Nainital (same as Uttaranchal rate) and in rural area it is 75.3. Of this the female mortality rate is 87.4 and male mortality rate is 65.4 (1999).
- Child birth rate is 19.6 per 1000 persons in Uttaranchal (1999).
- Child death rate 6.5 per 1000 person in Uttaranchal (1999).
- Women with full ANC rate 16.9 in Nainital.
- Safe delivery rate 55.7 in Nainital.
- Rate of children with full immunization is 81.6 in Nainital.
- Rate of children with no immunization is 6.9 in Nainital.
- Rate of females with symptoms of RTI is 25.30 in Nainital.
- Rate of males with Symptom of STI is 10.00, in Nainital
- Contraceptive Prevalence Rate (CPR) is 40.5 in Nainital.

Source : CHIRAG report on Concept MCC 2002.

3.2 HEALTH SERVICE PROVIDERS

A. Government Organization's Infrastructure

Existing Health Services of Nainital District

The following information was collected at an interview with the Deputy Chief Medical Officer of the Nainital District on a field visit by the author to Nainital.

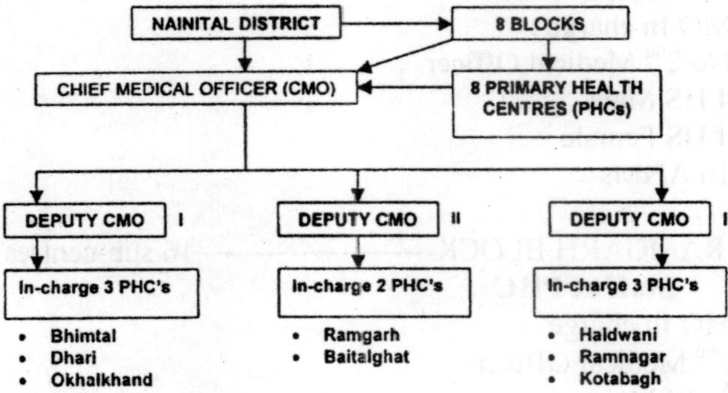

1.

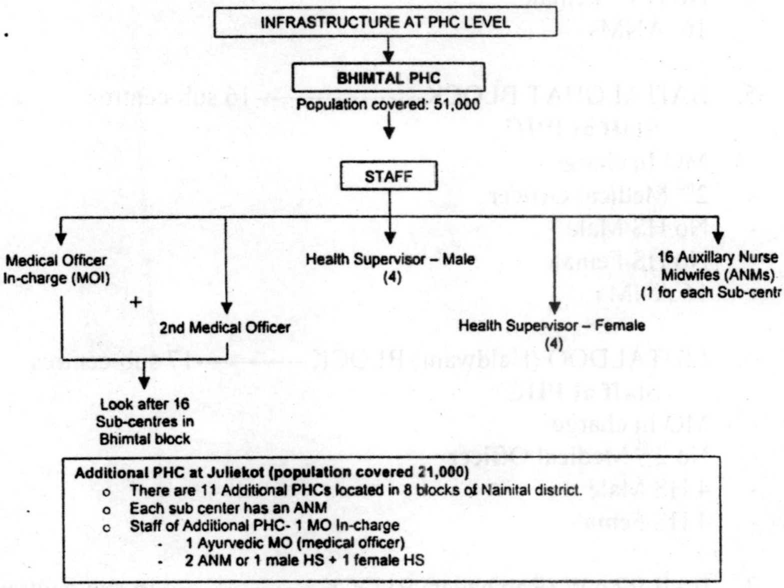

Fig. 3.3 : Information collected at an interview with the Deputy Chief Medical Officer of Nainital District

2. DHARI BLOCK ---------------16 sub centres

Staff at PHC

- Medical Officer In charge
- No. 2nd Medical Officer
- 4 HS (Male) 1 charge (MOI) for 4 sub-centrres
- 4 HS (Female) 1 for 4 sub-centres
- 16 ANMs

3. OKALKHANDA BLOCK----------------16 sub-centres

Staff at PHC

- MO In charge
- No.2nd Medical Officer
- 4 HS Male
- 4 HS Female
- 16 ANMs

4. RAMGARH BLOCK---------------------- 16 sub-centres

Staff at PHC

- MO In charge
- 2nd Medical Officer
- 2 HS Male
- No HS Female
- 16 ANMs

5. BAITALGHAT BLOCK-------------------16 sub-centres

Staff at PHC

- MO In charge
- 2nd Medical Officer
- No HS Male
- No HS Female
- 16 ANMs

6. MUTALDOO (Haldwani) BLOCK ------------17 sub-centres

Staff at PHC

- MO In charge
- No 2nd Medical Officer
- 4 HS Male
- 4 HS Female

7. BAILPRAW (Ramnagar) BLOCK -----------------16 sub-centres

Staff at PHC

- MO In charge
- No 2nd Medical Officer
- 2 HS Male
- 3 HS Female
- 16 ANMs

8. KOTABAGH BLOCK -----------------------------16 sub-centres

Staff at PHC

- MO In charge
- 2nd Medical Officer
- 3 HS Male
- 3 HS Female
- 16 ANMs

Role and Function of Staff

- At the PHC the Medical Officer In-charge (MOI) + 2nd MOI, alternate between 3 days of fieldwork and 3 days OPD (out-patient department). Fieldwork involves monitoring work of sub centres
- Health Supervisor, Male and Female---- Look after 4 sub-centres each and supervise the ANMs work at sub-centre. Their educational level is intermediate plus two years Health Visitor's training at Barielly or Lucknow.
- ANMs Role – ANC/PNC Registgration, Immunization of mother, Iron tablets, Safe Delivery, Immunization of child, Family Planning work, IUD, Copper T, etc. Counselling. High risk cases referred to PHC. Assist in National Camps, Pulse Polio, AIDS, Leprosy. Vit. A solution for 3 years is given. Maintain cards. Attend RHC camps held at every PHC run by a lady doctor.

Since this research was conducted in the Dhari and Ramgarh blocks of Nainital district, the PHC infrastructure at these blocks is presented below. This information was collected on a field visit to the two PHCs by the author in 2002.

Primary Health Centre, Padampuri, Dhari Block

(a) Staff at PHC

1. Medical Officer In-charge I – Dr. Mathur

2. Medical Officer In-charge II – Dr. Sandeep Nigam
3. Health Education In-charge – K.B. Pathak
4. 14 ANMs

(b) 13 Sub-centres 14 ANMs

	Sub-centre	Name of ANM
1.	Padampuri (I)	B. Singh
2.	Padampuri (Sarna)	Parvati Bargali
3.	Gunia Lekh	Chandra Maural
4.	Palara	Bina Bisht
5.	Daduli-Bawiyar	Savitri Bisht
6.	Dhari	M. Nisha
7.	Dhanachuli	Ganga Arya
8.	Dini	Bhagirathi Padiyar
9.	Pahar Pani	Jivanti Arya
10.	Sunderkhal	Rajinder Kanwar
11.	Parabara	Aster
12.	Chaukota	Mangala Thapa
13.	Buribana	Jaya Pande/Prabha Pande

(c) PHC – Padampuri – Dhari block works with

- 3 Nyaya Panchyats
- 35 Villages
- 35 Gram Sabhas.

(d) Primary Health Centre - Ramgarh Block

Staff at PHC

1. Medical In-charge - Dr. H.C.S. Martolia
2. Health Education Officer – Mr. B.S. Negi
3. 18 ANMs at 15 sub-centres
4. Optometrist – Dr. D.K. Mishra

15 Sub-Centres located at :

1. Ramgarh Malla
2. Nathuakhan.
3. Peora.
4. Satboonga.
5. Ramgarh Talla.
6. Gahna.
7. Pokhri.
8. Sirmoli.
9. Mona.
10. Suyalbari.
11. Kool.
12. Pathri.
13. Hartola
14. Darima.
15. Shyamkhet.

Notes from the Field

Besides visiting Nainital to meet the CMO and visiting the two PHCs at Dhari and Ramgarh, I interacted with about 8 ANMs at a family planning camp held at the Sargakhet clinic of the NGO, CHIRAG.

Rajinder Kanwar the ANM of village Sunderkhal said that on the 5th and 16th of every month they had a meeting at the Padampuri PHC with the medical officer in-charge. On the 5th the agenda was to decide their detailed tour programme, develop a time schedule, fix dates for family planning camps and take the required medicines and vaccines for immunization. At the 16th meeting, she continued, the focus was on MPR reporting (monthly progress record) which includes number of children in 0-1 age group, number of pregnant women, eligible couples (18-45), total population, number of deliveries, follow-up, health education, family planning counselling, patients referred to hospital and so on. Interestingly, she said, "I have a very good equation with CHIRAG, wherever I cannot reach to provide health services, the health team of CHIRAG reaches".

There was a lot of hectic activity at this camp, as each ANM had brought 2-3 women from her respective village for family planning, the whole focus it seemed was on achieving the target. I asked some of the ANMs present there, what were their major constraints and they said it was the problem of mobility and procuring educational materials from the PHC. Mangala Thapa, the ANM from village Chaukota said that she covered a population of 2,800 and conducted a house to house survey to keep her records up-to-date. She said that for each village they have to make a weekly report. She admitted that a lot of their working time goes in keeping records and meeting targets. She also said that they had in-service training for the ANMs, at the Padampuri PHC where they were given training in RCH in two batches.

According to her there is great job security in a government employment, the salary structure is also very good, she earned about Rs. 7,000 per month. On my visits to the 15 villages which were in the CHIRAG outreach programmes, I rarely met an ANM in the field, perhaps they were so confident of the services provided by CHIRAG. It is not that the government health care infrastructure is not in place, as I found that both the PHCs at Padampuri and Ramgarh were well equipped for taking care of the health needs of the population.

What emerges is how to make the ANMs who actually put the entire programme into action at the grassroots level more accountable. The objective of an NGO is not to replace the work of the government, but to strengthen and support the programme wherever required.

B. Health Service Providers — NGOs

(i) Central Himalayan Rural Action Group (CHIRAG)

1. Introduction

As stated in Chapter 2, the Himalayas are one of the youngest mountain ranges on earth, with a fragile, delicately balanced mountain ecosystem. The ever increasing rate at which this spectacularly beautiful region is being mercilessly exploited and the resulting environmental degradation casts a grim shadow not only over the lives of the inhabitants of the region but also over the lives of the millions who live in the valleys below.

The vast majority of the rural households in this mountainous region are heavily dependent for their survival on the fuel, fodder and water they collect from the forests in their immediate surroundings. The suffering of these people is thus directly linked to ecological degradation and the maximum impact of this is borne by women, because the collection of these bare necessities for the family is their responsibility.

The situation is further compounded by the lack of health care services in the area. The visible result in many communities is a highly degraded physical environment and an undernourished, over-worked female population with an increasingly bleak future. (Lall, K.: 1987)

According to Rajesh Thadani, the present Executive Director of CHIRAG, Central Himalayan Rural Action Group (CHIRAG) is a non-profit grass root development organisation working with rural communities in the Central Himalayan state of Uttaranchal. CHIRAG made a modest beginning in 1986 when it initiated forest management and health service related work in some villages of Ramgarh block of Nainital district.

In its sixteen years of close association with local communities CHIRAG has come a long way. Today, the intervention programmes of CHIRAG are being carried out in more than 150 villages of the five hill blocks of Nainital district. In 2002 CHIRAG extended its intervention out of Nainital district for the first time since its inception, to work in socially and environmentally degraded areas of Bageshwar district.

The apex body of CHIRAG is the Board of Governors which meets four times a year to review the performance of the organisation. The day to day running is left to the staff of the organization headed by the Executive Director. At present, CHIRAG has 105 full-time employees and about 150 part-time employees.

Since its inception CHIRAG has grown not only in terms of geographical spread of intervention and resource base but also in terms of range of activities. The intervention areas can be put into four broad categories. (CHIRAG Annual Report courtesy Rajesh Thadani).

(a) Natural Resource Management

In this area, CHIRAG is involved with forest management and reforestation, water management, agriculture, horticulture, animal husbandry, alternate energy and integrated watershed management.

(b) Social Programmes

CHIRAG's social programme is carried out through a number of different village level institutions and community groups. Areas of intervention include preparatory schools or *balwadis*, a Primary School Support Programme with thrust on environmental education, village libraries, science labs, centres for adolescent girl empowerment, preventive and curative health programmes, and a Panchayati Raj programme.

(c) Income Generation

Realising that social empowerment means little without economic empowerment, CHIRAG set-up a separate centre dedicated exclusively to exploring ways of boosting the income of local population, especially women. Kumaon Grameen Udyog (KGU) runs a weaving centre where shawls, mufflers, scarves and tweed are made on handlooms using local raw material, designs and patterns. It also has an apricot oil extraction unit and groups of knitters and weavers, and has three retail outlets at the moment. In addition many of the interventions of the agriculture programme and activities carried out with women's groups are aimed at boosting local incomes.

(d) Training and Communication

Training and Communication is the latest component of the spectrum of activities that CHIRAG is involved with. After sixteen years of accumulated experience and expertise we feel the time is ripe to share our experiences with like-minded individuals and organizations so as to forge mutually rewarding ties. In addition, we feel that the time has come when CHIRAG should give its inputs on policy formulation and implementation.

With these ideas in mind CHIRAG has initiated the exercise of training ten grassroots development organisations in the area of watershed management. In addition, trainings are being carried out for village level institutions in Panchayati Raj training and agro-horticultural techniques.

(e) Headquarters and Infrastructure:

The organisational headquarters are located in a rented building in village Sitla. The founders of CHIRAG felt that permanent infrastructure and buildings were unnecessary for an organisation with a mandate to be a catalyst for development. However, given the constraints of finding appropriate office space in rural areas – and our commitment to be headquartered in a rural setting to remind us of our roots, we have now taken on the construction of a small office and training centre in Orakhan, a settlement quite close to Sitla.

Additional facilities include two experimental farms – one in Ramgarh block (Nainital district) and the other in Bageshwar block (Bageshwar district), a 30-bed training centre in Dhokane (Ramgarh block of Nainital), two primary health care centres, and two veterinary clinics. Offices are situated in all are project areas including Sitla and Sargakhet (Mukteshwar working area), Naukuchiatal (Bhimtal area), Suyalkhet (Suyalbari area) and Dewaldhar (Bageshwar project area).

AN OVERVIEW OF CHIRAG's ACTIVITIES

(ii) CHIRAG – Health Care Programmes

(i) Brief background

CHIRAG, in 1986, under its various schemes started the first Community Health Care Programme in Ramgarh block that was funded for three years by the Canada-India village aid.

The success of this grassroots organization has been its aim of optimizing resource utilization and restoring the eco-system in a sustainable manner, for which the development of skills and attitudes at every point within the total system, i.e. the base on which the whole system depends is proper and scientific land-use management by the local inhabitants.

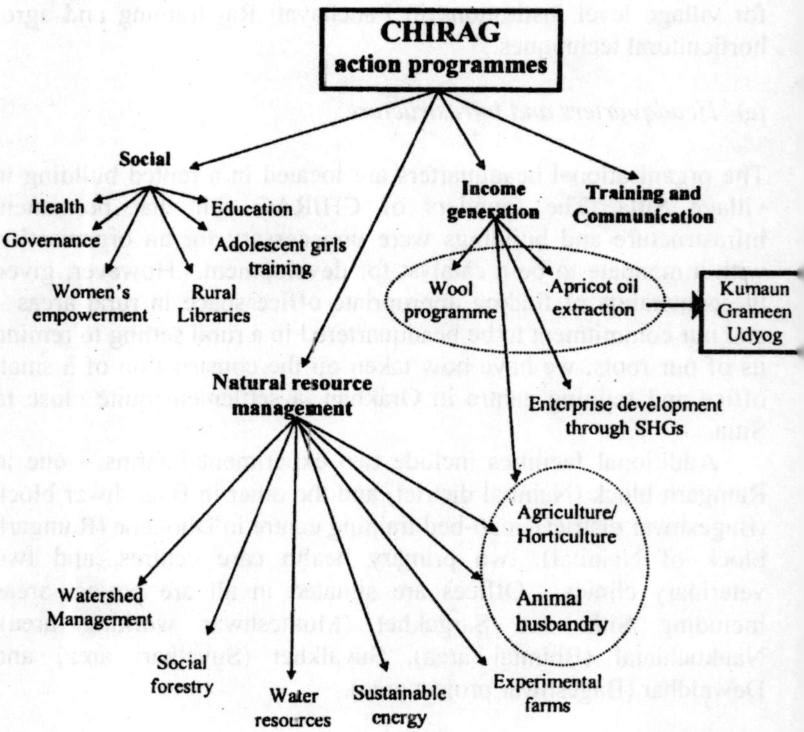

Fig. 3.4 : An Overview of CHIRAG's Activities

The main thrust was to move away from a narrow sectoral approach and set up more specific job descriptions and delegation of responsibility. The various sectoral activities were combined into two broad groups, viz. Land-use and social programmes, each under a team leader.

Later on, linkages with the government (at block, district and state levels) were maintained and strengthened; so also linkages with other NGOs in the region with the object of sharing experiences and expanding certain programmes on a wider scale in the Central Himalayas.

CHIRAG's aim from the very beginning has been to build an institutional framework in a rural setting where young, motivated, trained professionals (belonging to the region as far as possible) can work for the holistic development of these regions, especially by a methodology of 'learning by doing'. These are the essential strengths of a grassroots NGO.

By the year 1991 in CHIRAG, most of the new 'professional' staff were from a Hindi-speaking background, while the development professional were products of English-medium education, so that the internal working language continued to be English. As a result, many of the junior staff were unable to participate in internal meetings and discussions. Some significant questions emerged at this point of time, viz. communication with the outside world, especially with resource and funding institutions which requires English language skills for transactions. Truly bilingual professionals were difficult to come across. These were the ones who would be required on the board. Perhaps this experience has been felt by most other NGOs in the Social Development sectors. While communication in the local language enlists greater participation in the community and is therefore an important determinant for the success of any grassroots programme, it is seen that people who belong to the region and do not articulate in English find themselves handicapped, and in a way are unable to move to higher levels within an organization.

Community Health Programmes - A Profile

Systematic health-care work started in the villages of two blocks of Nainital district, namely, Dhari and Ramgarh, from April 1988, and this project was conceived as an entry point. An old house given by its owner free of rent was converted into a well-equipped Rural Health Centre (RHC), after major renovation with facilities for minor surgery, a diagnostic laboratory and drug store. The outreach programme has by now spread to many villages. The thrust areas of this programme have been to train Community Health Workers (CHWS), monitoring growth of children up to six years, immunization, ante-natal care, health education, community organization and curative services. On the environmental health front, the few demonstration latrines were installed initially in selected homes. Later on, this motivated others to have these at a cost sharing basis and has including expansion of the progamme into many other villages.

In 1990 the Community Health Project (CHP) which had completed two years since its inception in 1988 was broadly speaking divided into two categories, viz., curative and outreach.

In 1990 four of the senior-most CHWs spent a few days with the Health team at the renowned Community Health Project at Jamkhed in Maharashtra, where Dr. R.S. Arole had set up a unique programme to demystify the entire process of Health Care and give it a family approach. This training helped a great deal imparting participatory skills to the visiting team.

CHWs since then have continued to dispense basic medicines in their villages as well as performing their primary role of education and motivation in preventive cure. Their use of these drugs is regularly reviewed. Each village is visited at least once a month by a HEW for meetings, education, vaccinations, ante-natal care and supervision of CHWs. They play a complementary role to that of the 'dai' whose responsibility is traditionally only during labour.

(a) Curative

The RHC which started functioning at Sitla in 1988 was the nerve centre of the curative work. This was housed in a renovated old village building. The number of patients in 1990 was 4567, and significantly villagers were now coming from distant villages out side the project area. A programme for bringing outside consultants to hold camps at the RHC made a modest beginning during this year. Two family planning camps were held in collaboration with the district authorities at which eight tubectomies were carried out. The idea further was to move towards developing an annual calendar of visits by specialist doctor friends which was to be of considerable help to the local people but which also provided invaluable experience to the staff.

In due course the dispensary continued to stock all the essential medicines, and this was also to be a necessary service. The question of payments became a problem initially, so that later on a cooperative store was started whereby the dispensary became a part of the community which became responsible for ensuring that its members are not defaulters.

(b) Outreach

The outreach activities have expanded considerably since 1990, and its essential components being health education, community organization, training of CHWs, monitoring growth of children up to six years, immunization and ante-natal care. By 1990 the programme covered nineteen villages and the CHWs had become the mainstay of the outreach effort. This initiated the formation of the women's groups in their villages, where regular monthly meetings were held. The health team organized slide shows, talks, demonstrations at these meetings with the objective to use this forum to initiate changes in the prevailing health and child-rearing practices and give a boost to the other preventive measures such as immunization, nutritional monitoring, family planning, ante-natal check up etc. Interaction with eligible couples towards encouraging family and ante-natal care were the other activities, for example, 100 pregnant women were identified for this purpose and given anti-tetanus coverage and iron/folic acid supplements.

After two years of the CHP it became apparent that staffing would be a major problem run by NGOs as trained medical personnel in this type of work are rare. Realising this several training programmes were started for local girls in the skills of practical nursing. There were then volunteer nurses who came from the U.K. through the help of Action Health 2000 who were of tremendous help in training these girls. The training continues in a formalised sense so that HEWs have sufficient knowledge.

The outreach and preventive emphasis of the community health programmes have continued as before. Many teaching sessions have been carried out for both HEWs and VHWs and at mother's meetings in villages, to outline the new protocol and re-educate about prevention and treatment of malnutrition. Today the greater awareness of all these problems amongst the HEWs, VHWs and mothers; so also the concept of ante-natal care continues to grow slowly and covering many villages for health care of pregnant.

(c) *Mother and Child Care*

After working for about eighteen months in the CHPs, CHIRAG realised that it was essential to broaden its scope to achieve the stated goals in respect of the main target groups, viz. Children below six years and mothers. Thus, were started Mother and Child Care Centres to provide an integrated package of services at the village level comprising health care for children under six and pregnant and lactating mothers, non-formal pre-school education, mother education, formation informal women's groups and extra-curricular activities for school children. Ten Anganwadi teachers were selected in 1990 for this training and it was envisaged that this would become an integral part of the Health Care programme of CHIRAG.

As we see from the above description, CHIRAG has been working at the grass-roots level in the region for over a decade to improve the quality of life of the villagers – particularly the women and children. Thousands of patients have been treated in CHIRAG clinics and many hundreds transported to hospitals in nearby cities in CHIRAG's ambulance. Notwithstanding the usefulness and importance of these interventions, it is, however, amply clear that something vital remains lacking at this juncture.

Instead of reacting to repair the damage that has already taken place, the focus of development work in the region had to shift to pro-active, preventive and promotional activities, i.e. what the community does for itself to remain healthy and keep its environment healthy. This was imperative to make the process self-sustaining and sustainable.

This pro-active approach could only be achieved through education, training and motivation in a systematic and sustained manner. Only thus would the villagers accept and participate in new approaches, attitudes and appropriate technology. Women are potentially the most effective community based agents to bring about this attitudinal change and awareness, because they occupy a crucial role in the subsistence economy of these isolated communities. Most important is the need to create a growing sense of self-confidence among women in their ability to improve the quality of their lives with the minimum of external assistance. (Compiled from Annual Reports of CHIRAG 1988-2000).

(iii) Health Status of CHIRAG's Work Area

(a) CHIRAG's health programme covers 24 villages of the Ramgarh and Dhari blocks of Nainital district. Emphasis is placed on mother and child health. Immunization, awareness camps, growth monitoring of children under five years of age, ante and post-natal care, safe delivery, counselling on family planning and daignostic services form the key components of the health programme.

According to the CHIRAG Annual Report (2002-03) a total of 1,781 out-patients were treated at the two rural health clinics at Sargakhet and Sitla.

Table 3.1(a) : Antenatal Care

	TT	Iron tablets	Abortion	Delivery	Safe Delivery	ANC
Sargakhet	291	20,240	2	132	98	166
Sitla	61	5,520	5	52	39	54
Total	352	25,760	7	184	137	220

Table 3.1(b) : Growth Monitoring (Under 5 Years)

	Villages	Total Children (0-5)	Weighed	Weight less than normal	Healthy	Still birth	Infant Mortality
Total	24	969	646	48	598	7	21

Table 3.1(c) : Immunisation

	BCG	DPT	DPT Booster	OPV	Measles	TT	DT	Vit. A
Sargakhet	187	495	168	394	131	207	84	451
Sitla	32	81	24	192	34	41	22	71
Total	219	576	192	586	165	248	106	522

Table 3.1(d) : Family Welfare

	Eligible	Couple	Tubectomy	Vascectomy	Condom	OCP	IUD
Total	1504	847	616	101	68	54	8

Source : CHIRAG Annual Report, 2002.

Goal

While the focus of CHIRAG's health programme so far had been community mobilization, confidence building and awareness generation coupled with providing services like ante-natal and post-natal care and immunization, some professionals in the organization felt that quantitative measurement of the work output would help in preparing data-base for decision making with reference to future action. At this juncture, two young professionals Anil Bajpai (Senior Team Leader) and Pratima Singh who joined CHIRAG in 2001 to work on the Adolescent Health Programme revitalized and revamped the Health Intervention Programme of CHIRAG under the able leadership of their Executive Director, Rajesh Thadani.

In view of the above facts, CHIRAG's primary focus is now on preventive health interventions and sustaining these activities, because without awareness about the preventive aspect of health, the general picture of the health status of women and children will remain grim and it will be hard to minimize the focus from the curative aspect.

Keeping this in mind, CHIRAG's goal in health care is to achieve the following quantitative targets over a specific time period :

- At least 80 per cent ANC / PNC of all the pregnant women in the target area.
- 100 per cent Safe delivery of all the pregnant women in the target area.
- 100 per cent Immunisation of children aged 0-5 in the target area.
- Awareness about the benefits of colustrum immediately after delivery.
- At least 10 per cent increase in the contraceptive prevalence rate.

In order to achieve the above CHIRAG has clearly defined its outreach policy with the following objectives:

Objective

- Ante-natal Care to all pregnant women.
- Safe Delivery and post-natal care, child growth monitoring.
- Immunisation and Vitamin A supplementation.
- Health and nutrition education for mothers.
- Regular home visits by HEWs and the supervisors.
- Strengthening and empowering the existing women groups.
- Community Mobilisation – formation of Village health committee (*Balwadi Abhivavak*) as a step to sustain the activities after project phase out.
- Family planning counselling and services.
- Social marketing of contraceptives and general medicines by the HEWs.
-

Target area

District	:	Nainital
Block	:	Ramgarh/Dhari

Number of villages : **32**
Health programme in : 24 villages

Infrastructure

CHIRAG's Health Programme in 24 villages is put into action from two clinics, one at Sargakhet, and the other is located at Sitla near the office.

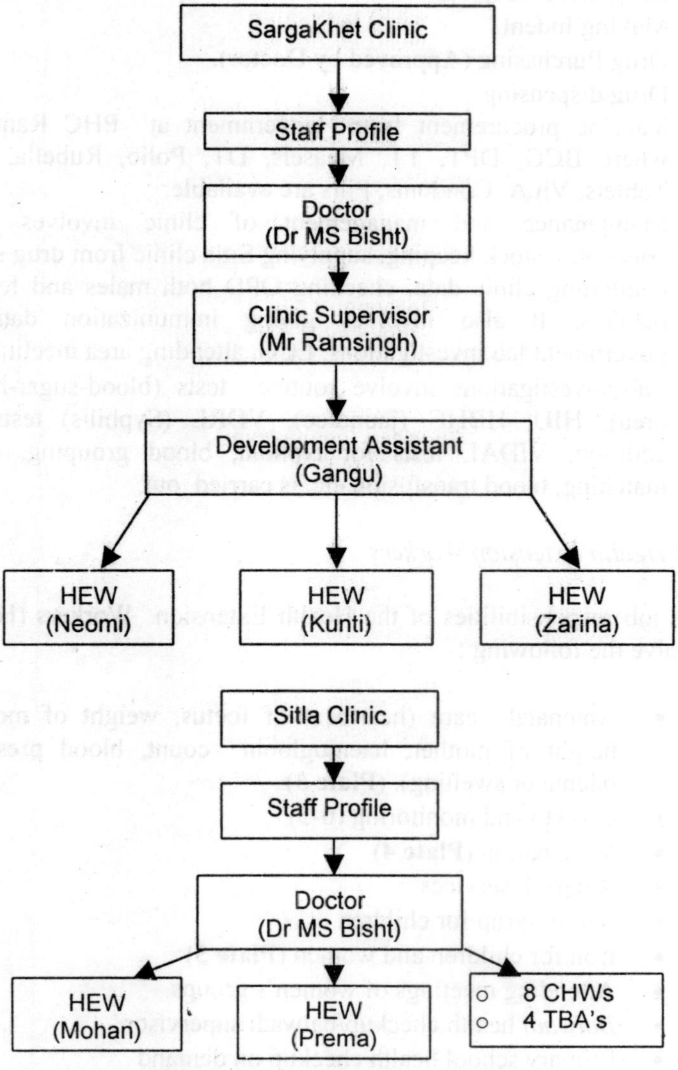

Fig. 3.5 : Sarakhet & Sitla Clinic – Staff Profile

Roles and Responsibilities

(i) The doctor is the overall In-charge of the Curative and Preventive aspect of the health programme at both the clinics.

(ii) Clinic Supervisor :

- Drug Store Keeping.
- Making Indent.
- Drug Purchasing (Approved by Doctor).
- Drug dispensing.
- Vaccine procurement from government at PHC Ramgarh where BCG, DPT, TT, Measels, DT, Polio, Rubella, Iron Tablets, Vit.A, Condoms, Pills are available.
- Maintenance and management of clinic involves cash collection, stock keeping, supplying Sitla clinic from drug store, combining clinic data, checking OPD both males and female patients. It also involves giving immunization data to government lab investigations, ECG, attending area meetings.
- Lab investigations involve routine tests (blood-sugar-blood urea), HIU, HBHG (jaundice), VDRL (Syphilis) tests. In addition, VIDAL tests for typhoid, blood grouping, cross matching, blood transfusion etc. is carried out.

(iii) Health Extension Workers

The job responsibilities of the Health Extension Workers (HEW) involve the following :

- Antenatal care (heartbeat of foetus, weight of mother, height of mother, haemoglobin count, blood pressure, odema or swelling). **(Plate 3)**
- Growth and monitoring (0-5)
- Vaccination **(Plate 4)**
- Referral services
- Vit. A syrup for children
- Iron for children and women **(Plate 5)**
- Attending meetings of women's groups.
- *Balwadi* health checkup/balwadi supervisor
- Primary school health checkup on demand

- Deworming programme every six months
- Family planning
- TT camps
- Community general health checkups
- Haemoglobin (Haeometer)
- Checking health workers record (Total population, total number of pregnant women, number of antenatal women, iron tablets, Vit.A received, eligible couples, no. of children and referral services
- Family planning
- Diarrhoea/vomiting
- 0-6 weight every month of child **(Plate 6)**
- Home visit/patient care/dispensing medicine
- Training other NGO health staff
- Attending area meetings, staff meetings, writing for Samvad, the news letter of Chirag
- Attending MCC meetings
- Post Natal Care (Home visit to see new born baby)
- Organize monthly meeting of CHWs and Dais at Clinic **(Plate 7)**.
- Nutrition education
- Family planning camp
- Dental camp
- Eye camp
- RCH camp at Kasialekh by inviting a government doctor.
- Adolescent girl education
- Educating mothers about the importance of immunization **(Plate 8)**.

HEWS Work Responsibility at the Clinic Level

- Auto claving
- Patient care/assisting doctor in patient care
- Assistance in delivery/DNC
- Doppler test
- ECG
- Vacuum
- Stitching
- All first aid procedures

- Care of patient and night duty
- Assisting doctor in minor surgeries
- Keeping room and clinic clean
- Vaccination at clinic level
- Child care/suction machine
- Monthly report (no. of OPD patients, in-patients, 0-5, antenatal and vaccination)
- Lab investigations (Blood HB, pregnancy tests, urine-albumen, sugar – ESR, Bile salts/bile pigment, Vidaal tests, Blood group, Water quality testing).

The Development Assistant, Gangu, prepares monthly reports, organizes camps, keeps drug store in the absence of Clinic Supervisor, taking care of patients, attends monthly meetings for the newsletter Samvad, he also prepares training material for health education at the grassroots level.

The HEW Dai (Zarina) does ante-natal checkup, delivery, and only if people call her then she goes to the field, takes care of mother and child after delivery, and provides specialized care in difficult pregnancies with complications.

Delivery involves, cleaning of mother, preparation of mother for delivery, using a rubber sheet, blade and thread, preparation of the room, performing the delivery lying down and cord-cutting by scissors, bathing the baby. **(Plate 9)**

On various interactions with the staff at the Sargakhet clinic, I collected the above information. When each one of them shared their work responsibility with me, I could see a sense of pride in them. The above is their perception and sharing of their own work and is presented exactly as they said it.

One question that concerned me was how the Community Health Workers and Dais were selected from a village and how did they become a part of the Community Health Outreach programme of CHIRAG. Gangu the Development Assistant with the Health Programme said, " the CHW was chosen by the village women at a meeting, the criteria for the selection being that she had some time off from her household duties to devote to this work, she had a good rapport with the community and interest in this work. Earlier it was not considered important that the Community Health Worker be literate, however now with the revamping of the programme the health team at the village meetings persuades women who are at least 8th class pass in order to take on this role." Regarding the Dai's

Gangu stated that the traditional Dai of the village in whose wisdom and knowledge the people had great faith was selected and given training in safe delivery methods; the CHW got a small stipend of Rs. 200 per month and the Dai's were paid Rs. 150 per month.

At several monthly meetings held at the Sargakhet clinic with the CHWs, Dais and the health team, I heard this issue of raising their stipend vociferously. Somehow my continued presence at these meetings gave them a feeling that I could reach their 'voice' to those whom they thought were the decision making bodies. Fortunately for me Rajesh Thadani walked into this meeting, and explained to all the women present that funding for the health programme came from CIVA (Canada India Village Aid) and it was becoming increasingly difficult for CHIRAG to explain to the agency why the CHWs and Dais intervention at the village level had not become a self-sustaining activity. This sharing from Rajesh Thadani, initiated a lively discussion and some crucial questions like, how do the CHWs and Dais perceive themselves and their role in the village community? How does the community see them? Do they see themselves as stakeholders in the process of health care? began to emerge in my mind? The answers to all these are not easy but perhaps significant for building the capacities of the CHWs and the Dais.

At a personal meeting with Bhagwati Pande who was in-charge of the health programme with the NGO Sahyog in Almora, I raised the same question about how did they pay the CHW and the Dai, and she said that from the beginning they had no remuneration for them. "The health worker and the dai are selected by a consensus at a meeting of the entire village, the CHW and the Dai are chosen representatives of the village community, they have great pride in them and also great respect for their work"(*inka chayan khud gaon vale karate hain ek meeting mein, yah gaon ki swasthya karyakarta aur dai hain, pure gaon ko inke kam par garv hai, aur inka gaon mein adar bhi bahut hai*). Perhaps, her sharing provided some answers to my querries above.

The detailed work responsibilities of the CHWs and TBAs are presented later on in this chapter.

Steps Taken to Achieve the Goal

In order to revitalize its community health programmes, Chirag envisaged a three year strategy for which clear steps have been delineated. During the first year, i.e., from May 2002 to May 2003 the following steps were taken:

First Year (May 2002 to May 2003)

- Informal discussion with the Health team
- Informal discussion with SHGs (Self Help Groups) in eight villages
- RCH status survey in six villages (which will be discussed in detail in Chapter 4.
- Clear under standing of health status of target area.
- Revised concept on the MCC (Mother and Child Care) programme.
- Formal area distribution among staff for intensive monitoring.
- Clarity of role and responsibilities of CHW, TBA, Supervisor and the Programme in-charge.
- Cluster approach for implementation.
- Improving communication and reporting channels between the
- Supervisors and the Extension staff.
- CHW / TBA ⟷ HEW ⟷ Supervisor ⟷ Program In- charge ⟷ E.D.
- Monthly action plan and report writing.
- Review existing reporting system and develop a new MIS.
- I.E.C. training every second month and collection of resource material by the Programme In- charge
- Collecting information on general medicines that can be given to the CHW/ TBA for social marketing.

Since monitoring is an integral component of any health care programme it was intended that special attention be given to the following :

- Monitoring Information System (MIS)
  - Ante-Natal Care.
  - Safe Delivery and Post Natal Care & Child growth monitoring.
  - Immunization and Vitamin A supplementation for Children up to 5 years.

- Health and nutrition education for mothers.

- Field visits, home visits and group meetings by the staff at community level.
- Cross-checking of data to establish correlation between various interventions.

Second Year (May 2003 to May 2004)

- Review of health status of target area.
- Capacity building training (CBT) of CHW/ TBA.
- Training on Family Planning method.
- Training on Social marketing of contraceptives and general medicines.
- Training on MIS of Family Planning

Special attention to be given to the following:

- Adoption of Family Planning.
- Social marketing of contraceptives and general medicines.
- MIS of Family planning.

Third Year (May 2004 to May 2005)

- Review of the programme and health status of target area.
- Establishment of health counseling and general medicines distribution depot at village level.

Special attention to be given to the following:

- Cluster approach of women groups.
- Community Mobilization – Village health committee formation (*Balwadi Abhivavak*)
- Withdrawal strategy.

(h) Programme Overview

Primary beneficiaries of the Programme

- Women who are pregnant.
- Women who are breastfeeding.
- All children under five years of age.
- All eligible couples (couples where wife's age is between 18 – 59 years)

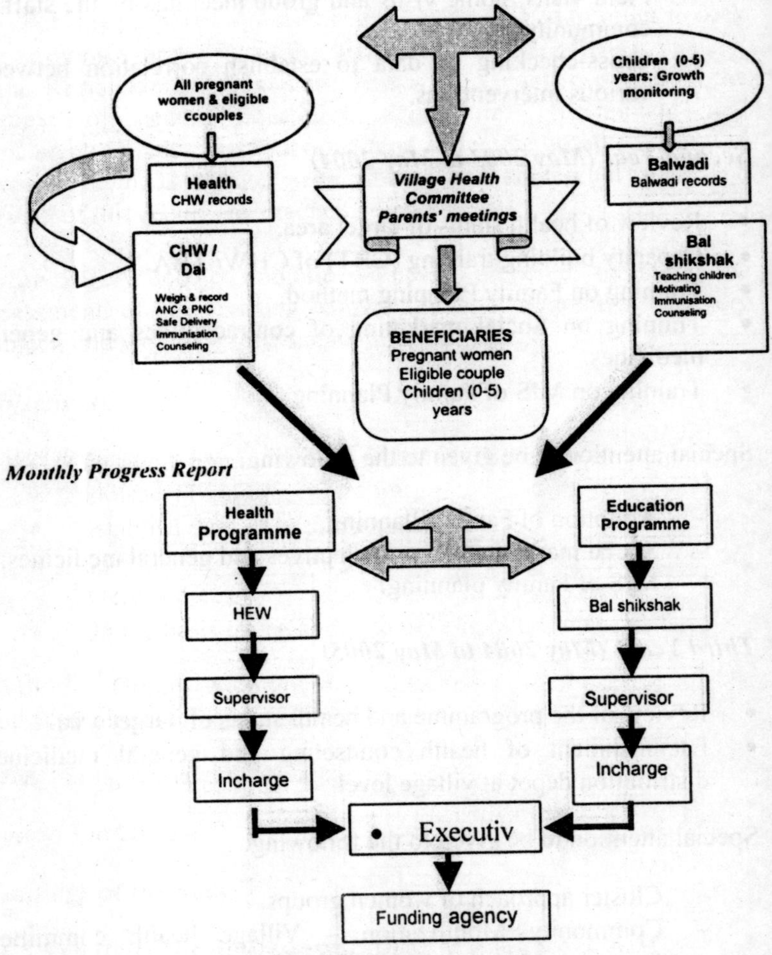

Fig. 3.6 : Programme Overview

Services Provided

Ante-natal Care ***Provided by***

- Minimum three ante-natal Checkups HEW

  (a) Weight
  (b) Blood pressure
  (c) Pallor
  (d) Odema
  (e) Foetal growth

- Two doses of tetanus toxide injection (TT) HEW
- At least 100 tablets of Iron Folic Acid (IFA) CHW
- Preparation for Safe delivery CHW
- Maintenance of "Mother- child card" HEW
- (to be kept by the mother)
- Counselling on proper food intake and reduction
- of workload CHW

Safe Delivery and Postnatal Care

- Deliveries by Trained Birth Attendants (TBA) TBA
- Advance preparation for possible emergency CHW
- Mothers motivated to initiate breast-feeding
- Immediately after delivery TBA
- Birth weight to be taken and recorded on Mother Card within 48 hours of birth CHW
- Post-delivery visit by the CHW within 7 days to all women CHW

Growth monitoring and Immunization

- Every child aged 0-5 year to be weighed and recorded every month CHW
- Weight of every child to be plotted on the growth card CHW
- Counselling for malnourished and unimmunized child CHW
- Counselling for children not attending balwadi Bal Sevika

Health and Nutrition Education for Mothers

- Counselling and sessions on these topics will be conducted by the HEW / TBA / CHW in SHG meetings and *Abhibhavak (parent)* committee meetings of the *Balwadis* at least ones a month.
- Every mother of child aged under five to be enrolled as *balwadi* member and motivated to attend the *Abhibhavak* meetings. In case of non-conformity this should be followed by CHW/TBA/B. S.

Issues to be discussed in the community meetings

For Pregnant Women

Ante-natal Care

- Importance of ANC and early enrollment
- Importance of IFA
- Importance of Tetanus Toxide
- What is complete Care
- Danger signs during pregnancy
- Importance of nutritious diet

Safe Delivery

- Preparation for safe delivery
- Danger signs

Postnatal Care

- Immediate breast feeding (colostrum)
- Importance of postnatal check-up

For women with children

- Breast feeding – merits of colostrum
- Complementary feeding practices
- Management of diarrhoea
- Immunization
- Vitamin A deficiencies
- Growth monitoring
- Iodine
- Iron

Importance of balwadi by Bal Shikshaks

Main focus during home visits by CHW / TBA

- Care of pregnant women
- Women who have recently delivered (7 days)

- Children nearing 6 months of age (for appropriate dietary practices)
- Cases of malnutrition in children
- Children who missed immunization
- Children not attending *balwadi*
- Eligible couples for family planning
- Dropouts from family planning

Monitoring by Supervisors

- MIS at the extension level
- Field visit to verify the records
- Identifying the required needs at the field level.

Vaccination Programme

Vaccinations centres are there in each cluster of villages where HEW does the vaccination. In these centres counselling will be done by the CHW.

Monitoring and Evaluation

Every year an evaluation of the project impact will be done by either the internal or external agency to determine the merits or demerits of the implementation methodology.

Monitoring Information System

- Mother Child Card
- Growth Chart
- Child Register
- Pregnant women register
- CHW daily diary
- Monthly Report
- F P client Register
- Stock Register

Table 3.2 : Monitoring of services by the MIS(Table 12)

	Mother & child card	CHW DD	Child Register	Pregnant women Register	Client Register	Stock Register	M.P.R.
ANC Care	*			*			*
Safe delivery and PNC	*			*			*
Growth monitoring	*		*				*
Immunization and Vitamin A Supplement	*		*				*
Health and nutrition education for mothers		*					*
Home visits and community meetings		*					*
F.P.					*		*
Social Marketing						*	

Roles and Responsibilities of the key workers of the programme

(i) TBA (Trained birth attendant)

- Counselling on food intake and reduction of workload during pregnancy
- Preparation for safe delivery
- Safe delivery
- Motivate mothers to start breast feeding immediately after delivery.

(ii) CHW (Community Health Worker)

- 90-100 iron folic acid (IFA) to pregnant women.

- Counselling on food intake and reduction of workload during pregnancy.
- Preparation for possible emergency during delivery.
- Regular home visits.
- Health education session in SHGs, Abhivavak meetings and vaccination camp.
- Taking birth weights and recording them in Mother Card within 48 hours of delivery.
- Post-natal visit within 7days of delivery.
- Weighing every child aged 0-5 year every month.
- Plotting the weight taken on the growth card and recording in the child register.
- Counselling for malnourished and un-immunised children.
- Motivating parents to send their children to *balwadi*.
- Maintaining the MIS.

(iii) HEW (Health extension worker)

- Immunization and record keeping.
- *Balwadi* Health Check up and record health status of *balwadi* children.
- Minimum three ante-natal Checkups
  (a) Weight
  (b) Blood pressure
  (c) Pallor
  (d) Odema
  (e) Foetal growth
- Two doses of tetanus toxide (TT)
- The mother-child cards should be given to mother
- Training to CHW/TBA
- Assistance to CHW/TBA in conducting health education session, home visits, counseling and record keeping / checking
- Cross checking through home visit
- Reporting to supervisor at the end of the month.

(iv) Supervisor

- The Supervisor will be responsible for complete monitoring of the programme.
- Monthly action plan and monthly reporting to the person in-charge of the programme.
- Will be responsible for need identification and problem solving at the field level.
- Will be the essential link between the extension and senior management level.

(v) Programme In-charge

The person in-charge of the programme will be responsible for maintaining the quality of the programme interventions, compile the monthly progress report and will report to the Executive Director.

Since I worked closely with the health team at the Sargakhet clinic, I observed that before the revamping of the Health care intervention programme, the Development Assistant, Gangu, and the HEWs Neomi and Kunti (all three as a team) visited the 15 villages in their outreach area at least once a month. While two of them handled the ante-natal and post-natal checkups and carried out the immunization, one would go to the community for individual home visits and counselling. Besides this, they had immunization camps at Kasialekh and Sargakhet, and the rest of the time they assisted the doctor in the clinic. This strategy was changed and each HEW was given total responsibility of five villages. It was envisaged that this would strengthen the MIS system and provide for greater accountability.

At an immunization camp at Kasialekh where I was present in March, young women from neighbouring villages had come dressed in colourful sarees with their children neatly dressed. I could sense a commitment in them to keep their children healthy. Some of them shared with me that they looked upon this day, as an 'outing' and had great faith that the vaccines would protect their children from disease. **(Plate 10 and 11).**

Table 3.3 : Area Distribution

HEW	Villages	CHW	DAI
Neomi Pal	• Kamola • Dubkhad • Buribana • Naveen Sunkiya • Lodhiya	Bhagirathi Devi Radha Devi Kunti Devi ------- Parwati Devi	----- Bhagawati Devi Jeewanti Devi Baculi Devi Kamla Devi
Kunti Bisht	• Gajar • Gahana (Gadejer) • Kaniyager • Supi Kafli • Kapuwa	Munni Devi Mohini Devi Kala Bisht Pushpa Devi Parwati Devi	Ganga Devi ------ Radhika Devi ------
Ganga Singh Bisht	• Pata • Supi Talla • Deratana • Supi Bhatelia • Supi Digger • Majhera • Pokhrar	Gobindi Ganga Mehta Bhagwati Devi Laxmi Devi ------ Munni Devi Beena Devi	Jamuna Devi ------- ------- ------- Bachuli Devi ------- Beena Devi
Prema Tiwari	• Meora • Simayal • Nath.kh. Bunaula/K.F • Chor ni Dhar	Mohini Bisht Shanti Raikwal Geeta Bisht. Jamuna	Laxima --------- Bhawna Bhawna
Devki	• Gargaon • Chataula I • Chataula II • Nathuwakhan • Tanda	Leela Devi Janki Devi Janki Devi Kamla	--------- Anandi Nandi ---------

Source : CHIRAG. Concept paper on Mother and Child Care Programme, 2002.

Vaccination Programme

Immunisation day	:	Wednesday
Centres	:	5 in Sargakhet, 2 in Sitla
Immunisation team	:	HEWs - 5 Sargakhet, 2 Sitla
Counselling team	:	CHW / TBA

Finally, one may state that it was important to outline CHIRAG's Community Health Programme in its entirety and also present in detail the new strategies for improved Health Care intervention before proceeding to study the traditional health-care practices of women especially during their reproductive phase. My journey of listening to the women's voices began with a daily field visit along with the health team to their scheduled village. Sometimes the strategy was to visit the Community Health Workers' home, establish contact with her and then wait for the women to come with their children. While the health team continued with their routine work, I would initiate a dialogue with the women present there and so many aspects of their lives would begin to unfold – their work roles, position in the family, decision making powers, their major health concern, how they took care of their children, rituals and ceremonies related to different phases of their reproductive life, their access to health care and their knowledge and wisdom regarding these aspects. (Fig. 3 in Prologue).

It was these sessions that gave me insights for developing the questionnaire comprising forty questions the findings of which are presented in the following chapter.

4

UNHEARD VOICES OF KUMAONI WOMEN : Reproductive and Child Health Management Practices

In the context of the general area of women and health, this chapter describes the research which was carried out by the author to ascertain traditional and current health care practices of women and the effect of Community Health programmes on rural health care in the Kumaon Hills. Before developing a training module on reproductive and child health for adolescent girls in Uttaranchal (see Part II of this book), it became imperative to ascertain the existing health practices of women and children in this area.

The objectives of the present study were:

1. To understand the health practices of women in the Kumaon Hills with special reference to Reproductive and Child Health.
2. To compare the health status of women and children in CHIRAG assisted and non-assisted villages.
3. To assess the relationship between levels of access to health care, heath-seeking behaviour, information, and facilities; and current health practices.
4. To find out the major health concerns of women and children in this area.
5. To see patterns of continuity and change in health care practices.
6. To discover in what ways indigenous knowledge and modern medicine can be integrated to create sustainable and effective health care.

Six villages were chosen for the field study. Out of these, two villages (Almori and Kwedal) have received no health assistance, either from CHIRAG or government agencies. The four remaining villages, Kafli, Chataula, Simayal, and Buribana, were selected from the CHIRAG assisted outreach health programmes. Of these four, Kafli and Chataula were considered to be moderately successful, while Simayal and Buribana were considered some of the most successful of the extension programmes.

For this purpose, ten women were selected from each of the above six villages making the total sample of women surveyed sixty. Women's ages ranged between 18 and 45, equally distributed within villages. To each village one health extension worker was assigned to perform the questionnaire. Health workers were chosen, because of their community rapport and knowledge of health related questions.

The data was collected from 60 women respondents. In order to get a representative sample the following structure was adopted to draw the sample.

NAINITAL DISTRICT

DHARI BLOCK	RAMGARH BLOCK
1. BURIBANA Chirag assisted village where the health outreach programme is very effective. • 10 women respondents	1. SIMAYAL Chirag assisted village where the health outreach programme is very effective. • 10 women respondents
2. KAFLI - HARIJAN BASTI Chirag assisted village where the health outreach is not so effective. • 10 women respondents	2. CHATAULA CHIRAG assisted village where the health outreach is not so effective. • 10 women respondents
3. KWEDAL A village where no health intervention programme exists. • 10 women respondents	3. LOD ALMORI A village where no health intervention programme exists. • 10 women respondents
TOTAL 30	TOTAL 30

GRAND TOTAL : 60

Grand Total : 60 Women respondents for survey

To get a holistic picture of the health management practices with special reference to women and children in the Kumaon Hills a semi-structured interview schedule was developed which focused on the following aspects:

SECTION – 1

A. DEMOGRAPHIC INDICATORS IN SIX VILLAGES IN RAMGARH AND DHARI BLOCK, NAINITAL DISTRICT

RCH SURVEY REPORT

Villages : 6

Sample Size : 60 Married Women

Table 4.1 : Demographic Profile with focus on Reproductive Health Issues of Women of the six villages under study

Village	No Health Programme		Health Programme Moderate		Health Programme Very Active		Total Average
	Almori	**Kwedal**	**Kafli**	**Chataula**	**Simayal**	**Buribana**	
Sample Size	1	10	10	10	10	10	10
Average Age	29.2	32.1	28.7	34.6	34.1	34.9	32.3
Average Age of Marriage	16.4	16.4	16.7	17.9	17.3	15.1	16.6
Average Age of First Pregnancy	18.6	18.8	18	20.1	19.8	18.2	18.9
Parity	2.5	3.9	2.4	4	3.4	3.8	3.3
Total No. of Pregnancies	2.9	5.3	4.2	4.9	3.9	4.8	4.3
Live Births	24	4.9	3.4	4.1	3.2	4.6	3.8
Abortions	1	2	3	5	4	3	3.0
Currently Pregnant	3	1	4	0	0	0	1.3
Child Death (0 –1 year)	0	10	10	6	2	0	5.8
Dead Born	3	1	1	1	2	6	2.7

Average Age of Women selected for the Survey

The women interviewed were in the age group of 18-45. The reason for taking this wide age group range was to analyze and to assess the changes that have taken place in the last 15-20 years in comparison to the practices today. The average age of 60 women was 32-33.

The figures available from the survey indicate that the average age of marriage for women was between 16-17 years. There was no major difference in the age of marriage of women between the villages where there was no health intervention and where the health programmes were being carried out. In Almori and Kwedal the average was 16.4, whereas in Buribana which is supposed to be the most advanced village in the area of health awareness, the average age of marriage was 17.9 and in Simayal 17.3 years.

Average Age of First Pregnancy

The average age of pregnancy according to the data was between 18 and 19 years of age. This links up with the average age of marriage which was found to be between 16-17 years. Only in two villages Chataula and Simayal (both of which are a part of the health programmes of CHIRAG) the average age of the first pregnancy was 20.1 and 19.8 respectively. There was no significant difference in the status between the villages Buribana and Kafli and Kwedal and Almori (where no health intervention was happening).

Parity

The average number of children per family was 3.28. Interestingly in Almori the average number of children was 2.2 per family whereas in Kwedal it was 3.9 (both villages with no health intervention). In Kafli and Chautala the two villages where the programme was not so effective the average number of children was 2.4 and 4.0, whereas the difference between Buribana and Simayal was not so significant, being 3.4 and 3.8 respectively.

From the above data one can see that the least average for the number of children per family was in a village where there was no health intervention at all (Almori 2.2) followed by Chataula 2.4 where the programme is not so effective according to the CHIRAG health team.

In order to link these figures to the intervention of health care assistance alone and arriving at conclusions would not be of any value, because other factors like education, occupation and economic status of the families would have a bearing on the size of the family.

Total Number of Pregnancies

The data from six villages clearly reveals that there is a distinct difference between the total number of pregnancies and the number of children per family. This leads to the fact that the access of women to maternal and child care services, facilities is still very limited.

In Almori the total number of children is 2.7 and the average number of children per family is 2.2. In Kwedal the difference is 5.3 and 3.9. Even where the health intervention programmes are successful like in Buribana the difference in total number of pregnancies and the number of children per family is 4.8 and 3.8 respectively. The figures clearly reflect the need to step up access to health care in the area of maternal and child health.

Live Births

There is also a significant difference between the total number of pregnancies and the number of live births. The average number of live births for all six villages was 3.9, against the average number of total pregnancies which was 4.3.

Almori 2.7 — 2.3
Kwedal 5.3 — 4.9
Buribana 4.9 — 4.6

These figures again indicate that women are losing their children because of the lack of appropriate health care facilities that support infrastructure and information.

Abortion

The total number of abortions from the sixty women respondents was eighteen. In Almori out of ten women interviewed only one reported that she had an abortion, while in Kwedal the number was two. In Chataula and Simayal the number of abortions (out of ten women interviewed in each village) was five and four respectively.

Currently Pregnant

Of the sample interviewed thirteen women were currently pregnant. These belonged to the villages of Almori, Kwedal and Kafli.

Child Death (Infant mortality rate IMR)

From the available data it in clear that the IMR is quite high. In Kwedal ten children had died out of 49 live births. In Kafli it was ten out of thirty-four. In Buribana where the health programme is very effective, out of forty-three children six died within the first year. These figures indicate a high IMR that necessitates further study as to the causes of death. (Uttaranchal 26/100 IMR, Garhwal 40/100).

Source : CHIRAG Report 2002, Sargakhet Clinic.

B. WOMEN'S PERCEPTION OF GOOD HEALTH

Women's perception of the definition of 'good health'

For a majority of the women respondents good health meant absence of disease, freedom from worry. A person who is happy is healthy stated some, while others said, "anybody who is walking around, performing their daily tasks well is healthy". "A healthy body is good health", according to most of the women interviewed in village Almori, where there is no health intervention. Another woman added to this definition and said, "A healthy body and a healthy village is my perception of good health".

Shanti from village Simayal said, "To be healthy in every way is good health". When I asked her to elaborate her statement she said, "If the body is healthy and mind is sad, if there is illness in the family or the children keep falling sick, then how can there be good health; all this is interconnected". Thus what comes across from the perception of women about 'good health' is that they are aware of the fact that not only the body, but the environment, village, family – society in general – are all interlinked in the creation of good health. Their ideas in a way reflect the WHO definition of health which takes into account the physical, emotional and spiritual well being of people.

Food consumption patterns and changes, if any, in the past decade

A majority of the women respondents stated that their daily diet consisted of – *Dal, Roti, Chawal, Sabji,* Milk, Curd. A few women also said that they had eggs and meat sometimes. When asked about where they purchased the food items for daily consumption, the women said that they supplemented the produce from their fields with products from the local bazaar or market. In order to obtain in depth information of the food consumption patterns, an attempt was made to understand from the women, whether there had been any significant changes in the food pattern over the past decade. The answers to this question varied to a large extent. Some women stated that there had been no change at all in their food consumption patterns, while others from the CHIRAG assisted villages opined that they eat a more wholesome diet now. "Vegetable production has increased to a large extent, our dependence on this as a source of economic sustenance has also led to our eating more vegetables" said Kalawati Devi of village Buribana (Dhari Block).

"There is more cleanliness now, and more knowledge about our environment – CHIRAG works well, our pregnancies are monitored and our children are vaccinated" said Deepa Bisht of village Buribana.

However some women from the villages Kwedal and Lod Almori stated that earlier they ate *mandua* and *jau*, the coarse grains that were rich in calcium and minerals, now they ate mill made wheat flour which has no strength. They felt that they were healthy earlier and had none of the diseases that women were inflicted with in the present times.

"The shift from traditional agriculture to 'cash crop economy' wherein there is more emphasis on growing potatoes and cabbage and vegetables has changed the food consumption patterns greatly in this region", said Pritam Singh Mehra, an elderly resident of this area. "Women had great knowledge about grains like *mandua*, *jhangora*, legumes and lentils like *gahat*, *bhatt*, which were extremely rich in calcium and protein. The consumption of these items in the Daily food intake has reduced considerably, and these have been replaced by 'commercial *atta*' and polished *dals* and vegetables. Earlier we used organic manure/compost *khad* in the fields, now the use of chemical fertilisers like urea has increased the produce per *nali* (220 sq. yds.), but it has depleted the nitrogen content of the soil, and when we grow potatoes on a field where cabbage was grown in the previous year the yield of the potatoes is much less from that field", said Kunti Bisht from village Buribana. "All this has affected the nutritional quality of the food we eat, even though one eats a stomach full, the body feels as though it has no energy", she added.

Women from village Chataula in Ramgarh block said that the coming of NGOs like CHIRAG and Aarohi had changed their food habits a lot. "Now we are more conscious of what we eat, there is more awareness and more information related to health", said Anandi Devi.

Dietary Patterns during festivals, marriages and fasts

Festivals and marriages are celebrated with the preparation of special food items. The community prepared food items on festivals and marriages were : *Puri, Aloo, Dal, Chawal, Gutka, Halwa, Mithai*. When asked what was the significance of preparing the above, the women said "It is auspicious. It gives us happiness to feed guests – we want to give them a special welcome, guests are the embodiment of god in our culture".

During fasts the commonly prepared dishes were *Suji ka Halwa* and *Kheer*. " It is a practice not to eat salt during fasts – only sweet things are allowed" stated Tulsi Devi of village Buribana. Foods like onion, garlic are also avoided during fasts as they are not conducive to the creation of peaceful thoughts. That is why eating fruits and sweets are considered more efficacious.

During death ceremonies the consumption of onions, garlic, meat and eggs is avoided. These are considered inauspicious and tabooed for their ill-omen. Adding another dimension to this question, Tulsi Devi of village Buribana said, "Dietary patterns are also influenced by the seasons. In the month of *Sawan* there is no intake of alcohol, or meat products in the Kumaon hills, this has both religious as well as health significance since during rainy season infection is very likely in such products. Moreover, during this period there is an abundance of fruits, vegetables and flowers in this region, the consumption of these items is efficacious for good health". These insights in a way show the interconnectedness of food ↔ culture ↔ environment ↔ health.

Foods avoided by women during menstruation, pregnancy and post-delivery

Menstruation	Pregnancy	Post delivery
1. Milk	1. Potato	1. Corn Chapati
2. Curd	2. Radish	2. Rice
3. Mandua	3. Rice	3. Fried foods
4. Tea with milk	4. Lauki ki Sabji	4. Green vegetables
5. Meat, eggs	5. Peanuts, walnuts	5. Oily foods, chillies
6. Almonds	6. Water	
7. Garlic	7. 'Basi' food, dahi, onion	

In India, as in many areas of the world, health is a balance between hot and cold states of being. While some foods and healing practices coincide with an actual temperature, it is not necessary for an item to be logically deemed hot or cold. For example, citric foods are "hot" and dairy products are "cold". At first this may seem arbitrary, until one has ever seen milk, tea, curd at the mixing of a squeeze of lemon (Pugh, 2000). Blood is considered to be a hot agent, and during menstruation when the woman is losing blood, she can become "cold". Health workers and trained *Dais* advise women not to ingest "cold" foods, such as curd and milk.

The reasons given by the women for not consuming milk and curd during their menstrual cycle were outside the realm of their decision making process. "The cow is worshipped in our *Dev bhumi* – if we eat curd or drink milk, the cow will stop giving milk – that is why we are given only black tea to drink for 4 or 5 days", stated a women from village Kafli in Dhari Block. This is a traditional belief and is still being continued. Also foods like meat, eggs, etc., were not consumed during menstruation as these were considered 'hot' food and would cause more bleeding.

As regards the foods women commonly avoided during pregnancy, the reasons given by most women were that they could not digest these items, and that they made them feel sick and heavy. Foods like meat, eggs were also avoided as it was believed that the baby might abort due to their consumption. After delivery all the women stated that they avoided fried foods, spicy foods, rice, green vegetables as they created trouble for the delicate digestion of the new born baby.

During pregnancy foods like peanuts, walnuts, almonds are avoided because it is believed that a whitish layer called *parat* in the local language will form on the head, shoulder-blade and back of the baby. It is because of this that it will become difficult for the child to move in the vaginal passage, causing great problems at the time of delivery. This belief was corroborated by Zarina, the *Dai* in the Chirag clinic who said that elderly women in the family often advised pregnant daughters or daughters-in-law to avoid these foods. According to the doctor at the Chirag clinic there is no scientific basis to this myth or belief, but certainly *Dais* in the village do say that delivery of a child with this white layer is certainly not easy.

A lactating mother avoids fried foods because the baby can get pneumonia or boils may erupt on the tender skin, stated some women from village Buribana. Post-delivery consumption of water which is considered a life source is also highly restricted. The women from village Kwedal believed that the body temperature reduces after drinking water, therefore some women hold their breasts and drink water. They believe that the child would get *habba-dabba* (pneumonia) if the mother drank water.

On further probing it was revealed that these traditional practices must have had some value and meaning earlier but now changes had taken place regarding the consumption of water during post-delivery especially in villages where there was health-care intervention, and women were aware more than before that there was no correlation between drinking water and getting pneumonia. Tara Devi from village Almori in Ramgarh block said that during pregnancy and after the birth of her first child many rituals and myths were observed regarding food intake. Her first child was a son, but for the second child during birth who happened to be a girl, the same precautions were not observed. Interestingly she turned out to be healthier than the boy, according to her!

The women respondents from village Simayal where the health programme of CHIRAG is very effective said that they no longer observe many dietary restrictions or avoid consumption of certain foods during menstruation, pregnancy and post-delivery. Shanti Devi from this village said, "I have opposed the members of the family and attended meetings on health and nutrition in the village to gain more information. Earlier we only depended on Gods and Goddesses, now we have other knowledge also".

SECTION - 2

MENSTRUATION

In this section following heads are discussed :

(i) Introduction.
(ii) Quantity of food intake during menstrual cycle.
(iii) Physical work during menstrual cycle.
(iv) Sanitary practices during menstrual cycle.
(v) Place where women stay during menstrual cycle.
(vi) First menstrual cycle after marriage.
(vii) Interviews with women and resource persons
(viii) Other Research
(ix) Highlights
(x) Summing up

Introduction

Menstruation is a crucial biological factor for women in their life. However, it is significant to note how it is placed in the socio-cultural context and it is here that various traditional practices need to be studied. This section examines these areas, including the psychological aspects as seen within the cultural context that affect women. For instance, how many women are able to menstruate with dignity, without feeling guilty, ashamed, polluted during this time?

These are some of the basic issues that one faces during fieldwork when meeting community women in the Kumaon hills of Uttaranchal, irrespective of their social status, i.e. it mattered little whether the women were non-literate or post-graduates, rural or urban, upper or lower caste women, or school teachers. It was clear that the socio-psychological attitude towards menstruation remained the same.

Food Intake during Menstrual Cycle

The data collected from the six villages from 60 women respondents with special reference to food intake clearly reflects that 35 per cent of the women respondents eat less than their normal diet during their menstrual cycle. The most commonly stated reasons for the above were " we don't feel hungry" or "we cannot digest the food" or "we feel sick", or there is severe pelvic and back pain. 28.3 per cent of the women who ate more food during this period said that they liked to eat food cooked by other women in the family since they were not allowed to enter the kitchen. 36.7 per cent of the respondents ate their normal food during this period, a higher percentage of these women were from the villages where CHIRAG had its health intervention programmes.

Table 4.2 : Food Intake and Physical Work during Menstrual Cycle

	Food Intake						Physical Work					
	Menstrual Cycle			Pregnancy			Menstrual Cycle			Pregnancy		
Villages	Normal	More	Less	Normal	More	Less	Normal	More	Less	Normal	More	Less
Almori	2	5	3	5	1	4	4	5	1	4	2	4
Kwedal	3	3	4	1	1	8	4	3	3	2	1	7
Kafli	5	1	4	4	2	4	4	1	5	5	2	3
Chataula	6	2	2	4	2	4	5	1	4	7	0	3
Simayal	2	5	3	4	2	4	5	1	4	6	1	3
Buribana	4	1	5	5	1	4	2	6	2	6	0	4
Total	22	17	21	23	9	28	24	17	19	30	6	24
Percentage	36.7	28.3	35.0	38.3	15.0	46.7	40.0	28.3	31.7	50.0	10.0	40.0

Physical work during Menstrual Cycle

According to the Survey of 60 women it was observed during menstruation that 40 per cent of the women respondents performed the some quantum of work during their menstrual cycle. Even though they were segregated and were not allowed to do any work inside the house, 28.3 per cent of the women stated that they performed more work outside the home, like bringing fuel wood and fodder and putting cowdung manure in the fields. Women from the village of Almori and Kwedal were not aware that carrying heavy loads during this period was harmful for the back and the pelvic region. "We do not think about ourselves – there are no choices, we have to perform all these tasks", said a woman from this village.

Interestingly, some of the elderly women from the same village told Kunti the HEW of CHIRAG that women were kept separately to give them rest during this period. The work roles performed by women in no way reflect this concern. In fact a mother-in-law of a women respondent said that the latter did more work during menstruation since she had no work inside the home, "we send her to the forest twice to get fuel wood and fodder".

For 31.7 per cent of the women respondents who performed less than their normal work during menstruation the reasons were: "We are not allowed to enter the kitchen or do other household work, we are also not allowed to milk the cow, so our work roles are reduced during this period".

During menstruation a woman may experience regular problems such as cramping or excessive bleeding that would be exacerbated by increased physical labour. More women from assisted villages perform less work during their menstrual cycles, however, most women continue to perform the same tasks and even a heavier work load during menstruation. Socially women are often subjected to increased isolation during menstruation. Some men believe that if they touch a woman during that time, boils will develop in their mouth. Even some employees of CHIRAG believe this and chose not to come to work for two days out of every month. Others, however, continue to work consistently without telling the men when they are menstruating, and so far have not caused any outbreaks. Women's lives are very difficult in the hills. While on the one hand, an excuse to relax from the drudgery of extreme physical labour may be desirable, most women do not have that luxury. If she does have the opportunity to refrain from work, she is isolated in the cow shed or an enclosed room.

Sanitary Practices during Menstrual Cycle

Table 4.3 : Sanitary Practices and place where women stay during Menstrual cycle

Sanitary Practices during Menstrual Cycle						Place where Women stay		
Villages	Any Specific Problem		Use of Cotton Cloth		At Least for 4 Days	Alone	Cattle Shed	Reason (Untouch-ability)
	Yes	No	Yes	No				
Almori	5	5	3	7	3	0	10	10
Kwedal	7	3	3	7	7	0	10	10
Kafli	7	3	2	8	7	3	7	7
Chataula	6	4	7	3	7	10	0	9
Simayal	3	7	7	3	6	7	3	10
Buribana	4	6	8	2	8	0	10	10
Total	32	28	30	30	38	20	40	56
Percen-tage	53.3	46.7	50.0	50.0	48.3	33.3	66.7	93.3

About half of the women surveyed reported that they experience some specific problem during menstruation, and half also use no type of sanitary cloth. Disposable sanitary napkins are expensive and are difficult to dispose, however there are alternatives that are inexpensive, made of local material, and are simple to reuse or dispose. They are pads that women can stitch together using a muslin cloth, stuffing them with ash to increase absorption. Women claim that yeast infections are the most common female ailment. Yeast infections can be induced by the creation of a moist environment around the vagina, which the use of cotton cloth or ash pads may help to reduce. But more importantly, using pads will allow women to move about freely during their menstrual cycle.

53.3 per cent of the women respondents, stated that they experienced a lot of problems during their menstrual cycle. These ranged from excessive bleeding to severe pain in the lower back, pelvic region and legs. 50 per cent of the women said that they did not use anything to contain the flow, they just walked around like that and washed their saree after a few days. 50 per cent however reported that they used cotton cloth. The percentage of respondents from CHIRAG assisted villages where the health programme was effective was much higher in the case of women who were using cloth to protect themselves. These women were more aware of the cleanliness and hygiene practices associated with keeping themselves clean during this period.

The HEWs of CHIRAG during their monthly meetings give information on the importance of using cloth-Spads, changing them frequently, washing and drying them in the sun. A majority of the women from the CHIRAG assisted villages were using cloth. Of those who used nothing at all a high percentage belonged to the two villages where there was no health intervention.

Place Where Women Stay during Menstrual Cycle

One of the significant findings of this survey was that of the sixty women surveyed, all of the women were isolated during menstruation, with 100 per cent of the women from non-assisted villages and half of the women from assisted villages being placed in the cattle shed. The half from assisted villages who were not put in the cattle shed were still in some form of isolation. When I asked why all women were isolated during menstruation, almost all of the women said that it was because they were unclean at that time. Some members of the CHIRAG health team shared with me during this survey, that because the hills of the Himalayas are considered to be the abode of the gods, perhaps restrictions due to untouchability are especially strong. The risk of infection increases by staying in the cattle shed without any sanitary cloth. Also, most cattle sheds are not made for protecting the cattle but for keeping them secure. Therefore, they are often made without ventilation, and cattle dying of carbon monoxide poisoning is not uncommon. When a woman is subjected to these living conditions every time she menstruates it is indeed detrimental to her emotional and social well-being.

When asked about the place where they stay during this period, 66.7 per cent of the women stated that they were segregated from the other members and stayed in the cattle shed of the house. 33.3 per cent of the women respondents said that they stayed in a separate room in the house, but were also segregated in the sense that they did not come out of the room or enter the kitchen for five days.

In the villages of Almori and Kwedal all the 20 respondents (i.e., 100%) stayed in the cattle shed during the menstrual cycle. In Chataula village where the health programme was not so effective none of the women stayed in the cattle shed. Other facts like nuclear families where women were alone influenced this practice. In Kafli village, Hema who was a member of the SHG group formed by CHIRAG said, "I live alone with my husband, there is no one to cook for and look after my children, so I do not observe any restrictions. However, because I live in a community, I sit separately in a room during this period because the sensibilities of women from neighbouring households would be offended."

The reasons given by 93.3 per cent of the respondents for these practices were that women were considered as untouchables during this period, (*choot lagti hai, isiliye hame alag rakha jata hai*) said Shanti Devi of village Buribana. On probing further, to understand this cultural practice the women shared that "*Kumaon is Dev Bhoomi.*" These traditions and practices have been observed from time immemorial. We only follow them blindly because that is the 'Niyam' (rule)".

"The Gods will be angry, our husbands will get infection, the elders in the family will get boils on their faces....Kumaon, the land of the abode of the Gods will become impure." These were some of the other reasons given by the respondents for staying in the cattle shed during this period.

While respondents from the villages where CHIRAG's programme was considered effective understood the unhygienic aspects of this practice, at least in Buribana village all the women interviewed nevertheless still continued to stay in the cattle shed, perhaps because of social pressure.

Tulsi Devi from the same village said that cow's urine is used for purification of any person who comes in contact with a menstruating women. On the fifth day the woman after her bath is purified by sprinkling cow's urine and only then allowed to enter the kitchen. The type of family, education level, age and exposure to the outside world seem to influence women's perceptions regarding this practice. While some said, "we blindly follow these practices", the younger women with higher education level said, "we know how to keep ourselves clean, so we have started staying in a separate room in the house, instead of the cattle shed. But we hope that our daughters and daughters-in-law will not have to observe these practices."

Incidently, it may be pointed out that in the Garhwal region I observed that women were not confined to the cattle shed during their menstrual cycle. This difference in tradition in the two areas would need further research.

The First Menstrual Cycle after Marriage

The first menstruation after marriage is considered a special event and is celebrated on the 11th day with a *puja* performed by the priest. The interviews with sixty women from six villages also revealed that this tradition is followed even today. Kaladevi from village Simiyal in Ramgarh block said, "for eleven days the woman is kept in the cattle shed, for the first two days she is given very good food to eat like *puri, halwa* and then normal food is given until the 11th day.

On the 11th day the family makes a *"panchgab"* (*panch* = five) of *dahi* (yoghurt), *ghee*, milk, sesame seeds and cow's urine. This is sprinkled to purify the woman after her bath. She is also given new clothes to wear. The priest is called to perform a *'namkaran'*, naming ceremony. A baby made of a coconut is placed in her lap, and she is called 'narve ki maa', the mother of a coconut. Relatives are invited, special food is cooked and this is considered an important event in the life of the new 'bahu'. According to Anandi Devi of village Chautala "some changes like keeping the girl in a separate room instead of the cattle shed for eleven days are now in practice." She said also that now-a-days it is no longer necessary to cook in an iron vessel.

The symbolism of this ceremony is to celebrate the possibility of the daughter-in-law becoming a mother. The continuity of these traditions and their cultural significance reflects the deep-rooted connection to women's lives particularly events that mark her reproductive phase.

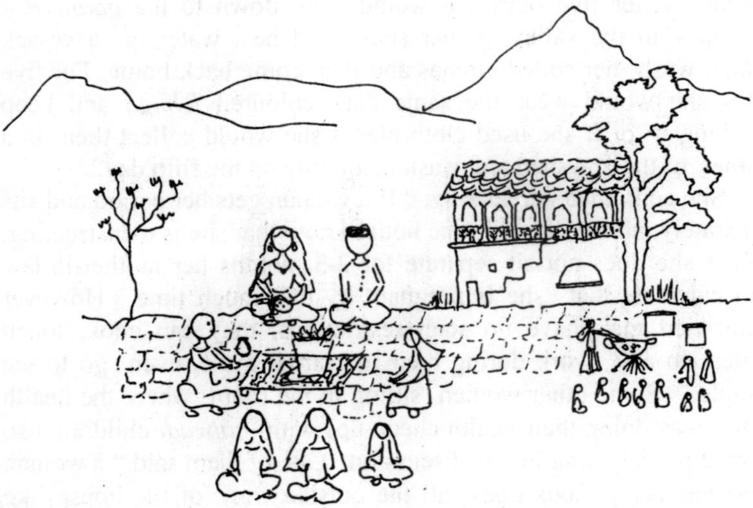

Fig. 4.1 : On the 11th day after the First Menstrual Cycle after Marriage – A ceremony is performed placing a Coconut in the Woman's lap in celebration of the 'Possibility' of her becoming a 'Mother'

Interviews with Women and Resource Persons

During a visit with the health team of CHIRAG to village Tota Banj – Parabara, I had the opportunity to speak with several women:

Interview with Radhika Devi

"Earlier girls were married off before their first menstrual cycle (12-13 yrs), if for some reason she was visiting her mother's home and got her first period there (after marriage), she does not see her brother's face or does not look up towards the ceiling and has to leave immediately for her in law's home. During the first menstruation in her in-law's home she is kept separately either in the cow-shed or in a room in the house."

"About 30 years ago", Radhikadevi, the Dai of this village, continued, " the women were made to stay in caves far away from the house in the jungle, or a separate mud thatched room was constructed for her, where she would stay for five days with only a small oil lamp. ..the food was given to her there by another woman in the family, and sometimes if the evening meal had not yet been cooked they would leave *channa* and some quantity of *gur* for her to eat. After five days she would walk down to the *gadhera* – stream – in the valley, gather sticks and heat water in a vessel, bathe, wash her soiled clothes and then come back home. For five days she would wear the same dark coloured *lehnga* and keep washing it or if she used cloth pieces she would collect them in a corner of the cowshed and wash them only on the fifth day".

She continued her sharing, " If a woman gets her period and sits separately, all the elders in the house know that she is menstruating, and if she does not sit separate for 2-3 months her mother-in-law can calculate that she is pregnant by that much time. However unmarried girls have no such restrictions, they can cook, touch water, do any work during their menstrual cycle, even go to the temple." Some other women sitting in the room where the health team was doing their health check-ups with *balwadi* children also started participating in this discussion. One of them said " a woman who has her periods does all the outside work of the house like bringing fuel wood and fodder from the jungle, collecting the cow dung and putting it in the fields, but she is not allowed to milk the cow, as the cow is worshipped and is a symbol of purity. If she has no help to milk the cow, either they release the calf for 4-5 days or she can milk the cow, but the milk can be drunk only by the children of the house and not by the elders who will get boils in their mouth if they drink milk taken out by a menstruating women." said Radhika Devi.

"A woman with periods is not allowed to touch certain plants or a fruit bearing tree...the squash will dry up or the mirchi will dry up if a woman touches the plant", said Radhika Devi. Neomi, a trained Health Extension worker from CHIRAG who was also present at this meeting said that "all of us walk through your fields abundant with vegetables when we come for the health checkups during our periods, nothing happens to your fields, so why do you believe all this?" Also, she continued, "you go to the jungle to cut grass and bring fuelwood for the house, how the jungle is green even when you touch the trees?" Some women said to this, we have no explanation for all this, it has come down to us from generations. Others said the trees in the jungle are evergreen, they are not fruit bearing, this restriction is only for fruit bearing trees.

No clear answers were emerging from this discussion. However, what is significant is that all their taboos, rituals and practices are linked to the notion of purity and pollution which is linked to their world view. These have a 'scientific' basis, said Malti Devi, "Blood at this time is impure, the woman has to shed it for 4-5 days to become pure once again, that is why she is made to sit separately, this also gives her rest".

It was interesting to note from the above discussion that while a woman is given rest from light household work like cooking and cleaning utensils she does all the heavy work of walking to the jungle bringing fuelwood and fodder in a condition when she needs rest. Some significant issues emerged from this discussion, and when I asked the women the following question: –

Why are only married daughters and daughters-in-law considered impure during menstruation when the same treatment is not given to adolescent girls (*kunwari*)? An elderly woman wearing a 20 yard traditional *'lehnga'* said, "After marriage a woman becomes a *'Suhagin'*, she has relations with her husband, she can procreate and therefore she is considered impure (*ashudh*)...when she is a *kunwari* (virgin) we do not consider her impure. Our ancestors believed in this and these practices have come down from generations, Kumaon is *'devbhumi'*, the abode of the gods. My mother use to say "When a woman is menstruating, the earth can get burnt for seven layers, if we do not observe these traditions and practices our gods will be angry". Continuing her dialogue, she further said, "Now the age of marriage has changed, earlier girls were married at the age of 13-14, so they had their first period in their in-law's house. This is celebrated in a big way in the sasural (in-law's house)."

The discussion then moved on to rituals associated with first menstruation in the in-law's family. " I was 11 years old when I got married," said Radhikabehn, " they kept me in a cowshed, when I got my first period at 13, I was cold, but they would not allow me to sit near the fire. On the fifth day I was sent to the river to bathe in the icy cold water, I would cry with fear, but today I heat up the water for my daughter-in-law, I do not make her sit in the cowshed but in a room in the house, she bathes everyday." She went on to narrate the story of her son in the context of the above conversation, who is a priest in the temple in the village, "My son studied till class 10, but failed his 11th class examination twice, he did not want to leave me and go to the plains for a job, so in the month of *Sawan*, he stayed in the temple, bathed three times a day and ate only *vibhuti* for 11 days, for the next 7 days he ate half a *roti* and would do *puja* in the temple at 4 p.m. After the 18th day he ate one *roti*, on the 22nd day he ate 2 *rotis* and on the 23rd day a full meal. After that he became a *pujari*, that is why I do not allow my daughter-in-law to touch the food to be served to my son. If there is a *'jagar'* in the village they call my son to perform the jagar ceremony. A menstruating woman is not allowed to go there, in fact it is believed that if such a woman is sitting in the audience the person will not get possessed and the *'jagar'* ceremony cannot proceed" said Radhika Devi.

Her sharing all this was in a way drawing up a broader holistic picture of the rituals, taboos and practices of the people with reference to women during menstruation period. "After marriage when the woman gets her first period she is kept separate in a cattleshed for 11 days", said Bachuli devi of village Leitibunga, Dhari block, " During this period the woman is given good food to eat for the first five days. On the 11th day the Pandit is called and there is a ceremony in celeberation of the fact that she can now become a mother. During the ceremony the Pandit keeps a coconut in her lap and on that day she is called *'narwe ki ma'*, mother of a coconut. *'Panchgab'* a preparation of *Dhub* grass, cow's urine, yoghurt, *Til* (Sesame) and a copper coin is sprinkled to purify the girl when she comes out of the cattle shed after 11 days. Even now-a-days they sprinkle cow's urine to purify the woman when she enters the house after 5 days. If a sister-in-law goes to the cattle shed to give the woman her food, she too is purified by sprinkling cow's urine. Because of the importance and significance of the first menstrual cycle after marriage for the in-law's family, a daughter visiting her parental home is immediately sent to *sasural* on getting her periods as it is believed that now this flower belongs to her in-law's home and there is a celebration in the hope that she is ready to bear fruit." Interestingly another woman sitting next to Bachuli devi said *"Rasta khul gaya, yeh khushi ki bat hai"*. The way has opened, now for her to become a mother. There was laughter all around in the room in this sharing.

Interview with Bachuli Devi, the Dai of village Navin Sunkhiya

According to Bachuli Devi, earlier the hygienic practices with reference to menstruation were not at all conducive to keeping a woman in the household. Women wore dark coloured *lehngas* or *sarees* and just sat in them in the cattle shed, often they walked to the jungle with their clothes all stained and legs soiled, they were given no water to keep themselves clean, so the question of allowing them in side the house did not arise." The doctor working at the Sargakhet clinic of the NGO CHIRAG also reiterated the above and said, " The hygiene precautions they were taking were not at all adequate to allow women to participate in household activities. No tradition is to be denigrated, it has some meaning". "Now-a-days", said Bachuli Devi, "because of the presence of CHIRAG, in these villages the daughters-in-law and young adolescent girls have become more aware of the importance of cleanliness during this period. Women bathe everyday with hot water and wash the cloth they use with soap and water and dry it in the sun. Some women also use sterilised ash and wrap it in an old cloth because it soaks the blood".

Neomi, the health worker from CHIRAG, used this opportunity to share with the women present, the importance of menstrual hygiene. She explained to them that blood can have bacteria which can lead to reproductive tract infections if a woman does not keep herself clean and does not use clean cloth. She suggested that they should soak the cloth after use in warm water and surf with a little salt, which makes them clean and they should be dried in the sun so that all the bacteria die.

Giving value to their traditions and practices, Neomi said, "you value purity, cleanliness, earlier all these facilities were not available but now with changing times and availability of more water a woman can keep herself clean." She was urging the mothers-in-law not to keep their daughters-in-law in the cattle shed as cowdung has bacteria which can enter the vagina and travel to the cervix, if a woman sits on the cold floor with no undergarment or pad.

I could see the women listening to her with rapt attention, a more active and educated woman, Hema said, "I live separately as a family with my husband, and he does not expect me to sit separately or not cook for the family. But I have to hide and do all this from neighbours and other women in the community because the elders regard this as completely inappropriate."

The two most important reasons emerging from the above discussion being, (i) Giving women some rest, and (ii), withholding her participation in household chores like cooking and fetching water because she was not clean.

I observed a lot of changes in the outreach areas of CHIRAG's Health programmes, but perhaps that is not representative of the interior regions of Kumaon.

Interview with Reetu Sogani and Bhagwati Pande, NGO Aadhar, Buniyad (Units of Sahyog), Almora District

Food Intake during Menstruation

During menstruation milk and milk products, tea with milk, *dahi,* butter milk, etc. are not given to the woman. It is believed that the gods will be angry; particularly in Kumaon they believe that *'aidi devta'* who is the god for protection of animals will become angry if milk is given in any form to a menstruating woman. It is also believed that the cow or buffalo will get sick or their milk will dry up if a menstruating woman milks the animals or drinks the milk even in tea. Black tea is given to her for 5 days, now-a-days however they have started using powdered milk in some areas. A woman is also not allowed to eat the *prasad* from the temple or any form of non-vegetarian food. She is also not to touch pickle, or plants and trees bearing fruit as these will dry up or die if she touches them.

For five days during the period, the woman cannot cook food or touch water, water is drawn from *"naulas"* or springs which are treated as places of worship as many of these water sources have a shrine attached to them (add other reasons). The utensils used by the woman during times are kept separately in the cattle shed, food is put into them from a distance by another family member who is purified with cow's urine before entering the house.

Not only are there restrictions for movement within the house, a menstruating woman is not welcome or allowed in community spaces, the village temple, neighboring households and her presence is absolutely forbidden on social or religious occasions like marriages, prayer meetings, *jagar* ceremonies and other religious festivals.

According to Bhagwati Pande after bathing on the 3rd and 5th day the house is cleaned with a *'lipai'* (coat) of a fresh coat of cowdung and *bhusa* mixture, and only after the fifth day is a woman allowed to enter the kitchen for preparation of food. Regarding their menstrual hygiene practices in the villages, in Almora district the pattern was quite the same, some women used nothing at all, others used old cloth, they felt since blood is impure it is not necessary to use clean cloth at all. Even the mattress or quilt which they would be given to use in the cattle shed would be old and not clean. In some communities women sit in the cattle shed on a *'paral'*, a mat made of grass which can be thrown later if it gets soiled.

Evidently, women have very little knowledge about their reproductive organs coupled with that they do not have the resources to adequately take care of themselves in terms of plenty of water or clean pads. Even the cloth that they use and wash has to be hidden in some dark corners to dry, so that it does not catch the eye of any other member of the family. It is believed that even if they set eyes on such a cloth they will get boils on their face or fall sick.

Elderly people particularly women believe that any illness related to menstruation cannot be cured by the gods, as menstrual blood is too impure to be linked to the benediction of a god. Only when a woman is suffering seriously is she shown to a doctor.

Not only is this a difficult time for a woman in terms of physical work, food intake, restrictions of movement, a woman in this state also undergoes a lot of emotional tension. When I asked some women at a meeting in Tota Banj how they felt during these days, what did they experience, the older women said " we felt like untouchables – lesser human beings – the whole episode is a nightmare". The younger women some of whom did not have to sit in the cattle shed any longer but stayed separately in a room in the house, said that "all this has to change, and it will slowly go, nothing goes on for ever."

"Some day the daughter-in-law will become aware, and in some cases the mother-in-law will also change to bring about transformation said", Kunti Bisht, a health worker of village Buri Bana.

Some major and minor problems related to menstruation are as follows :

- irregular periods, backpain, white discharge, excessive bleeding, itching and burning.

Kishni Devi of village Sargakhet, Sunkiya, age 65 years said, "During any illness related to menstruation earlier we did our own treatment. Rice soaked in water and made into a *halwa* either salty or sweet is very effective for white discharge". She further said that her mother-in-law had cured her by giving her this twice a day when she had severe leucorrhoea (strained with blood).

Zarina the trained *Dai* of CHIRAG who works at the clinic, said that if one soaks rice and grinds it to a paste and then mixes it with small pieces of coconut and eats this in the morning on an empty stomach it is extremely helpful in curing the problem of white discharge. For excessive pain during menstruation, Zarina said that if gur boiled with water and ajwain is given it relieves the stomach cramps and pelvic pain greatly. Bhagvati Devi the health worker of village Kamola on a visit to the village told me that when women had severe back pain and pelvic pain during menstruation she would heat a brick till it was red hot and then wrap it in wet sack/gunny cloth and give fomentation. This was very effective. Now-a-days some women use a rubber hot water bottle.

Highlights of Other Research

To add to the body of knowledge, the findings of other research in this area are given below :

A field study by Das (1998) entitled "The Status of Women's Health in Uttaranchal", made an attempt to look at the issue of menstruation within a socio-cultural context, in terms of the following headings :

1. Women's morbidities.
2. Socio-economic factors affecting health.
3. Health seeking behaviour.
4. Reproductive Health Practices.

This study was conducted in pockets of 250 households over ten locations in all the districts of Uttranchal in 1996-97. It was done through discussions, individual interviews and key informants, culminating in diagnostic camps. All in all, there were individual interactions with over a thousand women across the length and breadth of Uttaranchal, ranging in age from 14 to 70, and including community birth attendants, herbal healers and women with special problems. (Das, Jashodra, 1998).

Field research about menstruation ranged from perceptions and knowledge about the process, attitudes towards it, ritual and practices related to it, morbidities arising from it, and related health seeking behaviour.

Highlights

Beliefs and practices related to the menstrual cycle :

- Nearly everywhere, women withdraw from society and go into seclusion for 5-7 days of the menstrual cycle. Women generally stay in the house but in a separate corner. However, they are not exempt from work in the fields or forest, that is, heavy work. This practice is more common in Kumaon and in some places women are made to stay in a cowshed. In a community every women's period is a matter of public knowledge and is kept track of. If a young bride does not go into seclusion soon after marriage it becomes a matter of public speculation.
- During this period women are not allowed to enter the kitchen and places of worship. She is not allowed to touch anybody or pass on any object. Whatever 'shutouts' must be purified by sprinkling cow's urine. They cannot travel, participate in meetings or social gatherings. Cooking during menstruation is strictly prohibited special when there are elders in the family. A woman can cook only for her children and herself. If there is no one else in the family, the husband has to do the cooking or help is sought from the neighbours. In Kumaon, a woman is not allowed to have

milk, yoghurt, buttermilk, etc. The common belief is that if a menstruating woman is given milk or milk products the animal is infected and stops lactating. In one place, meat eating and touching the sacrificial lamb is prohibited. Women are not allowed to cohabit with their husband for fear of his becoming impotent.

- When asked for the reason behind these oppressive practices, women said these customs had been followed for generations. It is believed that when these norms are defied, people are possessed by spirits and others who have been defiled, and in the process develop rashes and allergies.

Some Myths related to Menstruation

Several myths related to menstruation common in the hills (probably common throughout India) are as follows :

1. If the shadow of a menstruating girl touches her father or brother, it is disastrous.
2. Anyone who touches a menstruating woman, falls ill. Menstruation is an infection, and its symptoms are rashes, inflammation of the skin etc. In order to protect yourself, sprinkle cow's urine on everything she touches.
3. The infection spreads faster through water.
4. If a menstruating woman touches pickle or other perishables, they are spoiled.
5. Animals stop lactating if a woman is given milk during menstruation.
6. Consumption of milk increases blood loss during menstruation.
7. If a menstruating woman touches a tree, it dries up and its fruits rot.

Menstruation in Unmarried Women

Generally, the menstruation of girls is a carefully concealed event. Once the community acknowledges it, it is because society frowns upon girls remaining unmarried even after puberty, so everyone has to pretend that the daughter is still pre-pubescent, even if she is eighteen. The girls use underwear and rags to soak the blood, but cannot wash or dry them in public. Girls do believe they are polluted, and would not go to a place of worship during menstruation.

Hygiene during Menstruation

Generally women do not use cloth during menstruation. Only those who bleed excessively do so. Some women use underwear while others don't. They bleed in their clothes. If at all cloth is used, it is either disposed of or washed and used again. But as menstrual cloth is considered very polluting and infectious, this cannot be done publicly.

Generally women bathe on the fifth day of menstruation as bathing before that day is prohibited. Young women however bathe everyday. A menstruating woman can enter the kitchen only on the fifth day after bathing and sprinkling cow's urine. Since a quilt cannot be washed, a woman may only use blankets during menstruation, despite the bitterly cold winters in this region.

Traditionally, although menstrual blood has frightfully polluting properties, there is no organized way of soaking or disposing of it. Women generally bleed into their clothes or a piece of sacking they might be sitting on. Since they may not touch water or utensils, they cannot wash themselves or their clothes until the period is over, for someone would need to pour out water for them. Younger women who own a pair of knickers would surreptitiously wash the mat at some water source while working in the forest organizing cattle, dry them out on a bush and re-use them. If this is not possible, the knickers or rags used are washed and dried covertly – under a petticoat that is drying on the clothes line, or stuffed under a mattress, or under the roof eaves. The lack of direct sunshine in drying the menstrual cloth means that there is a great risk of bacterial growth on the cloth, and the attendant risk of reproductive tract infections. Although we do not have conclusive evidence to prove that this lack of hygiene is responsible for the high incidence of white discharge in the area, it might be interesting to look at some figures. Among the women contacted during the study, 73 (29.1%) out of 251 women (15-45 years contacted in the community) reported suffering from white discharge, and in the diagnostic camp 104 out of 397 women (26.2%) reported white discharge. On medical examination of 105 women, 83 (79%) were found to have a serious problem. (Das, Jasodhara, 1998)

Special Customs

In some parts of Kumaon, in a certain community, there is a special custom when the unmarried girl is sent away to another village during her first menstruation, usually her maternal grandparents for 20 days. It is believed that if she sees her father and brother during that time, it is a bad omen.

There are special customs related to a married woman's first menstruation after marriage, which is considered polluted for eleven days and seven days in the second menstruation. In some places, a priest is summoned to perform a religious *'Ganesh Puja'* ceremony, after which coconut fruits are placed on the woman's lap and *tilak* is applied on her forehead.

Change in Customs

Older women have described changes in customs over the years. Earlier, they said, all five days of menstruation were considered polluting but now women do not even disclose their periods. Earlier they walked with downcast eyes so that they would not see the temple; earlier they were married before they reached puberty, now they are married much later.

Correlations

There many reasons given behind such various customs, but a major one was fear of the *Ishta devta*, i.e., if a menstruating woman or someone whom she touched visited a place of worship, or participated in any rites, the chief deity would be furious with the entire village stating this pollution as *'Aghoor ho gaya'*. These chief deities include, Golju, Harju, Semju and others. However, nowhere is there a mention in life histories of these deities about incidents related to menstruation cycle and who are supposed to have been superhuman characters who were deified after death. Nonetheless the mediators of these deities, shamans, who were possessed by them consistently express the wrath of the deity if any of the taboos were broken. Strangely enough there is an absence of female deities with such potency except in Pithoragarh and some parts of Garhwal.

It may be noted that when the same women migrate with their men outside of Uttaranchal, they do not maintain several of these restrictions except when entering a place of worship. However when they return to their own home they again maintain the beliefs and practices since now they are, as they say, back in the '*devbhumi*', or holy land.

It is interesting to note the various taboos for menstruating women; not to touch fruits, pickles, milk or milk products, meat, and water resources; prohibited to own any luxury item and things which are in short supply; all this as if to punish them for menstruating. Yet there is no pollution of her tools, like hoe and sickle, probably because her labour is essential for farm work and she is not allowed to rest. While on the one hand this event is an extremely public one she is isolated and kept separate (*alagh*), on the other hand there is no public discussion of this issue or open conversation, so that it remains a mystery especially for young girls.

On an examination of the beliefs and practices related to menstruation in the region, it became evident that in her segregation, her prohibited entry to places of worship, her polluting properties, she becomes, for a few days every month, the lowliest of lowliest, irrespective of the caste she belongs to and her education. Women themselves firmly believe in this phenomenon, and enforce this belief in other women. For instance, women themselves would describe how they break out in rashes or allergy, when a 'polluting' woman is around. As with all other forms these superstitions leading to gender violence, women have internalized it to the extent that despite being victims, they seem to be perpetrating the same ideology.

An extension of the 'untouchable' status is the sanction imposed on women's mobility. A woman who is menstruating may go into the fields and forests for arduous back-breaking work, but she may not enter anybody's house (or for that matter, her own), visit or even pass by any place of worship, sit in on any public gathering like a wedding or a village meeting or travel. This directly affects women's participation in community activities, including developmental interventions. Further it dispossesses her from her own home and ensures that her power is also regulated. Moreover all village paths are always considered potentially 'polluted', in the sense that a menstruating woman may have passed through them at sometime or the other. So in the case of any sanctified procession (like the transfer of an idol of the deity from one house to another), it would be preceded by man sprinkling cow's urine on the way to purify the entire path. Thus, any movement at all by menstruating women is an inconvenience to the community at large. All this then is associated with religious rites and rituals, through a fear which has been mentioned earlier, whereby it permanently distances women from the deities, and disempowers them even with regard to their reproductive capacity.

What happens if a woman has a reproductive health problem? At free listing sessions of women's health problems, the illnesses ended at the waist, eye problem, throat problem, headache, toothache, body ache, stomach ache,etc. However, it took a lot of coaxing before women would admit to having gynaecological problems. Consequently, this denial and acknowledgement of these problems even does not allow them to seek help and is generally termed 'dirty things'. Thus, in any sense, women are so alienated from their own reproductive system that they prefer to ignore their reproductive health.

The question of menstrual hygiene has already been described above, women are unwilling to use clean rags, or wash out their pad and sun-dry. There is a prohibition on bathing, so willy-nilly women have to remain unclean. The implications of this outlook leading to reproductive tract infections is obvious.

Apart from the physical aspects stated here, all these discriminations affect the mental health of women, because she is constantly a reminder of her low status with in the social system. With this state and a sense of low worth, and not a positive self-image, this is one area that needs serious consideration for transformation.

Statements of some women interviewed in Almora district by Sahyog health team

1. I am considered infectious and polluting for five days.
2. I am kept segregated; often in the cowshed.
3. I cannot bathe for five days.
4. I hardly have anything warm to cover myself and I am given a straw pallet and sacking to lie on.
5. I do not use any pad or cloth.
6. I cannot say with my husband – he will become impotent.
7. I cannot go inside the house, more so inside the kitchen.
8. I cannot milk the cows, I cannot drink milk, curd or ghee.
9. I cannot touch water, I cannot touch fruit trees, I cannot touch pickles.

10. But I still have all the hard work to do – get the fodder, get the fuelwood, look after animals, work in the fields.
11. When I was unmarried I did not have to tell anyone – now the whole village must know when I have my periods.
12. The first time I had my periods after marriage there was a *'puja'*, I got gifts; but look what I got after that!

Gender and menstruation is thus deliberately brought into the public sphere, denying their privacy, suggesting a low status, and the punishment meted to her that follows makes her an untouchable beast of burden, both inside and outside of the house. Of course, women voluntarily accept it as a curse, as polluting rather than life giving, which is explained away because of the notion of *dev bhuṃi*, and so on.

Summing Up

Menstrual discrimination is a manifestation of gender violence because it reduces women to a class of untouchables, restricts their mobility with the threat of community inconvenience, uses religion to disempower women about their reproductive capacity, prompts women to neglect their menstrual hygiene and suppress reproductive health problems, and prevents women from developing a sense of self-esteem. This violence is mediated through religion, through shamans, and through women themselves.

Although the case of this area may seem to be an isolated case, but it is not so since in reality menstruation discrimination is widespread all over India, and there are a few places in India where a menstruating woman would freely enter a place of worship, except it may not be now so in urban areas.

An interesting parallel is the belief about pregnancy and puerperium. After the third (in some cases the fourth or fifth) month, a pregnant women is also considered 'impure' and therefore she may not actively participate in worship rituals. In some places in Kumaon she would not even be allowed to cook for or serve food to senior family members. Similarly, after childbirth women are considered equally impure for about three weeks.

There appears to be an underlying assumptions that all processes which manifest women's fertility are polluting and unacceptable to the Hindu gods. There is an overwhelming negativistic outlook on the special role in procreation, which woman as a biological entity is endowed with. Could it possibly be an urge to enforce patriarchy?

What can be done today for women to overcome their personal sense of impurity, and to restore their faith in themselves in the processes of fertility, without a sense of guilt? As women, being one of the prime mediators of this particular form of gender violence is it not for everyone to take the first steps ourselves, to reassert our pride as women, to work together, with men, and to realize the fundamental right of womanhood, the right to menstruate with dignity?

SECTION - 3

ANTENATAL PRACTICES

Table 4.3 : Food Intake and Physical Work during Pregnancy

Villages	Food Intake			Physical Work		
	Normal	More	Less	Normal	More	Less
Almori	5	1	4	4	2	4
Kwedal	1	1	8	2	1	7
Kafli	4	2	4	5	2	3
Chataula	4	2	4	7	0	3
Simayal	4	2	4	6	1	3
Buribana	5	1	4	6	0	4
Total	23	9	28	30	6	24
Percentage	38.3	15.0	46.7	50.0	10.0	40.0

Food Intake during Pregnancy

Pregnant women in the developed world often humorously remark that they are "eating for two." Though partly in jest, health professionals in fact encourage women to increase their normal food intake during each trimester of pregnancy. However, for many women in Uttaranchal, social and cultural constraints make this an unlikely option. Our survey reveals that only 15 per cent of women increase their food intake during pregnancy, while 85 per cent ingest the same or a decreased amount. Of this amount 46.7 per cent women eat less than their normal food intake which is indeed alarming. It is understandable that women who are not informed about the benefits of eating more during pregnancy would continue to eat the same amount of food. However, the survey indicates that almost half of the total women surveyed eat less. Local *Dais* informed us that although women may eat more during the second trimester, they often feel nauseous during the first and third trimesters and choose to decrease their food intake. It is also possible, as has been shown in other areas of India (Werner & Bower, 1995), that women are fearful of producing a large baby that may be difficult to deliver, though a strong mother and a strong child actually decrease complications. Out of 46.7 per cent women who eat less food during pregnancy, a majority were from the village Kwedal (8 out of 10) where no health education programmes was on. The reasons given for eating less were, "Don't feel like eating.... feel sick during the first months...cannot digest food...there are so many restrictions for the type of food we can eat during pregnancy". Some women from village Kafli also said that if we eat more the baby will be large, and there will be problems during delivery.

Radhika Devi a *Dai* from the same village said that the consumption of high protein and high calcium content foods (eggs, peanuts, walnuts, meat) produces a big head and leads to complications during delivery. This traditional belief is still held by the elderly women in the family. 15 per cent of the women who ate more food belonged to the villages of Simayal and Chataula in Ramgarh block. The reasons they gave were, " Both the mother and child will be healthy" some of them also said that not only do they eat more quantity, they also eat nutritious food. The two women from each of the above village said that they were educated and attended the meetings and talks on health and nutrition held in the village by the Chirag Health Extension Staff. 38.3 per cent of the women who stated that they ate the same, said that they ate less during the first three months, and then ate their normal diet in the second and three trimester.

It is interesting to note that access to extension health programmes caused no differentiation in the proportion of women eating normal, more, or less amounts of food in all of the six villages. From this observation one may conclude that most villages in this area would benefit from increased education on food intake during pregnancy, that would be different from current nutrition intervention programmes. I also wish to express the urgency of nutrition education here. Recently a woman living in a CHIRAG assisted village died after giving birth due to anaemia and possibly jaundice. These are two diseases that could have been prevented with better nutrition during her pregnancy.

Table 4.4 : Care During Pregnancy

Villages	29 WOMEN WHO DO SOME KIND OF ANC							No ANC
	Registration of pregnancy	Medical check-up	Routine blood test	Routine urine test	Weight taken	T.T. Vacc.	Iron ablet	Do nothing
Almori	0	0	0	0	0	1	0	9
Kwedal	2	1	1	1	1	3	2	7
Kafli	1	1	0	0	0	2	2	7
Chataula	7	7	2	2	7	7	7	3
Simayal	7	6	1	1	3	7	6	2
Buribana	7	7	5	3	6	7	7	3
Total	24	22	9	7	17	27	24	31
Per cent (29 women)	82.8	75.9	31.0	24.1	58.6	100.0	82.8	
Per cent (60 women)	40.0	36.7	15.0	11.7	28.3	48.3	40.0	51.7

Care during Pregnancy

One of the largest causes of female mortality in India is lack of ante-natal care and monitoring (Mukhopadhyay, 1992). Of the sixty women surveyed, slightly more than half (51.7%) do not make use of ante-natal services.48.3 per cent of the women who go in for ante-natal check up belong to the villages where CHIRAG had its ante-natal programme. These services, provided monthly by CHIRAG extension workers, include registration of the pregnancy, medical check-ups, haemoglobin tests, urine analysis, weighing, tetanus toxide (TT) vaccines, and iron tablet distribution. Ante-natal and vaccination camps are held monthly in a central location for those villages within its proximity. For more distant CHIRAG assisted villages, health team members make monthly visits. Our survey reveals that most women receiving ante-natal care do some combination of services, usually registration, medical check-ups, weighing, and iron tablets. Amazingly, 100 per cent of these women have received TT vaccinations, which not only protects the mother but also the unborn child. Of those who do not take advantage of ante-natal care services, the majority are in non-assisted villages. However, approximately one-third of women who have access to ante-natal care do not take advantage of CHIRAG's services. It may be concluded that while accessibility is a strong factor in determining whether the woman will receive care, increased awareness of its benefits and availability is also a key factor. (Huff, E.: 2002)

Out of the 51.7 per cent of the women who do not make use of ante-natal services, a majority belonged to the non-assisted villages of Almori and Kwedal. Some of them also belonged to Kafli, where the programme is not so effective. The reasons given by the women for not availing of any of the antenatal services was "we do nothing, our family does not allow us to go for a check up, they consider it inauspicious". One elderly woman in Kafli said, "pregnancy is a normal state, why do you people make so much fuss about it...we did nothing and I produced thirteen children". Of course she missed the significant issue that seven of her thirteen children died during the first two years of birth.

It is difficult to establish linkages between ante-natal care and safe pregnancy in the minds of people who have been working in a different tradition. Kunti a HEW from CHIRAG who visited village Kafli with me said, "The greatest opposition to ante-natal care comes from the mother-in-law". I thought about her remark and felt that a 'family-oriented approach' to maternal and child health care which took the whole family along needs to be developed and strengthened. This could become an integral aspect of the pro-active health care strategy.

What is emerging from this survey is that there is a need to build a matrix where in the traditional health care practices intersect with the modern medicine systems in order to provide a more holistic health care strategy to women and children in the community. In this view, the family is sacred and every member has a role to play – it is a question of living together for fulfilment of the values of the family which signifies the notion of strong family bonds in this culture.

Table 4.5 : Problems during Pregnancy

Villages	Backpain	Weak-ness	Swelling	Bleeding	Deformed foetus	Others
Almori	7	9	1	0	0	0
Kwedal	8	7	2	0	0	0
Kafli	5	6	1	0	0	0
Chataula	4	4	1	2	0	4
Simayal	5	6	1	0	0	0
Buribana	5	8	1	1	0	0
Total	34	40	7	3	0	4
Percen-tage	56.7	66.7	11.7	5.0	0.0	6.7

Physical Work and Problems during Pregnancy

Although the initial intention of this survey was to discover what kinds of problems women experience specifically related to pregnancy, it inadvertently or as a peripheral fall out reveals patterns of overwork for pregnant women. Few women claimed that they had swelling, bleeding, or other specifically ante-natal problems. However, most women experienced backpain (56.7%) and weakness (66.7%), which are more likely caused by the sustained and even increased workload that 60 per cent of women stated that they endured during pregnancy.

The work roles performed are also linked to the family structure and the economic level of the family. 10 per cent of the women who performed more work said, "we have no help at home, we live alone, if we do not go to the forest to get fuelwood, fodder and water our family and animals will go hungry."

Out of the 50 per cent women who performed their normal tasks; some of the women from village Buribana and Simayal said, "it is good to be active and do all the work, this helps us in the delivery". The reasons given by 40 per cent of the women who performed less than their normal work during pregnancy were 'it is dangerous for mother and child'... 'family does not allow us to do more work'.... 'it is difficult to walk especially during the third trimester...other women in the family come forward to support and help'. Linked to the roles performed are the problems women shared that they had during pregnancy with 56.7 per cent women stating that they had severe backpain and 66.7 per cent women experienced weakness. These findings can be linked to the earlier discussion on food intake during pregnancy which is reduced by 46.7 per cent of the women. It is not that being active and performing the household tasks is not recommended during pregnancy, it is the back breaking nature of the work and the heavy load (a head load varies from 20-40 kg) is the cause.

At a meeting in Kasialekh some of the women from village Kafli said that in order to avoid going to the forest twice they increase their head load, not realising how harmful it is for the back and the pelvic regions. This is why the special conditions in the hill economy have to be focused on, while planning health care interventions. With very little or no support from the men in the family the tasks women perform become even more crucial for the sustenance of the family household. (Fig. 4.2)

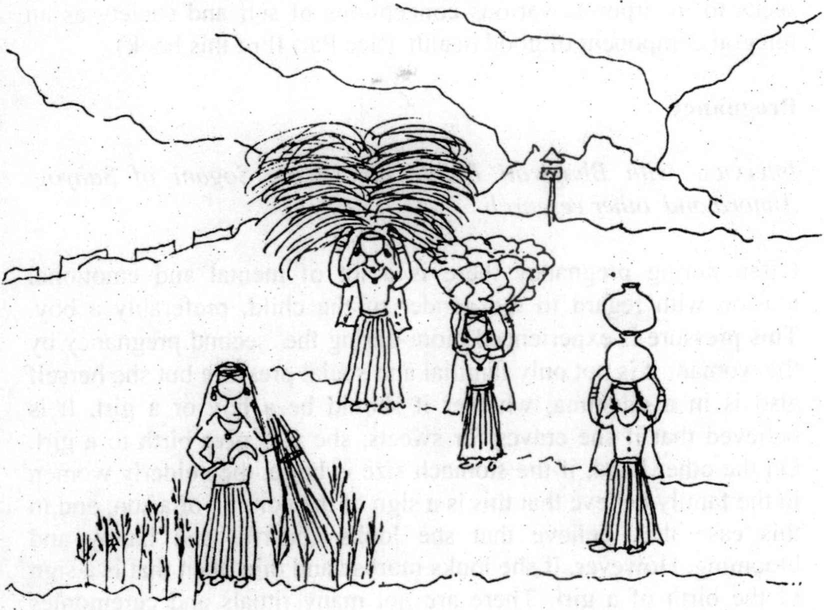

Fig. 4.2 : Apart from Household and Farm Work Women perform back-breaking tasks like Fetching, Fuelwood, Fodder and Water from Long Distances.

Culture ←→Work ←→ Environment ←→ Health

The above factors are all closely inter-linked.

Therefore, it is clear that health education should focus on patterns of work distribution in the family and especially during the reproductive phase of a woman's life cycle. As is typical throughout India, women are the sustainers of the family. Though they often have no monetary income, from adolescence to adulthood they tend the fields, feed the livestock, cook for the family, wash the laundry, care for the children, and provide for the elderly. I have seen women close to term carrying headloads of wood and fodder so heavy that they barely have the strength to lift one foot in front of the other. She feels every stone through her thin sandals. She can only manage to swagger her hips, swinging side to side as she climbs the steep road home. According to local health workers, carrying headloads is the number one cause of miscarriages. For a pregnant women even performing the normal amount of work can become too much for the unborn child to bear, and risks the mother's life as well. This is why the adolescent health module seeks to incorporate various conceptions of self and society as an integral component of good health. (See Part II of this book).

Pregnancy

Interview with Bhagwati Pande and Reetu Sogani of Sahyog, Almora and other research

Often during pregnancy there is a lot of mental and emotional tension with regard to the gender of the child, preferably a boy. This pressure is experienced more during the second pregnancy by the woman. It is not only familial and social pressure but she herself also is in a dilemma, whether it should be a boy or a girl. It is believed that if she craves for sweets, she will give birth to a girl. On the other hand, if the stomach size is large, then elderly women in the family believe that this is a sign of the coming of a son, and in this case they believe that she looks cheerful and happy and blooming. However, if she looks morose and thin, then that is a sign of the birth of a girl. There are not many rituals and ceremonies associated with pregnancy except that after the fifth month elders do not eat food cooked by her, or drink water which has been brought by her from the water-source, and she is not allowed to go to the temple because she is considered impure.

Food Intake during this time

During this time a woman is prohibited to eat yoghurt, rice, potatoes and 'hot' foods like peanuts, meat, fish, and eggs because it is believed that the child will get lazy in the sense that it will not emerge easily from the womb at the time of delivery. Drinking hot milk and eating yoghurt makes the lips of the new-born baby to become black. If the pregnant woman unduly rests too much, the size of the baby will increase so much that there will be difficulties at the time of delivery.

Care during Pregnancy

It is mostly the *Dais* of the village who are consulted if any problem arises during this period. The *Dais* often give a massage to the woman with mustard-oil and believe that by doing so they are able to change the baby if it is in a breach position. However, according to Kishni Devi, a *Dai* from village Sargakhet "this is not possible, since a child changes position on its own, and if child has to be borne with its feet first then no *Dai* in the world can change that since nature must follow its own course."

Problems during Pregnancy

During this period the woman has itching in the body and there is a white discharge also. There are no remedial treatments given for these problems. If a woman aborts it is generally believed that it must have been a boy since he is generally considered of a weak constitution. However, if a woman aborts or is not able to bear a child then it is linked to gods and goddesses. A pregnant woman is not allowed to carry cowdung on her head, however she may carry fuelwood and grass and water, but no reasons for this distinction are given.

Highlights

- The average age of a mother during her first pregnancy in Kumaon hills is 18 years.

- A majority of the women become pregnant five times, of which at least one child dies.
- Seven out of ten women do not get any ante-natal check up during pregnancy, neither do they get a tetanus injection or eat iron tablets.
- Village *Dais* are generally called in the eight or ninth month to assess the condition of the child.
- Women until the delivery time go to the forest to bring fuel wood, fodder and water.
- Because of a lack of separate bathing facilities women are not able to give special attention to their personal hygiene.
- It is believed that during pregnancy :
- women should not be given too much to eat because the baby will grow big causing trouble during delivery,
- if a woman is given meat, eggs and fish to eat she may abort her child.
- Because of a lack adequate rest and diet five out of ten women have problems during pregnancy.
- About 70 per cent of pregnant women complain of giddiness, weakness, swelling and about 10 per cent have more serious complications like bleeding, etc.

Even in the Ramgarh and Dhari block villages of Nainital district where I worked and had several interviews with women, health workers and *Dais* the above findings hold true, except in the villages where the NGO CHIRAG had its health programmes 80 per cent of the pregnant women had complete ante-natal check ups. Neomi a HEW with CHIRAG said that during pregnancy women avoid high protein food like peanuts, yoghurt and walnuts because it is believed a child will develop a white layer on the skin and it would be difficult to move easily through the canal. Interestingly Kunti another HEW also added that a pregnant woman is not allowed to sit in the entrance (*dehleej*) of the door, because they believe that if a woman sits there, the birth of her child will be delayed. It will keep moving in and out in the passage.

Kunti also added that those men who perform the *'jagar'* (a religious ceremony) only eat food cooked by their pregnant wife or daughter-in-law until the 4th month. From the beginning of the 5th month until 22 days after delivery either some other woman in the house cooks the food or they cook themselves.

What emerges from all this sharing is that the pregnant woman because of traditional beliefs about certain foods and their effect is denied adequate nutrition during this period when she most needs it. There is so much fear about producing a big baby, a lazy baby – all of which are linked to problems during delivery – that women eat less, do the same amount of work and suffer from headaches, giddiness, weakness and other dangerous symptoms. Both Neomi and Kunti HEWs shared with me that even though women come for their tetanus injections and ante-natal check-ups, and eat iron tablets the restrictions about food intake during pregnancy and after delivery are still strictly observed. All this reflects in the low weight of the child at birth.

SECTION-4

TRADITIONAL PRACTICES RELATED TO CHILD BIRTH AND POST-DELIVERY

Village Dais and Safe Delivery – Secondary Data Review

Dais, traditional birth attendants, are known by this name in many parts of India because they are respected members of the community known for their skill and knowledge available for women who need them. They may be considered as the link between the formal health service and village women thereby bridging the gap between the biomedical system and their traditional medical practices. They need to be put back on the map of the health care system as they are providers of their traditional knowledge and skills that celebrates their culture of birth. Despite poverty, prejudice and lack of support, they continue to serve the vast majority of poor Indian women.

This section deals with myths and rituals associated with safe delivery and the role of the *Dais*, her status, training and changes in methods due to the intervention of health services, both at the NGO and governmental level.

Studies conducted in many parts of India by such authors as Bajwa, 1991; Jeffery, 1989; Kaur, 1981; Sandhu, 1980; and Srivastva, 1971, have recognised the key role of *Dais* in the village community broader health programmes. For example, Dr. Ashok Dyalchand of the Institute of Management, Pachod, Maharashtra has involved *Dais* community health workers since the 1970s, creating a model for other NGO programmes in India and elsewhere in the world; and, similarly in Gujarat the NGO Chetna has developed a programme for Dais to be incorporated into the childbirth practices and training programmes, so also the VHAI has also been actively promoting the role of Dais in maternal and child health programmes.(Kumar: 1990)

Dais are usually older married women who have borne their own children, and are mostly illiterate having learnt their skills from another older Dai and through personal experience. *Dais* may come from any of the three major social groups – Brahmin, Rajput and Scheduled Castes, in contrast from other parts of India where they are mostly from the Scheduled Castes. *Dais* work in two or three villages at the most and this is why the number of deliveries conducted by them is low, averaging one or two a month. Other *Dais* who have conducted more deliveries who tend to be more experienced often have undergone training programmes through the NGOs, and these specialised Dais are called in for difficult cases. Besides their health work with women they are often involved also with the care and treatment of young children since they also have considerable indigenous knowledge about herbal treatments in many types of illnesses. This is why it is important to study traditional beliefs and practices, indigenous concepts of health and illness that *Dais* use to classify and understand the process of pregnancy and childbirth. Taking all this into account, health programmes in training health workers may become more understandable and relevant to the *Dais* themselves, as well as others.

Matrika

Matrika is an organization, whose objective is also to reflect on ways for bridging the gap between the biomedical and ethno-medical system, restoring medical personnel's respect for the *Dai*. Working with Dais it has evolved a broad outline of what may be called "Good Practices": practices that promote the well-being and safety of mothers and children-practices which are congruent with Indian cultural ideas about the body, health and the place of the human body in the cosmos. These experienced traditional *Dais* form a part of indigenous body and health knowledge. Their good practices are culturally appropriate since these maximise the use of locally available resources, thereby providing a palpable life force energy, and assume the naturalness of birth. In this way these practices work at bodily, emotional, social and sacred levels. The

Dais use these time tested modalities, nevertheless are open to new inputs and willing to adapt if they see value to the new methods.

Dais practice the following traditional ways which make them "mother friendly". The following are a sharing of the Dais present at a workshop held by Matrika in New Delhi

- We are always available for the *'Jacha'* (pregnant women), be it day or night.
- We pray to the gods to help us handle the delivery.
- We open all the windows and boxes and locks of the house. The *Jacha's* hair is also opened.
- We wash our hands before examining the *Jacha*.
- We put our ear to the mother's stomach to listen to the baby's heartbeat. If there is still time, we make the *Jacha* walk around a little. We tell the *Jacha* how to breathe correctly.
- We do *'maalish'* (massage) around the *'shareer'* (body) to make it maximally flexible.
- *Dai* gives *'aidi'* on the *'shareer'* (presses the vagina with her heel).
- In all these regions the *Jachas* are told to lie with their ankles crossed so that no *hawa* (cold air) can enter.
- If *bachadani ka munh* (mouth of the uterus) is open three fingers, the *Bacha* is likely to be born soon.
- When the *Jacha* is ready to give birth, she begins to sweat a lot and her thighs begin to tremble and her passages begin to loosen. This is when we give her *shakti* and *sahara* (strength and support).
- When the child is ready to born, the upper part of the stomach becomes loose.
- When water and a little blood comes out, we know that the birth will take place very soon.
- We tell the *Bacha* how to breathe correctly.
- Roasted cloves, *jaiphal* (nutmeg) and *ghee* in milk is given to increase the contractions. *Methi ka pani* (fenugreek decoction), *ajwain ka pani* (thymol concoction), warm milk with *shakkar* (brown sugar), all these help in increasing contractions.
- *Chuara* and *badaam* (dates and almonds) is given to help in opening of the *bachadani ka munh*. *Ghee* in milk is also given to facilitate birth.

- After the birth, *nariyal* (coconut) with *gur* (jaggery) and *ghee* is given. Also, sonth (dried ginger), pipar, *haldi, ajwain. Pinni* (rich sweet) is made with five *magaz* (seeds) *suji* (semolina) and *ghee. Laddoos* with *methi, sonth* and *gond* is given in some places.
- Incidently, in Rajasthan, the human body is understood to be divided into three parts. *Bemata* lives underground in *narak* – which corresponds to the lower part of the body, those parts involved in reproduction. *Bemata* lives under the ground and signifies the force which generates babies, but also trees, crops, etc. (Matrika Report)

Sahyog

Sahyog, another NGO in Almora also lays emphasis on the traditional *Dais* in the village. They conducted a survey of 50 *Dais* and trained them to keep clean and how to move ahead in their work, and to encourage them to carry on with traditional practices. For example, making a woman sit/squat to give birth, which in this way takes less time as it is working parallel to gravity. This method is not only easier but it does not get a perineum tear. The government training programme stresses the lying position which is difficult and women end up by getting a tear during childbirth. This NGO also validates massages, the taking out of the placenta by putting the woman's hair in her mouth. The training also enables to give respect to the *Dais*.

Practices during Labour and Delivery in Kumaon Hills

The *Dai* during labour encourages the woman to walk, and when the pain is getting to be intense she gives a body massage using warm oil. When the pain becomes regular she encourages the woman to bear down (*jor lago*), in order to hasten the delivery. During the active second stage of labour, when the woman is bearing down, the *Dai* goes behind the woman and presses down with considerable force of the fundus of the uterus in order to prevent the foetus from moving upwards. Sometimes the *Dai* presses one knee into the small of the back so that it prevents any abnormal position of the baby as it moves down the birth canal. Often many *Dais* carry out vaginal examinations, and sometimes even ruptures are done with a finger nail. Massage of the vagina is commonly carried out, in order to 'open the path' for the baby.

Delivery

The woman traditionally delivers her baby in the squatting position, often holding on to another woman for support, with the *Dai* kneeling behind her and pressing on the fundus of the uterus or her lower back. When the actual birth occurs, sometimes they do not observe the emergence of the baby's head, others massage the perineum to ease the passage of the baby's head, and usually support the perineum to prevent tearing. Some *Dais* support the perineum with one of their feet, and others support the perineum with the left hand.

Traditionally, *Dais* cut the umbilical cord with a sickle (*dranthi*) and the thread to cut the cord which is often a piece of jute extracted from a mat on the floor. The care of the cord has been a major focus of *Dai* training programmes, and significant changes in practice have occurred in recent years. It is now tied with boiled thread and the cord is cut with a boiled razor blade, while the umbilical stump is left dry. While some *Dais* have learnt this in their training others have also learnt it with informal meetings and discussion with trained *Dais*.

Many *Dais* squeeze the cord blood away from the baby in order to avoid contamination of the baby's blood with placental blood, thereby avoiding the polluting effects of the latter on the baby. Many *Dais* do not cut the cord until the placenta is delivered because they fear that the placenta might shift from its normal position. After the placenta is delivered, it is carefully disposed of, usually being wrapped in a cloth and buried in the forest or in the nearby fields, often under a green fruit bearing tree. If a green fruit bearing tree is not available nearby the placenta is buried under the projecting lentil of the ceiling of the house thereby symbolizing that just as the roof protects the house it will protect the new born baby as well.

Postpartum Period

Practices during this period are directed towards protecting the mother for this a particularly vulnerable period. Although rest is advised, the duration of it is variable. However, the woman is not permitted to cook or touch water for a number of days after the birth, due to beliefs about the polluting effects of the childbirth process. (Diet is discussed separately, during this period.)

To conclude this section, while most traditional practices associated with labour and delivery are appropriate, a few of them can cause problems. Bearing down before the cervix is fully dilated, it can lead to exhaustion and later to a uterine prolapse especially as excessive pressure on the uterine fundus during labor can be harmful. Rupturing the membrane with a finger nail and repeated vaginal examinations introduce infection. The squatting position is generally appropriate as it is important for the *Dai* to observe the emergence of the head, so that she can support the perineum which then prevents tears. The hygienic care of the cord is an essential part of a safe delivery, and finally there is a need to promote the practice of giving the first breast milk to the new born baby.

Indigenous Concepts about Health and Illness

According to Karen Trollope Kumar (1990), the major explanatory models of folk concepts that may be identified are, humeral, supernatural and purity/pollution notions. Humeral theories evolved during the 5th-6th centuries B.C. according to her, following the Ayurvedic system, which is more than just a system of healing, it has philosophical way of leading one's life. That is, there has to be a balance within the human organism and the environment that are organized around the five basic elements (*bhutas*) of the universe, namely, ether (*akasha*), fire (*agni*), wind (*vayu* or *vat*), earth (*prithvi*), and water (*ap*). Furthermore, health is conditioned by the balance between the three primary body humours (*dosa*), namely, *vata* (wind), *pitta* (bile) and *kapha* (mucus). The five elements are the constituents of all life, and are made of up the three humours and the seven physical components (*dhatus*) of the body. (Kutumbiah, 1962)

Humeral Theories

The influence of these humeral theories of illness is clearly evident in the therapeutic practices of *Dais*, in Kumaon, as the interviews with the *Dais* revealed as is given above. Thus pregnancy is thought of as a heating condition, so that a diet which is composed of cooling food is recommended, for hot foods are a danger for both the mother and the child. Similarly, the *Dais* say that 'rog' or disease in the new born, while in the foetus, occurs when the woman is exposed to hot food, which includes meat, eggs, peanuts, several forms of lentil, and several types of vegetables. What are the nutritional significance of these tabooed hot and cold categories is not clear and requires further studies.

Immediately after child birth, the woman is given hot foods, since she is supposed to be susceptible to sudden cooling, such as ghee, *gond,* and nuts. An *anghiti* is lit in the confinement room so that the woman is protected from wind (*vayu*) which is considered harmful. Karen Trollope Kumar (1990) further states that the therapeutic practice associated with humeral models of illness are usually helpful. These theories of harmony and balance stress the importance of adequate rest, attention given to diet in the context of an ecological concept of health rather than the doctor and medicine-centred concepts of modern medical practices. However, being dogmatic can be disastrous since a delay in giving antibiotic treatment is possible when *Dais* often interpret fever associated with puerperal sepsis with merely a condition of overheat that is treated with cool compresses and cooling foods. Similarly, a neonate with fever due to septicemia may also be diagnosed as suffering from overheat. Here it is thus important to look for early referral cases to allopathic practitioners, and this needs to be included in the training of the *Dais*.

Supernatural Theories

Belief in supernatural causes for illness was prevalent everywhere in the world, and more so in India, such as that disease is believed to be caused by visitation of punishing gods or the evil work of demons, so that a pregnant woman must observe certain behavioural rules during pregnancy in order to protect herself from evil forces. For example, she is not to visit cremation grounds, or go near cross roads where ghosts (*bhuts*) are likely to be found; she must avoid seeing an eclipse which can cause deformities in the baby, avoiding ritual pollution rules such as room is shuttered and closed so that ghosts, etc. do not enter the room, or placing an iron knife near the door of the confinement room [as noted by Karen Trollope Kumar (1990) in Garhwal]. Such complications as trimester bleeding, obstructed labour, etc. are wrongly attributed to supernatural causes and given the relevant (*jhar-phuk,* apart from sacrificial rituals of animals, the use of charms, talismans, spells, curses, etc.) treatment which may often prove fatal. (Kumar: *ibid.*)

Supernatural theories are often ridiculed by allopathic practitioners, yet their psychological effects must be looked deeper as these govern the lives of the villagers, in terms of the forms of healing practices that play a crucial role in their psyche and it is in this context that the woman might heal herself through her ordeal. A judicious application of the cultural context to healing needs to be taken into account, so that hospital care is also not neglected. In this context P.C. Joshi makes a distinction between *bimari* and *dosh* which according to him, the former refers to natural causes whereas the latter is generally a collective and transgressional cause rooted the supernatural behavioral norms of the society. Therefore, both are empirically speaking to be considered for healing to take place. Healing rituals, he rightly says, are needed to be linked to the microcosm of an individual's life and also to the macrocosm of wider supernatural forces. (Kumar: *ibid.*)

Purity and Pollution

A system of socio-cultural taboos concerning contacts and dietary habits is most clearly stated in the ancient texts. Without going into details, this may briefly be stated into two types of pollution, (i) Permanent related to birth into a caste, and (ii) That which arises from normal functions of everyday life, covering blood, faeces, saliva, urine and semen which are ritually impure and breaking these taboos can result in both ill health and misfortune. (Kumar, 1990)

In Kumaon, as elsewhere, child birth is considered ritually polluting while at the same time also very auspicious. It is the role of the *Dai* to maintain the ritual purity, such as by maintaining ritual pollution rules when ranging from a period of 11-22 days after child-birth women are not permitted to cook for their families. It is on the fortieth day that a purification ceremony takes place with a *hawan* and it lasts up to one day and one night, depending upon the wealth and status of the family; after which a woman is once again normal and pure. Perhaps these rules allow a women to rest, even though these represent a negative image of women. However when blood is considered to be polluting even in the case of a haemorrhage, blood is allowed to be let out and postpartum treatment is delayed.

Folk Knowledge about Health

A popular form of folk healing is *jhar-phuk* in which *mantras* are recited while a sweeping feather is moved over the afflicted individual, in the direction of the feet, which sometimes can become quite hurtful at times. There is then the common way of massaging the body in the management of pain, and for correcting malpositions of the foetus, including the version of breech foetus into a vertex one; this specialized skill is known to a only a few of the *Dais*. Manual removal of a retained placenta is sometimes done by *Dais* after trying initial measures such as the administration of the uterine fundus.

Thus, when *Dais* choose a therapy, it is based more on availability and affordability and efficacy of the treatment rather than on the underlying basis for that therapy, i.e. it is pragmatic as she will use the medical system in case of a serious obstetrical indication. However, biomedicine is seldom the first choice, particularly when the problem is believed to have a natural cause. This is why it is crucial to train Dais to negotiate a complicated case by referring it to the hospital care. Of course one has to keep in mind that economic and other infrastructural barriers to a high quality care are seldom available. Another significant barrier to complicated deliveries is the notion of shame *sharam* because of which women do not get to be examined, and often even a Dai is unable to overcome these powerful feelings.

To sum up this section, the research about the beliefs and practices of the *Dai* in Kumaon reveals that while a great many of the practices are appropriate and she is the key health resource person in the village, any training programme will have to take into account these various socio-cultural aspects of the *Dais* themselves, so that areas of conflict can be explored. Such a training programme can be rewarding for both the *Dai* and the trainer, as each can benefit from the other's experience.

Safe and Unsafe Deliveries

A safe delivery is one in which the trained Dai or health worker will use five safety precautions; a plastic sheet, sterilized blade, clean hand with short nails, sterile gloves, and a string to tie the cord. *Dais* are women of great wisdom concerning pregnancy and deliveries. They often have the delicate skill that only comes with experience, such as being able to turn a breached child without damaging the womb. While visiting a village under CHIRAG's assistance, I was able to glance at a trained *Dai's* record of deliveries. She must have overseen the delivery of over a thousand children! However, untrained *Dais* are unaware of the invisible microbes that exist everywhere, many of which can enter the mother or child during the birthing process from using some traditional methods. For example, often the harvesting sickle is used to cut the umbilical cord because no other blade is available. Yet some traditional practices are beneficial. Most *Dais* use a metal coin placed opposite the blade while cutting the cord to protect the infant. Using a copper coin is especially auspicious, but use of any coin is a benefit. CHIRAG holds a monthly training of *Dais* to ideally utilize these beneficial or neutral practices, while improving some of the more harmful ones. They also provide these five safety precautions for a safe delivery. It is interesting to note that 100 per cent of women in villages where there is no outreach programme used untrained Dais for their last pregnancy, while 25 per cent of women within access to CHIRAG health programmes chose to use untrained *Dais*. This shows that while access to CHIRAG health care programs is the most discriminating factor, even in areas where women have access, a large portion continue to use traditional methods. Therefore, it is imperative that access to health care and education be combined.

Table 4.6 : Safe and Unsafe Delivery

Delivery Status				
	Safe Delivery			Unsafe
Villages	Trained Dai	A.N.M.	Hospital	Untrained Dai
Almori	0	0	0	10
Kwedal	0	0	0	10
Kafli	5	1	1	3
Chataula	8	0	0	2
Simayal	7	0	0	3
Buribana	7	1	0	2
Total	27	2	1	30
Percentage	43.3	3.3	3.3	50.0

It is interesting to note here that the ANM who is the representative of the government primary health care infrastructure at the village level has very little role in ensuring safe delivery. In the villages of effective CHIRAG assistance the role of the ANM seems to be almost negligible in ante-natal care and in directing women to have their deliveries from trained *Dais*. Wherever the NGO outreach programme is effective the government infrastructure in providing health care seems to recede. However, a more effective interface between the two would go a long way in changing the status of mother and child health in the country.

Since 93.3 per cent of the deliveries are performed by *Dais* (43.3 per cent by trained and 50 per cent by untrained) the role of *Dais*, their indigenous knowledge and wisdom has to be strengthened and integrated in the training provided to them. Matrika an organization in Delhi has done some path-breaking work in this direction, as stated earlier.

The *Dai* belongs to the community and owns responsibility for the well -being and health of the women in the community.

As a care giver and provider she has natural affection while the ANM who is appointed by the government to perform a task is an outsider.

Table 4.7 : Five Safety Precautions during Delivery

Villages	Five Safety Precautions observed during Delivery							
	Yes	No	Things applied on the cord after cutting				
			Metal coin	Talcum powder	Medicinal tube	Nothing	Dettol
Almori	0	10	8	0	2	0	0
Kwedal	0	10	4	0	0	5	1
Kafli	3	7	10	0	0	0	0
Chataula	4	6	10	0	0	0	0
Simayal	3	7	9	0	0	1	0
Buribana	8	2	2	2	0	6	0
Total	**18**	**42**	**s43**	**2**	**2**	**12**	**1**
Percentage	**30.0**	**70.0**	**71.7**	**3.3**	**3.3**	**20.0**	**1.7**

Use of Five Safety Precautions during Delivery

Only 18 (30%) of the women reported that the five safety precautions were observed during delivery. To reiterate, the five safety precautions are sterilized blade, clean hands, short nails, rubber sheets and a string to tie the cord. Considering that 43.3 per cent of the respondents used trained *Dais* for delivery there seems to be some in congruency in the buildup. This could be because, although the strained *Dais* know of the five safety precautions, some continue to practice harmful methods. For example, in Simayal seven women used trained *Dais* and three used an untrained *Dai*. Yet the latter the women were asked if they had used the five safety precautions and only three said they had. If seven women used trained *Dais*, then the number of women who used all five safety precautions should also be seven. In Chataula the same has occurred. Eight women used trained *Dais* but only four of these deliveries were fully sanitary. These incongruent numbers could indicate that not all trained *Dais* are consistently using all of the safety precautions.

It may also indicate that although the Dais were using safe methods, because of lack of health education the mother may not have been able to determine if the *Dai* had truly used the five safety precautions. Either way, the root cause is lack of education, either of the trained *Dai* or of the mother as to the use of the five safety precautions during delivery.

Table 4.8 : Practices related to Cord cutting during delivery

Villages	Data related to Cord Cutting								
	Cord cut by				Tool used		Place of Disposal		
	Dai	Mother	In-laws	Nurse	Blade	Unknown	Under tree	Under roof	Unknown
Almori	3	6	1	0	6	4	0	10	0
Kwedal	3	5	2	0	10	0	9	0	1
Kafli	3	4	0	3	9	1	4	5	1
Chataula	0	10	0	0	10	0	10	0	0
Simayal	6	3	1	0	10	0	10	0	0
Buribana	8	1	0	1	10	0	10	0	0
Total	23	29	4	4	55	5	43	15	2
Percentage	38.3	48.3	6.7	6.7	91.7	8.3	71.7	25.0	3.3

Twenty per cent women said that nothing was applied on the cord after cutting, a few used talcum powder, medicinal tube and dettol. All these seem to be very recent additions as traditionally nothing was applied on the cord after cutting. The fact that 70 per cent of the women reported that the five safety precautions were not used indicates that training of Dai's and educating mothers about the importance of using these precautions so that they can ensure that these are being practiced is crucial to safe delivery.

Cord Cutting

Who cut the cord ?

Of the total sample of 60 women, 29 (48.3%) reported that the mother cut the cord, 23 (38.3%) started that the cord was cut by the *Dai* and 6.7 per cent by the in-laws and the nurse respectively. According to the survey, more *Dais* than mothers cut the cord in most CHIRAG assisted villages, while non-assisted villages the tradition of the mother cutting the cord was still in effect.

One of the consequences of development is often cultural degradation. With increasing knowledge of safe delivery practices, there has been a decrease in traditional practices that did no harm and even had indirect social benefits. In this area, it is considered most auspicious when a mother is able to cut the umbilical cord of her own child. If the mother is too weak, the next best option is for an in-law, preferably the mother-in-law, to cut the cord. When the mother is able to cut the cord of her own child, she retains ownership over the health of herself and her family. Often when development organizations begin to educate about new practices, they put less emphasis on reinforcing beneficial traditional practices that allow the people whom they are assisting to remain in control of their own health. A partnership can be developed between the development organization and the local people by synthesizing local and scientific knowledge of health. Rather than stealing control of health knowledge, they should create a participatory atmosphere, which will lead to greater sustainability. Teaching the mothers as well as the *Dais* how to sterilize and bind off the umbilical cord allows the mother to participate in sustaining the health of her child. The example of *Dais* rather than mothers cutting the cord is just a shadow of the underlying problem this survey intended to uncover – that assisted villages have begun to shift from sustaining their own preventive health care to increasing dependence on curative health services provided by CHIRAG.

The significance of cutting the cord by the mother is that it is she who is separating the baby from the body and bringing it forth into the world. Modern health care systems are taking away this right of the mother to cut the cord, and are training the Dais to perform this task instead.

How ?

91.7 per cent of the women reported that the Dai used a blade for cutting the cord. 4 Women (8.3%) from village Almori said that they did not know what was used.

Table 4.9 : Time Taken by Placenta to come out

Villages	Immediate	4 hours	2 days	4 days
Almori	8	0	1	1
Kwedal	8	2	0	0
Kafli	10	0	0	0
Chataula	9	1	0	0
Simayal	8	1	1	0
Buribana	10	0	0	0
Total	53	4	2	1
Percentage	88.3	6.7	3.3	1.7

The Placenta

As described earlier in the section on traditional practices the placenta is buried under a green tree which can bear fruit is considered very auspicious and this practice is followed by 71.7 per cent of the women.

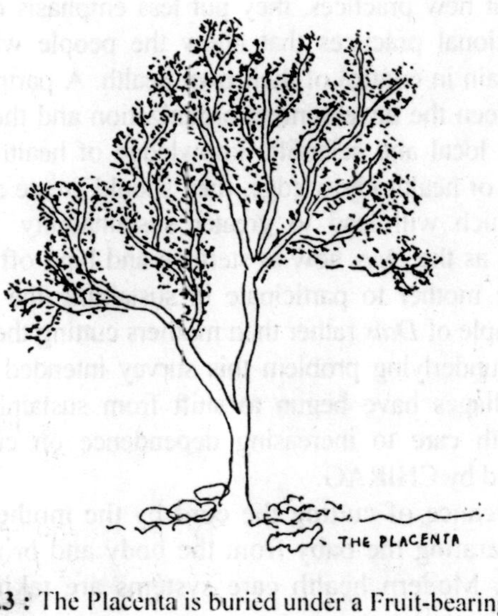

Fig 4.3 : The Placenta is buried under a Fruit-bearing Tree

Table 4.10 : Breast-feeding, reasons and period of rest after delivery

Villages	Breast-feeding		Post Natal Care Reason				Period of rest after Delivery					
	Same day (choles.)	After 3-4 days	Good	Harm-ful	No milk produced	No rest	3 days	11 days	22 days	1 month	2 months	3 months
Almori	0	10	0	10	0	0	0	5	0	1	3	1
Kwedal	1	9	S1	9	0	0	0	10	0	0	0	0
Kafli	2	8	2	5	3	2	1	7	0	0	0	0
Chataula	6	4	6	4	0	0	0	6	0	3	1	0
Simayal	7	3	7	3	0	0	0	6	2	2	0	0
Buribana	5	5	5	4	1	0	4	6	0	0	0	0
Total	21	39	21	35	4	2	5	40	2	6	4	1
Percentage	35.0	65.0	35.0	58.3	6.7	3.3	8.3	66.7	3.3	10.0	6.7	1.7

A woman from Simayal in Ramgarh block said, "the placenta is never buried under a dry tree because the mother's milk will dry up. Traditionally the placenta is buried under the *'dudila'* tree so that the mother will always have milk for the baby and the baby will be healthy." She also added that the buried placenta is not covered by a stone, because that symbolizes that the woman will not bear any more children. Rewati Devi from the village Almori where all the women reported that the placenta was buried under the roof said, "It is the placenta that has nourished the baby in the womb, that is why we bury it below the roof of the house, so that no animal will take it away to the forest. The significance of this is that the child will always remain with us in the *'angan'* (courtyard) of the house, it will protect the baby also."

These traditional beliefs give value and meaning to each phase of the woman's life. This practice of burying the placenta under a tree indicates their perception of the unity of life with nature. The tree and the environment are an integral part of the nourishment cycle which links culture practices and practical benefit.

SECTION-5

POSTNATAL PRACTICES

Breast-feeding (See Table 4.10)

While it is a simple thing to teach that, like the trained *Dai,* the mother can also in a sterile manner cut the cord of her newborn child, the breast-feeding issue confronts strong beliefs about cholestrum, or mother's first milk. Because cholestrum is thicker breast milk, women believe that it is better to allow another lactating woman to nurse her newborn child for the first three to four days. However, cholestrum is thicker because it contains more nutrients, antibodies, and immunities, which is a great benefit to the newborn during the first few days after delivery. The survey showed that 65 per cent of the women waited three to four days to breast-feed their child. Of this percentage almost all the women in non-assisted villages (19 out of 20) waited the traditional three to four days to nurse their child, while in assisted villages only half had decided to breast-feed immediately. When asked why they chose to wait, most (58.3%) said they believed the mother's first milk to be harmful to the child and a few said that they had not produced milk initially. For those women who claimed they had not produced milk (6.7%), it is a circular argument. Most likely they had not produced milk because they had not allowed the child to suckle and stimulate the nipples (Werner & Bower, 1995). However, it is disturbing that even in villages where there has been CHIRAG assistance for the past sixteen years, 50 per cent of women are still unaware of the benefits of the mother's first milk.

50 per cent of the women who breast-fed their child with in the first few hours belonged to the villages of Simayal, Chataula and Buribana where CHIRAG's health programme is effective. One interesting correlation was that these women were younger in age (20-30) than 50 per cent of the women from the CHIRAG assisted villages who were not breast-feeding immediately. Since CHIRAG's intervention into the health sector is about 16 years old, some of the older women may not have benefited from this knowledge. However benefits of the mother's milk should form an integral part of the health education programme and CHWs of CHIRAG as well as the ANM of the PHCs should promote this aspect of maternal and child health.

Period of Rest after Delivery

It is most common for women of the Kumaon Hills to rest for exactly eleven days after delivery (see Table 4.11). Eleven days seems to be an appropriate and even auspicious amount of time, as stated by 66.7 per cent of the women. Though professionals suggest rest for one month, this is often difficult to achieve because of the heavy responsibility women carry for maintaining the home. About 20 per cent of women reported that they were able to rest for more than eleven days, but about 10 per cent said that they either got no rest at all or rested for a mere three days. The reason given by these women was, no support at home, alone in the family. Though suggesting that women rest longer is medically correct, it is not simply education but social change that is needed to change this practice. Decreasing women's workload needs to be coupled with education about resting for at least one month after delivery. This can be done by educating the community about sharing the workload during a woman's pregnancy. Since it is unlikely that men will participate in "women's work" then local women's groups can organize to assist one another.

Table 4.11 : Other Practices related to Post-natal Care

Villages	Post Natal resting place coated with cowdung		Used Cotton for cleaning			Other means of cleaning Vaginal Parts			No. of days for cleaning				
	Yes	No	Yes	No	No answer	Soap	Brandy	Bath	2 days	7 days	11 days	22 days	Done nothing
Almori	10	0	4	6	0	0	0	0	0	1	2	2	5
Kwedal	10	0	0	1	9	2	2	5	0	1	8	1	0
Kafli	9	1	0	0	10	0	2	8	1	0	6	1	2
Chataula	10	0	9	1	0	0	0	0	0	2	7	0	1
Simayal	10	0	7	3	0	0	0	0	0	2	3	2	3
Buribana	7	3	0	5	5	1	9	0	2	2	4	1	1
Total	56	4	20	16	24	3	13	13	3	8	30	7	12
Percentage	93.3	6.7	33.3	26.7	40.0	5.0	21.7	21.7	5.0	13.3	50.0	11.7	20.0

Postnatal Resting Place Coated with Cowdung

Not all traditional practices are harmful, with the advent of new technology some practices may have become outdated but when they flourished these were based on knowledge and wisdom of the people. In fact it is important to see the value behind it, before denigrating it. 93.3 per cent of the women stated that they rested in a place coated with cowdung after their delivery. In Kumaon there is a tradition to coat the walls and the floor of the room where the delivery is to take place with cow dung. In most of India, a mixture of fresh cowdung, mud and water is considered to be a cleansing agent.

Kunti Bisht of village Buribana said, "a *bari* two inches high of cowdung is built around the resting place of the women who has just delivered, where she rests for eleven days. This is made to prevent insects from entering the space where the women is lying down. Also, the demarcated line is a symbol of protection. No one except one member of the family who is looking after the woman is allowed to enter this space". Perhaps, there is some sound rationale behind this practice. Though dung contains bacteria that can prevent the growth of some kinds of fungus, the risk of tetanus or bacterial infection is often greater than the benefit (Werner & Bower, 1995). Because this practice is so prevalent, accessible, and affordable, it has been difficult to change the tradition of coating the walls and floors of the home with cowdung mixture. Because the home must be cleansed after a woman has given birth, she often rests in a room that has a fresh layer of cow dung, thus increasing her chances of a tetanus infection. The Government of India has supplied tetanus toxide (TT) vaccinations free of cost to pregnant women. The vaccinations not only protect the mother but also the foetus invitro. Since it is unlikely that women will discontinue using the cowdung mixture to cleanse the home, and one may suggest that women be educated as to the causes of tetanus infection in conjunction with increased ante-natal care.

Postnatal Vaginal Cleaning

Traditionally the *Dais* did not use anything for post-natal vaginal cleaning. When asked whether the women were using cotton wool or sterilized cotton cloth for cleaning, 33.3 per cent women said yes, 27.6 per cent said no and 40 per cent of them did not give any answer. The survey revealed that other means of cleaning the vaginal parts were now being used by the *Dais* who had undergone training. 21.7 per cent of the women reported using brandy in hot water and, an equal number stated that they sat in a sits-bath.

50 per cent of the women stated that they continued this cleaning routine for 11 days, while 11.7 per cent said that they continued this routine for 22 days. Women from the village Almori were doing nothing for keeping themselves clean after delivery. Women who were using brandy with hot water said that this provided a lot of comfort to the sore area and also helped them to keep themselves clean. They were very conscious of this post-natal care, and particular in following this routine.

During a recent health worker and trained *Dai* meeting, the women were asked in what ways had they changed their traditional health practices because of CHIRAG training. One wise woman described how they used to do nothing to clean a woman after giving birth, but now they have discovered that a bath of warm water and a little brandy is not only a disinfectant, but a warm and comfortable relaxant for the exhausted mother. Because of the visible benefits, in conjunction with the scientific reasoning, many trained *Dais* have begun incorporate this new method into their birthing routine. Some of the women at the meeting had not yet heard of this new practice, but the question prompted the sharing of knowledge among health workers and trained *Dais*. In this participatory manner, with a simple question all the women became a little wiser by their own doing.

However, many women continue to use traditional practices or sometimes nothing at all, both of which have the potential to harm. It is not because the knowledge is not there. Many health workers and *Dais* are intelligent and well respected within their communities.

Table 4.12 : Problems during and post-Delivery

	Problem after Delivery			
Villages	Excess Bleeding	Late Placenta	Breach Delivery	No Problem
Almori	3	2	0	5
Kwedal	6	1	0	3
Kafli	3	0	0	7
Chataula	1	1	0	8
Simayal	1	2	0	7
Buribana	1	0	0	9
Total	15	6	0	32
Percentage	25.0	10.0	0	53.3

Yet there are those who are skeptical of new health practices. However, when another woman of equal standing explains to the other that she has tried the new method and discovered its benefits, even the skeptics must think twice. Thus, increasing awareness through health education is very important.

Problems during and post-Delivery

Problems during post-delivery are inevitable, but with the experience of a *Dai* trained in sanitary health care methods and a mother that is able to assess when a situation is normal or critical, post-delivery difficulties need not worsen. A little less than half the women (35%) experienced problems after delivery. Most (25%) experienced excessive bleeding, as well as delivering a deformed baby and slow placenta removal (10%). No problems were experienced by 53.3 per cent of the women during delivery which is an indicator that their active lives helped them during this process. It is important that mothers and *Dais* be able to differentiate between a normal amount of bleeding and excessive bleeding which can lead to death. Traditional methods of removing a slow placenta include sticking the woman's hair into her own mouth to cause her to retch. Although this method is not harmful, it also is not pleasant for a weakened mother after delivery. Some *Dais* know of massages that produce the same results, and have shared this insight with other *Dais* at training sessions. However, some women claim that the placenta was very slow to come out. Four claimed it took four hours, two claimed two days, and one woman claimed it took four days. Had these women known the dangers associated with leaving the placenta inside the womb, they could have at least attempted to retch or massage it out, or go to a nearby clinic for assistance.

The three women who reported they had delayed placenta four hours, two days and four days, were from the non-assisted villages of Almori and Kwedal. They had their deliveries from untrained *Dais*. The need to have training for *Dais* of all villages and not only NGO assisted villages is very important. It is surprising that these villages were not covered by the Government PHC in Dhari block. Those who experienced problems shared that they did not seek any medical or professional help but only consulted the *Dai*, who is very wise and has years of experience to support her knowledge and wisdom. This total reliance on the village *Dai* is a pointer again to the crucial role they play in the traditional as well as modern health-care scenario.

Table 4.13 : Treatment Sought after Delivery

Villages	Problem after Delivery		Kind of Treatment		
	Yes	No	Medical Doctor	Witch Craft	Did Nothing
Almori	1	9	0	0	1
Kwedal	4	6	3	1	0
Kafli	3	7	1	1	1
Chataula	0	10	0	0	0
Simayal	1	9	1	0	0
Buribana	3	7	3	0	0
Total	12	48	8	2	2
Percentage	20.0	80.0	13.3	3.3	3.3

Treatment Sought After Delivery

A majority of the women (80%) stated that they had no severe problems of post-delivery. 20 per cent however reported that they had some problems out of which 13.3 per cent sought help of a medical doctor who was either the RMP in Bhatelia or the CHIRAG doctor at the Sargakhet clinic. The kind of problems they had were fever, weakness and excessive bleeding after delivery. Two women from villages Kwedal and Kafli said they used their own traditional healing remedies to cure themselves, and another two said they did nothing at all, even if they had problems. On further probing out of the 80 per cent women who categorically said they had no severe problems it was ascertained that home remedies suggested by the mother-in-law or an elderly woman were used for dealing with minor problems after delivery.

Table 4.14 : Postnatal Food Intake (Up to Forty Days)

Villages	Post Delivery-food in take (40 days)								
	For 11 days			For 15 next days			For 15 next days		
	Nor-mal	More	Less	Nor-mal	More	Less	Nor-mal	More	Less
Almori	5	0	5	5	0	5	9	1	0
Kwedal	1	1	8	5	3	2	2	7	1
Kafli	6	1	3	4	4	2	6	3	1
Chataula	3	2	5	6	0	4	5	4	1
Simayal	1	3	6	5	3	2	5	4	1
Buribana	5	3	2	8	2	0	6	4	0
Total	21	10	29	33	12	15	33	23	4
Percen-tage	35.0	16.7	48.3	55.0	20.0	25.0	55.0	38.3	6.7

Postnatal Food Intake (Up to forty days)

There are many myths associated with food intake after delivery in Kumaon. While this aspect has already been discussed in the section on types of foods avoided after delivery (pp.107-08), this question focused on the quantity of food eaten after delivery. 48.3 per cent of the women reported eating less food for the first 11 days after delivery. Even women from CHIRAG assisted villages were eating less food than normal. The reasons given by the women were, "If we eat all types of food like rice, *Dahi*, green vegetables, the child will catch a cold and get pneumonia, or a loose stomach. We even avoid drinking water after delivery". Some others said they ate less because they did not feel like it, or because of restrictions imposed by the elderly women in the family. Another belief related to food intake after delivery according to Tara Devi of village Almori is, "..to give only salt, *roti* and *halwa* for the first 11 days to protect the child from cold; and not to give any water for 11 days and not to eat everything to avoid the child falling sick."

35 per cent of the women had their normal food the first 11 days, and 16.7 per cent even reported eating more in the first 11 days. The reasons given by the women for eating more were "because we are breast feeding we need more nutritious food to keep ourselves and the baby healthy……we feel more hungry after delivery………we have more knowledge now" (*Jankari*). Women from the villages of Simayal and Buribana who were eating more belonged to the age group 20-26.

The percentage of women who had their normal food intake during the next 15 days post-delivery increased from 35 per cent to 55 per cent. Most of these women were from the CHIRAG assisted villages where the HEWs have established a good rapport with the women. Also, as the women begin to feel better by the 11th day, their food in take also increases. It was heartening to see that in the next 15 days(25-40) the percentage of those eating more increased from 20 per cent to 38.3 per cent and the percentage of the women eating less decreased progressively from 48.3 per cent (1-11 days) to 25 per cent (11-25 days) to 6.7 per cent (25-40 days).

The reasons for eating normal/more were again, "the baby is growing and drinks milk, we feel more hungry". With education, health intervention, exposure to mass media, these practices of reducing food intake drastically have changed. However, in the more remote areas the beliefs that permeate the post-delivery food intake practices have to be seen in a context, wherein individual lived experiences find expression into a practice. It is critical that this aspect of maternal and child health is addressed by integrating the traditional practices with promotive health care strategies.

Just as during pregnancy, many women feel sick following delivery and therefore eat less. Women in assisted villages have been encouraged to eat more even up to 40 days after delivery, and a few have followed this advice. In the Kumaon Hills, women in traditional homes eat last after the men and children have had their portions, and they ought to be encouraged to eat more all the time, but especially during and after pregnancy. An example of a local food that is high in iron and carbohydrates is jaggery, which health workers and trained *Dais* instruct women to eat after delivery.

Table 4.15 : Post-natal Physical Work (Up to Forty Days)

Villages	Post-delivery – physical work (40 days)									
	For first 11 days				For next 15 days			For next 15 days		
	Normal	More	Less	No work	Normal	More	Less	Normal	More	Less
Almori	1	0	9	0	6	0	4	6	2	2
Kwedal	2	0	6	2	5	1	4	3	6	1
Kafli	2	1	4	3	4	2	4	5	3	2
Chataula	2	0	8	0	6	0	4	6	0	4
Simayal	2	0	8	0	6	0	4	7	1	2
Buribana	1	0	5	4	7	0	3	7	2	1
Total	10	1	40	9	34	3	23	34	14	12
Percentage	16.7	1.7	66.7	15.0	56.7	5.0	38.3	56.7	23.3	20.0

Postnatal Physical Work (Up to Forty Days)

In keeping with the tradition that women are allowed a period of eleven days rest following delivery, 80 per cent of women reported that they perform less or no work during that time. Yet after those eleven days, most women are expected to work with the same diligence as normal. It appears as though there is little difference between assisted and non-assisted villages in this respect.

The reasons given by 66.7 per cent of the women who were doing less work and 15 per cent who were doing no work were, "The mother is weak and has to take care of the baby… women are considered impure (*achut mante hain*) and are not allowed to do any work". According to Shanti Devi of village Simiyal, "the physical work post-delivery has a distinct pattern, 1-11 days no work, the woman is considered impure and she is also weak; 11-22 days after the ceremony on the 11th day she is allowed to do some work outside but cannot cook or touch the water as she is still considered impure; from the 22nd day she is allowed to cook and do all the tasks inside the kitchen and the house; after 40 days she is allowed to go to the jungle/forest."

Her sharing was so clear that it put the entire issue of post-delivery physical work in a well reasoned context.

Women performing their normal tasks increased from 16.7 per cent (1-11 days) to 56.7%σ per cent from 11-25 days. Many women who have no or less familial support have to perform their normal household tasks (except cooking for 22 days which is taboo). The survey reveals that from 25-40 days 80 per cent of the women are performing their normal (56.7%) and more (23%) tasks.

All of this does effect the women's health, but in the absence of alternate support systems and the nature of the work which has to be performed Daily (getting fuel wood and fodder; fetching water from the spring) the woman has little choice.

Focusing on her nutritional status that would give her energy to meet the pressure of her work schedule would go a long way in making a difference to the health of women in this region.

Table 4.16 : Medical Check-Up After Delivery

Villages	Medical Check-up after Delivery	
	Yes	No
Almori	0	10
Kwedal	2	8
Kalli	1	9
Chataula	0	10
Simayal	0	10
Buribana	1	9
Total	4	56
Percentage	6.7	93.3

Medical Check-Up After Delivery

A whopping 93.3 per cent of women do not seek a medical check-up after delivery. Following delivery, the woman is in some ways more vulnerable than when she was pregnant. There are some cases in which the woman may not feel the need for a medical check-up, but it would do her much good. For example, the woman may have lost a lot of blood during the birthing and can be at risk if she was already close to anaemia. Besides medical benefits, a post-natal check-up gives the health worker the opportunity to remind the mother to breast feed the child, take rest for forty days, increase her iron intake, and vaccinate her child.

Post-delivery Ritual Ceremonies

The interviews with sixty women indicate that on the 11th day after the birth of the child a special ceremony called *Namkaran* is performed by calling a priest. This ceremony has been described in detail in the section on Traditional Practices related to delivery.

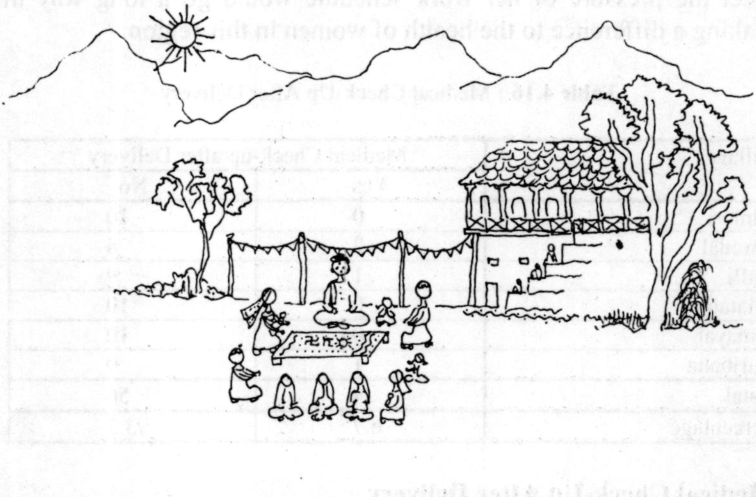

Fig. 4.4 : The 'NAMKARAN' Ceremony on the 11th Day after Child Birth

Basanti Devi from village Chataula said, "On the 11th day, the baby is shown the sun, new clothes are made for the baby and the mother. Cow's urine is sprinkled for the purification of the mother before she comes out into the courtyard for the ceremony. Family and guests from neighboring households bring gifts, a sweet called *'batasa'* and some milk to bless the child. A red tilak is put on the forehead of the guests as a mark of welcome, and *gur* is distributed to the guests. On this day the Dai who delivered the baby is specially invited, she is given a saree and some money as acknowledgement of her services."

Another woman from village Almori said, "An *'Uchani'* (a small platform) is made for the gods and goddesses and grateful offerings are made to them for their benediction and the presence of the new baby in the house. This is *'Dev Bhoomi'* we have to make offerings to the gods that reside in this land. A *'jagar'*, a religious ceremony where special singers come and perform from the epics of Mahabharata and Ramayana are also held in some households."

"All these ceremonies are in a way invoking the higher, the transcendental, the presence of the god and reiterate the sacredness of the culture, said "Kishni Devi a *Dai* of village Sunkhiya.

Culture → Lifecycle events related to women's life → Health →Development

From Kishni Devi's sharing one can see that life is sacred, therefore, all the rituals and ceremonies that mark the reproductive phase of a woman's life are a celebration or a manifestation of that sacredness.

Interviews about delivery and post-delivery with TBAs, CHWs, village women and resource persons

A. Interview with Deepadevi

Wife of Durga Dutt Dhani, Brahmin family, Village Kanarkha, block Dhari, Kumaon Hills.

Kanarkha is a village in Dhari Block, near Padampuri. I went to this village with Lata Harbola and Basanti from CHIRAG (who were initiating the formation of Self-Help groups here). This was one journey I will never forget, the village was at a height of 1500 feet from the road where the jeep left us. A stony path moving through dense oak forest weaved its way upwards, our brief stops interrupted by "be careful, there are bears in the forest..just the other day a woman's face was ripped apart". Lata and Basanti were, of course, not deterred, half way up a small pony appeared from nowhere as though 'gods' had listened to me. "I have seen you somewhere before" said the 18 year old boy who was carrying some grains to his house in Kanarkha. That was a wild statement I thought! On reaching his home (he turned out to be the son of Durga Dutt Dhani, whom Lata was intending to contact) a traditional Kumaoni house made of mud and stone, with carved pillars, I was introduced to his mother Deepa and his father who said, "Didi I have seen you somewhere". Some conspiracy is going on here, I thought, but before I could respond, he produced an album with a snap of me and my family standing outside an old house. "Don't you remember me I was the cook at Jilling Estate?" I had no idea that I was anywhere near Jilling Estate, which I had visited in 1995 with the family. What a small world, how do we come back to places and get connected with people, were some questions floating in my mind. We were soon fed the most delicious Kumaoni food, Mandua *rotis, bhatt* (lentil) and *jholi* (made of Yoghurt). This indeed was a special moment.

Deepa is an untrained *Dai* of village Kanarkha. She said that traditionally and in some remote villages even now, a rope is tied to a hook in the ceiling of a room in the upper story of the house for delivery. When the pain increases (i.e., the spasm becomes more frequent) the woman sits on her haunches and pulls the rope. The *Dai* sits behind her and gently supports her. When the baby is born the *Dai* ties the cord with a thread after leaving a distance of three fingers, she places a copper coin below and cuts the cord with a blade. Initially the blade and thread were not boiled, but now with more awareness this practice has changed. Deepa said that they put the blood that comes out while cutting the cord on the child's lips as it is considered to be the life source which has nurtured the child in the womb. In some homes the cord is cut by the woman herself. However, if she is too tired or listless and has little energy the cord is cut by the mother or by the mother-in-law. If they also do not do it then the *Dai* cuts the cord. If the mother-in-law cuts the cord then she is not allowed to cook food in the family for eleven days. Cow's urine is sprinkled to purify her as she moves in and out of the room where the delivery has taken place. Earlier the delivery would take place on a piece of *jute* mat which is thrown away. Now-a-days they use rubber sheets, specially where the *Dais* have been trained.

She shared with me that when her daughter was born the placenta did not come out for five days, but the mid-wife Kamla was skilled enough to take it out and no harm came to her. In medical terms this is considered a very serious thing as poison can spread in the body and a woman can die. When the placenta comes out, it is buried under a green fruit bearing tree. This is considered very auspicious the reason being that just as the tree is green and bears fruit, may the child grow healthy and the mother should keep bearing children.

A stone is never placed above the buried placenta as they consider this as stopping the way for more children. Some mud is dug around the fruit bearing tree and the placenta is buried there and covered with loose mud.

After the child is born the *Dai* with the help of the mother bathes the child with hot water. The mother is made to lie on the floor on a mattress and covered with a quilt. A small barrier made of cowdung called *'Bari'* demarcates her area for rest, from the rest of the room. This is about 2-3′ high. Traditionally the woman was not allowed to move from this area except for her bath which she takes on the 3rd, 5th, 7th, 9th, and 11th day. Odd numbers are considered auspicious in this environment. (Refer to *'ban-snan'* ceremony in Garhwal Himalayas where only *Suhagin* women in odd numbers are invited to the ceremony, Capila: 2002). The *'Bari'* is made to keep any insects from entering the area wherever the mother and child are lying down, it is also symbolic of 'protection' from infection. Bachuli Devi, a *Dai* from another village in Dhari block, had some interesting insights about the *'Bari'* or cowdung line. According to her just like Sita had a *'lakshman rekha'* to protect her which she crossed and Ravan took her away, the *'Bari'* is made to protect the woman and her child from infection and disease, also by linking this aspect to Goddess Sita, the creation of the cowdung *'Bari'* is viewed as divine intervention.

Any person entering the room to give food to the mother or see the baby is purified by sprinkling cow's urine which is left in a small vessel in the room. A women who has given birth to a child is considered impure for 11 days because she is bleeding *"uska pait kacchha hota hai"*, said Deepa Devi. Some other women from the neighborhood were asking why women were considered impure after childbirth when the child is considered a gift of the Lord.

The 11th day after child birth is a very special day and is called the *'namkaran'* ceremony. The *'angaan'* or courtyard is cleared and lipai is done with a mixture of green *gobar* and *bhusa.* A *'chowki'* decorated with a traditional *'mandala'* made with rice paste is specially constructed in the centre of the courtyard, around which the Pandit, father-in-law, mother-in-law and the mother and father along with the 11 day old baby sits.

The mother and baby are given new clothes to wear on this day. The priest enters the room where the mother has been confined for 11 days and gives the woman a purified wooden stick to hold from one end. The other end is held by the priest and her brings her out into the open courtyard. This is also the first day when the new born baby is shown the sun. When I asked Deepa Devi why this was important she said that by showing the child the light or *'prakash'* of the sun it is believed that the child will be as radiant as the sun, when he or she grows up.

Some Kumaoni women during group discussions related to the above ceremony, said that the sun's rays are important for the baby who has been confined to a dark, badly ventilated room for eleven days. The priest then puts the baby in the mother's lap and refers to the religious texts for the letter from which the name of the baby should start. After a name is decided by the family, he utters the name in the baby's ear through a *'shankh'* (conch shell), as this is considered auspicious. He then announces the name loudly to the whole gathering and flowers are showered on the new born child.

Relatives, friends and other people from the village are invited for this ceremony. They all bring gifts for the child. The *'buas'* (aunts) of the child are given gifts from their maternal family. They also give the child new clothes and some silver items. If it is a son he is considered to be Lord Krishna from this day until he is eleven years old. This is because he is absolutely pure and does not have the concept of mine and yours, till this age. He develops this identity later, according to Deepa Devi. A girl is considered to be a *devi* and she is worshipped like that. After her 12th birthday she normally gets her periods and is no longer considered pure. *Puri, halwa, pakori,* rice *kheer* are prepared on this auspicious occasion. After the *namakaran* ceremony the woman is allowed to enter the kitchen and do all other household works, but is not allowed to cook food for 22 days.

Interview with Bachuli Dev **(Plate 13)**

According to Bachuli Devi a Dai of village Navin Sunkiya in Dhari Block, "There are many restrictions with reference to food consumption immediately after delivery. The woman is given wheat *halwa* or *'mandua ka halwa'* prepared in pure *ghee* and a glass of milk on the first day. From the third or fourth day onwards she is given *dal, chappati,* honey, milk and some light vegetables. Foods like rice, potatoes, yoghurt are totally avoided because they are considered cold foods and produce gas in the stomach. Green leafy vegetables which are a rich source of iron are also avoided because the mother is feeding her baby, her stomach will start running and this will cause discomfort to the child, so we avoid giving any green vegetables to the mother.... the mother should preferably cut the cord herself, this is important because it is her baby." According to her, some *Dais* had received training from the Trained *Dai* Practitioners – TDP. When I asked Bachuli Devi what she had learnt she said, *"Hath to vahi hai, dimag bhi vahi hai, kya sikha, yeh to Bhaghwan ki Dain hai, mere hath se koi bhi bacchha nahin mara, 30 varsh mujhe yah kam karate hue"*, (i.e. "The hand is the same, the mind is the same, for 30 years not a single child has died from my hand"). There is an innate sense of confidence and pride in her work and her skill, all of which she considers as a gift of the Lord. However she said that after training she has started using a rubber sheet, a pair of gloves, a blade and thread (both of which she boils before use).

According to Bachuli Devi women in the village have been greatly influenced by the presence of CHIRAG working in the area of health in the villages of Ramgarh and Dhari block where this research was conducted. After the birth of the third child women were highly motivated to go in for an operation. Very interestingly she shared that earlier around 1975-80, there was a movement for the men in the family to go for vasectomy. Nevertheless, a number of women got pregnant and this created a kind of rift in the family, so they decided that the woman of the household would go for the operation. This sharing by Bachuli Devi during the federation meeting at Kasialekh initiated a lively discussion, with some women saying "even in this act the men have the upper hand", while some others said the operation gave them much freedom from the fear of getting pregnant.

Interview with Kishni Devi Dai of village Sargakhet, Dhari Block

"When nine months are complete and the pain starts, the mother-in-law calls the *Dai*. She examines the woman and puts her hand inside and sees if the mouth of the uterus is open. When the water bag bursts she spreads gunny bags on the floor and makes her lie on the floor. She then ties the cord after leaving four fingers, with the thread and boils the blade in hot water and asks the mother to cut the cord. The *Dai* then presses the stomach of the woman, to allow the placenta to come out itself. Some *Dai's* put the woman's hair in her mouth to create a sensation of vomiting. Then the woman takes her mother's name and the placenta falls off. They bury the placenta under a green fruit-bearing tree. If however she does not want any more children, the placenta is buried in the ground over which they place a large stone, and this acts as a symbolic barrier." According to Kishni Devi, "It is believed that if a woman who is having trouble conceiving puts the placenta of a women who has delivered a baby on her stomach, and if it fits around her, she will get pregnant very soon. The child is then bathed with hot water and given a *'gutti'*, of honey and some new clothes. Earlier they would not give the cholestrum, now they feed the child from the first day."

"Diet for the woman on the first day is thin *suji halwa*. They do not give *roti,* but one glass of milk, with one cap full of brandy for the first five days. They feel that by eating grain/wheat *roti* for the first five days, there would be unrest in the stomach and she would have to exert to pass stool. They give her less water to drink, and more butter-milk and vegetables. On the eleventh day, the pandit comes and gets the mother out of the room, and the child who is also not brought out for eleven days, is shown the sun (sun god). This is to prevent the child from getting infection. The pandit then utters the name of the child in the right ear. The relatives are invited for the ceremony and they bring gifts for the baby. She works after 22 days but does not do domestic work. I have never taken my children to a doctor, nor have I have been to one myself", said Kishni Devi very proudly.

"Today the greater the loss of religious value, the more problems are created for humanity (*jitana niyam-dharm chuta, utni hi kharabi hoti hai*). Agricultural practices have been totally spoiled, everything was pure earlier, we use to put *gobar* manure so that the vegetables and grains were pure, the forest had its own energy and when the woman went to the jungle, she would come back after eating berries like *'kafal'*, *'gungaroo'*, *'kilmora'*, etc. These were nutritious and we would drink clean water from the spring. Everything has changed with "development". When I was young I did not even get a stomach full, now people eat everything and still they are not healthy. Today people are so competitive that even in terms of knowledge, they say "I know more than you"!

Interview with Beena Devi, health worker and Dai, CHIRAG, village Pokhrar (Dhari Block) **(Plate 14)**

I visited the house of Beena Devi with the health team of CHIRAG. A vaccination camp was held in Beena Devi's house who is both the local *Dai* and the health worker of the village. The house is traditional, made of mud and stone, the living rooms are on the upper story and the cow shed and fodder store below.

Women from neighbouring households located at quite a distance from this house bring their young children (0-5) for their routine, vaccination and growth monitoring is done by the health team.

There is no separation between the forest and the house, in fact the forest seems a part of the house, in a kind of a symbiotic relationship. Sitting on the open verandah freshly coated with cow dung, hearing the sound of pine needles rustling in the wind one experiences or becomes present to the life of the people of Kumaon. There is stillness, broken by Beena Devi's query, "Didi, how did you become interested in understanding our traditional health practices? When I go for meetings to the Primary Health Centres in Padampuri (Dhari block) the medical officers give us information about vaccination and how to reach our target, but do not focus on our knowledge or wisdom related to health."

Beena Devi's question at once focused on the central theme of my work, listening to the 'voices' of women who have lived and taken care of other women's health related problems in their area. Some significant questions began to emerge as follows :

1. Why is it that when we talk of health care we do not include the knowledge and wisdom of people whose lives are inter-linked and interconnected with the culture of the region?
2. Is health care a service to be delivered or does it build on peoples knowledge, integrating that into the process of development of the health sector?
3. Why have we fragmented life and living from cultural practices, from health as though they are not connected?

All these questions were floating in my mind like the clouds that had just entered Beena Devi's home engulfing us, and obliterating the landscape, only to disappear a moment later leaving everything green and clear, as though in a way giving clarity to the ideas in the head. Beena Devi said, "The forest was green and full of trees, the air was clear and fresh, that is why people were naturally healthy in this area. We used to boil the water and drink it, especially in the rainy season. If some one fell ill they were given local herbs and medicinal plants prescribed by the Vaid. Today the reliance for well-being on the local Vaid has diminished because of the availability of the RMP's (Registerred Medical Practitioners) at Bhatelia a nearby market and the formal healthcare centers."

I asked Beena Devi to share her experiences as a *Dai* and what changed with the training she had received from the CHIRAG doctors (Abhijit and Yashodhra Das, and Diane a trained midwife from UK).

"Earlier I would make the woman sit on her knees and pull the rope hanging from the ceiling. I would support her buttocks from behind and facilitate the birth of the child. If the mother is healthy, I would encourage her to press downwards and then I would gently press her stomach downwards for the placenta to come out, or put her hair in the mouth to create a sensation of vomiting. This enables the placenta to come out. After training from CHIRAG I do not do the delivery by the woman kneeling and pulling the rope. But I make her lie down on a rubber sheet or a clean cloth and use sterilized gloves, a blade, thread and coin, all the three of which I boil for an hour. After measuring three fingers, the cord is cut and I allow the residue in the cord to flow towards the baby. (There is some difference of opinion on this practice as the doctor presently working in CHIRAG from AIIMS had discouraged the Dai's from doing this as he felt it could effect the heart of the child). The important thing is that I cut my nails, before the delivery and wash my hands with soap and water. I now use these new methods while delivering children in the village. These new methods do not in anyway undermine our skill or wisdom but help to make the delivery safe and free from infection."

Beena Devi is an amazing *Dai* and health worker, she understands the problems that women in the hills face with regard to menstruation, child birth. When I asked her what according to her were the major health problems faced by women in her village she was quick to enumerate them, as follows:

1. Repeated pregnancies, having a child every year.
2. Over-burdened with work, women here work in the fields, look after the animals, walk to the forest for fuel wood and fodder, cook for the family, take care of children and elders. All this poses a constraint on their health. If she has a mother-in-law at home, it is a great help as the grandmother, bathes the children and feeds them while the woman goes to the field and jungle. The socializing and meeting people in the village is done by the mother-in-law, this is also an important aspect of health care. Earlier about 30 years ago, the men of the family used to share all the work in the house, but now-a-days they help in the agricultural tasks and watch only television at home. In the context of the women of Kumaon and the participation of men similar situations were found in the Tehri Garhwal district of Uttaranchal (Capila, 2002).
3. Menstrual pain, excessive bleeding and fibroids, no rest.
4. White discharge, pain in the pelvic region, frequent headaches. Traditionally to cure white discharge we would soak rice, boil it and drink water while it was hot. This would give a great relief and stop discharge. I still recommend this practice to the women in the villages but it does not give them relief, I refer them to the doctor in CHIRAG.

Continuing our dialogue on women's health, Beena Devi shared with me her work roles as a *Dai* and health worker :

1. Keeping record of the weight of the children 0-5 in the village.
2. Informing the mothers about the vaccination-day, in case some children were left out, accompanying the mothers to the vaccination camp at Kasialekh, held once a month by the CHIRAG health team.
3. She does all the deliveries in the village and refers a complicated case to the hospital in Padampuri.
4. Care of pregnant women in the community which includes 2 tetanus injections after 5-6 months, monthly check up to see the position of the baby.
5. Refers women in the village to the family planning camp conducted by Chirag at Kasialekh, and also accompanies the women for an abortion to Haldwani or Nainital (no facilities for an MTP exist in this area).

Beena Devi earns Rs.200 per month as a health worker and Rs.150 per month as a *Dai* from CHIRAG. She strongly feels the need for a lady doctor in the region and an ambulance van which can facilitate access to health care. According to Beena Devi under the Swajal programme of CHIRAG which has a component of HESA (Health and Environmental Sanitation Awareness) the *Dai's* received a kit containing : (1) rubber sheet, (2) thread, (3) blade, (4) one dettol soap, (5) cotton wool, and (6) nail cutter.

Discussions with Bhagwati Pande and Reetu Sogani from Sahyog, Almora, August, 2002.

Bhagwati Pande has worked with the health programmes of the NGO 'Sahyog' in Almora district for several years as a Coordinator of their health programmes in Nainital. Discussions with her about traditional practices regarding delivery in the villages were indeed stimulating. According to her, the role of the *Dai* as a care-giver assumes great importance for the woman who is ready for delivery. The Dai massages the stomach with warm oil, she keeps talking to her so that she does not go to sleep. By giving her examples of other deliveries and her own experiences she gives her a lot of emotional support. At this time elderly women in the family and other women who have knowledge about these practices also come to the house where the delivery is to take place, not only do they give emotional support, but also assist in preparing the room by collecting the bricks and a rope. The mother-in-law brings warm milk with *ghee* for the woman to drink so that she has strength for what the *Dai* calls *'jor lagao'* (Push hard).

In documenting traditional birth practices, not much emphasis is given to this kind of support which is both nurturing and welcome. In the modern health care system this is lacking, i.e. familial and community support becomes peripheral to the presence of the doctor and the hospital. According to Bhagwati, the Dais believe that they have a major role in correcting the position of the baby while massaging the stomach even a baby in breech position is corrected by them, some *Dais* put their finger in the vagina to make sure that dilation has occurred or not and even put a few drops of oil to lubricate the area. Even when actual labour pains have not yet begun they urge the woman to press downwards with the result that by the time the actual labour pains start the woman is already exhausted and there is a chance of the uterus prolapsing, as stated earlier in another context.

The family and the *Dai* believe that the delivery should be at home and unless they see any life-threatening danger, or signals they try to appease their gods by performing some rituals. A complicated pregnancy according to them is a curse of the gods and in a way pleasing them would bring relief and comfort to both the woman's natal home and her in-laws home.

Generally delivery is done by most *Dais* in this region (Almora district) in the squatting position with knees resting on bricks and the woman pulling at the rope which is tied to the ceiling. Immediately after delivery the woman is given half a glass of brandy to drink for removal of the placenta, the same practice is followed in the villages of Almora also, i.e. putting hair in her mouth to induce vomiting sensation which induces the placenta (*awal*) to come out.

The mother mostly cuts the cord herself and after delivery the *Dai* does not touch the woman as she is considered impure (*ashudh*) or polluting. The Dai does not want to be isolated in her own home because if she cuts the cord then she cannot cook in her house or touch water for ten to eleven days.

The new born baby is not fed the first milk, it is not considered healthy for three days, and any other women in the neighbourhood (Dhrati Mahila) who is breast-feeding her child comes to feed the baby, or cow's milk is given for the first few days. If the mother does not get breast milk she is given some herbal medicines like *'karve ki jar'* (Asparagus root), which is ground to a paste and fed to the mother. This is believed to induce breast milk on consumption; also *Mandua,* a coarse grain which is rich in calcium, and rice are cooked together and given to the lactating mother.

During the first delivery whether it is a boy or a girl several precautions with reference to food consumption are observed post-delivery. These include no green vegetables, curd, meat, eggs, and certain *dals*. Drinking water standing and gulping it down is absolutely not allowed, the belief being that the water will go into the breasts of the mother, and will be harmful for the child.

Bhagwati Pande said that women in the villages in Almora district shared with her that if a women eats fish after delivery the tiny fish bones will come out of her breast milk and harm the baby; green vegetables would induce green stools in the baby and the consumption of fried food would give the child problems in the throat (*'chupra ho jaiga'*). For the second child these precautions are followed more rigidly for a boy than for the girl. Inadvertently this is good for the girl child as the mother is eating more things, the reasoning behind this is discrimination of course, so that no harm should come to the baby boy.

The new born baby is massaged with warm mustard oil and a pad made of *'atta'* is gently rubbed on the baby's body. Elderly women in the family generally do this massage. A woman who has other support in the home gets to rest more. Women entering the room where the baby and mother are resting are purified by sprinkling cow's urine. On the fifth day a preparation called *panch-gab*, five elements is prepared by the priest and kept in the corner of the room in a vessel for purification of anyone entering and leaving this room. This *panch-gab* contains cow's urine, milk, a copper coin, *dhrub* grass and *jau* a kind of millet.

According to Bhagwati a woman who has given birth to a baby girl is under a lot of mental tension because of the socio-cultural pattern of life in this region. She sees her own life reflected in a way in this new born girl, overburdened with workload, repeated pregnancies, frequent abortions, lack of access to health care, lack of decision-making in using contraceptives, and lack of freedom in mobility. All these factors pose a constraint on her mind and this tension manifest in a number of health related problems in women.

A research study concluded by Sahyog in 1998 on the status of women's health in Uttaranchal has been published in a report entitled *'Pahar ki cheli'*, the findings support the interviews and group discussion with *Dais* in this area.

Some of the highlights related to birth practices (delivery) are presented below :

1. Generally deliveries are performed in the cowshed or a separate room in the house.
2. Delivery is performed by untrained Dais, mother-in-law or a knowledgeable women from the neighbourhood.
3. Delivery is done generally done in a squatting position.
4. No preparation is done to deal with any problems that may arise during delivery.

5. Generally the mother cuts the cord herself with a *'daranthi'* (sickle) or blade. A coin, a piece of wood or a flat lump of mud is kept below.
6. The check ups are done immediately preceding delivery from a medical professional, ANM or *Dai*.
7. People believe that the process is *apavitra* (not pure) therefore a woman who cuts the cord becomes *achut* (polluted).
8. For eleven to twenty-two days after delivery the mother and child are kept separate room.
9. 50 per cent of the women have to face several problems related to the process of delivery.
10. If pre-delivery check-ups are done many problems like extended labour, breech position of baby, excessive bleeding or delayed placenta can be avoided.

Traditional Practices, Post-Delivery and Related Health Problems, according to the survey are listed below :

1. Many taboos related to food consumption and drinking water are observed. In remote villages women are given only *roti* and salt to eat.
2. After delivery for 11-22 days a woman is considered *ashudh* (polluted). She is not allowed to cook or fetch water for 22 days. If she is healthy she does all the outside work like going to the fields and the forest after the fifth day.
3. If a boy is born there are more restrictions on her diet, so that no problems are caused to him in comparison to when a girl is born.
4. During the first delivery the restrictions are the same for a boy or girl.
5. A baby is breast fed until about two and a half and three years.
6. Some misconceptions or beliefs in this region are that if a mother drinks water after delivery the child will get pneumonia.
7. Milk or milk-products, fatty and fried foods will cause *chupar* (throat problems).
8. Green vegetables produce green watery stools.
9. Out of ten every two women complain that their uterus comes out after delivery.
10. Out of ten every two women complain of weakness, giddiness which if not treated becomes a serious problem afterwards.

SECTION 6

FAMILY PLANNING

Table 4.17 : First Menstrual Cycle During Breast Feeding

Villages	First Menstrual Cycle during Breast-feeding				
	First year	Second year	Third year	6 to 8 months	Second month
Almori	4	0	2	4	0
Kwedal	5	0	0	5	0
Kafli	5	0	0	4	1
Chataula	4	3	1	1	1
Simayal	6	1	1	2	0
Buribana	5	0	1	4	0
Total	29	4	5	20	2
Percentage	48.3	6.7	8.3	33.3	3.3

First Menstrual Cycle during Breast-feeding

48.3 per cent of the women reported getting their first menstrual cycle during breast feeding after one year, 6.7 per cent had got it within the second year and surprisingly 8.3 per cent women reported that they were breast feeding the child until three years and did not get their menstrual cycle.

The above figures also indicate that breast feeding is a very important aspect of child care in this area, women from village Buribana said that "breast milk is highly nutritious and they continued to breast-feed along with the supplementary food".

Table 4.18 : The Gap Between Last and Second Last Child

Villages	The gap between last & second last child				Only one child
	1 year	2 years	3 years	4 years	
Almori	1	7	0	2	0
Kwedal	2	4	3	0	1
Kafli	1	2	1	3	3
Chataula	0	6	4	0	0
Simayal	1	2	5	1	1
Buribana	1	4	2	3	0
Total	6	25	15	9	5
Percentage	10.0	41.7	25.0	15.0	8.3

Child Spacing

Linked to the above question is the gap between the last and the second last child. Extended breast feeding is one of the oldest forms of child spacing. Not only do women suspend the onset of their next menstrual cycle, they are also providing a rich nourishment to their young child which contains specific antibodies and immunities that formula or solid food often lack.

A majority of the women (41.7%) shared that the gap between the last and the second last child was two years, 25 per cent stated that it was three years, 15 per cent said the gap was four years and only 10 per cent of the woman said the gap was one year.

These findings made it imperative to find out what methods besides breast feeding they were using to space the birth of their children.

Methods of Contraception

Table 4.19 : Methods of Contraception

Villages	Family Planning					
	Temporary Method			Permanent Method		No Method
	Oral pill	Con-dom	Copper-t	Tube-ctomy	Vase-ctomy	
Almori	1	0	0	1	1	7
Kwedal	0	1	0	7	0	2
Kalli	0	0	0	3	1	6
Chataula	1	1	0	6	0	2
Simayal	1	2	0	6	0	1
Buribana	0	0	0	6	1	3
Total	3	4	0	29	3	21
Percentage	5.0	6.7	0.0	48.3	5.0	35.0

Table 4.20 : Reasons for not using any family planning method

Villages	Reason for not using any Family Planning Method				
	Not aware	Objection by the family	Not available	Belief in natural process	Other reasons
Almori	2	2	2	1	0
Kwedal	1	0	1	0	0
Kalli	1	1	0	0	4
Chataula	0	1	0	0	1
Simayal	1	0	0	0	0
Buribana	0	1	0	0	2
Total	5	5	3	1	7
Percentage	8.3	8.3	5.0	1.7	11.7

Use of temporary family planning methods is abysmally low in the Kumaon hills, oral pills being used by 5 per cent of the women, condoms as a family planning methods by 6.7 per cent of the husbands and none of the women responded to using a copper-T. 35 per cent of the women mainly from the non-assisted villages of Almori, Kwedal and Kafli were not using any method at all. The reasons given by them were 8.3 per cent had family opposition to using any birth control methods, 8.3 per cent non-availability, 5.3 per cent belief in natural processes (one woman from village Almori) and 11.7 per cent of the woman reported other reasons for not using any birth control pills. These were vomiting, severe headache after having used oral pills for a month, wanting a child. One women from village Kafli said, "my religion does not allow me to use family planning methods, children are god's gift, who are we to try and stop this process."

Reasons for not using Family Planning Methods

Large families are still desirable for many reasons. Perhaps the greatest determining factor is the unsaid desire to have male children. Typically the family will continue to have children until at least one son has been born, and the more sons the better. For numerous reasons, the son is preferred over the daughter. For example, when the parents pass away it is the son who must light the funeral pyre, ensuring good transition into the next stage of life. Also, the tradition of dowry has spun wildly out of control in India, and to pay for a daughter's marriage can put a family into debt for years thereafter. What needs to be stressed is the use of temporary methods for child spacing, overall reducing the number of children, and the value of the girl child, needs to be stressed.

The survey also revealed that 48.3 per cent of the women interviewed had gone in for a more permanent method of birth control, tubectomy (ligatomy), but most of the women had gone in for this procedure after having given birth to a number of children. A large percentage of these women (21 out of 29) belonged to the villages where CHIRAG has it outreach programmes. The HEWs refer cases of tubectomy to the family planning camps held at the Sargakhet clinic and Kasialekh clinic. Many of these women had also contacted the local ANM and gone to Haldwani or Nainital hospital for their tubecotomy.

Surprisingly 7 out of 10 women in Kwedal (non-assisted village) had gone in for tubectomy. These women went in for this operation after having at least four children. They were accompanied by family members to Haldwani, Nainital hospital or a camp in Bhowali.

I was personally present at a family planning camp at the Sargakhet clinic which CHIRAG had organized with a government lady doctor from Nainital. The ANM's from 16 sub-centres of the PHC at Padampuri (Dhari block) were present with their prospective clients. In all the field visits that I had visited over the year to villages in Ramgarh and Dhari block, I had never seen the ANMs in the village.

Perhaps their most active role is to bring potential women for tubectomy as this is rewarded in their work performance.

SECTION-7

CHILDREN AND HEALTH

Supplementary Feeding practices for the child (0-6 months, 6-12 months, 12 months)

Child–rearing practices, particularly the weaning foods given to the child determine to a large extent the health of the child in the first year of his/her life.

All women (100%) reported breast-feeding the child from 0-6 months, only one or two who said they did not have enough milk said they fed the baby cow's milk after two months. After six months which is the time when the *"annaprashan"* (introducing cereals and other solid foods) ceremony takes place for boys, and for girls after the 5th month, soft foods like *dal* water, *suji, dalia,* banana, are introduced as reported by Durga Devi of village Almori. She adds, " until six months onwards the child is not able to eat or digest solid foods so we give soft foods. After 12 months when the child gets teeth and his digestion improves (*pachan shakti*) we give the child everything cooked at home, *roti, dal, chawal*".

As seen in the earlier table on first menstrual cycle during breast-feeding, mother's milk is fed along with the supplementary feeding. Children in this age group 0-12 months looked healthy in this area.

Table 4.21 : Immunization

Villages	Immunization	
	Yes	No
Almori	2	8
Kwedal	4	6
Kafli	2	8
Chataula	9	1
Simayal	9	1
Buribana	7	3
Total	33	27
Percentage	55.0	45.0

Immunization

Immunization programmes are provided by CHIRAG and the Government of India free of charge for all children, however the government run primary health clinic provides CHIRAG with all of its vaccines while administering very few themselves. This is why more children from assisted villages receive vaccinations than children from non-assisted villages under the government's responsibility. Yet even in assisted villages, only 67.5 per cent of mothers have had their children vaccinated. Of the 45 per cent women who reported not taking their child for immunization (14 out of 20) were from the non-assisted villages of Almori and Kwedal. The women from village Almori shared with us that the ANM does not visit their area at all, so they were not aware of the vaccination programme. The two women who did take their children went to a clinic in Nathuakhan, a village nearby which is more progressive and is on the road-head, and has a doctor in a clinic.

The four women from village Kwedal who took their children for vaccination were not aware of the complete immunization schedule, they stated "we have only been given the polio drops". Even in village Kafli where CHIRAG has its health intervention programmes 8 out of 10 women reported that they had not got their children immunized. These women were in the age group of, 35-40, and may not have had access to CHIRAG's outreach programmes earlier. What comes across alarmingly is the complete absence of the government infrastructure in providing primary health care to the community.

One of the most important duties of the health extension team of CHIRAG is to hold a monthly vaccination camp at a central location and travel to distant villages with vaccines. According to Ramsingh Bisht, CHIRAG laboratory technician, most organizations either do not have the capabilities or the knowledge to preserve vaccines. CHIRAG is one of the few in the area that can keep them in cold temperatures, thus preserving their effectiveness. In the past, organizations have provided warm or expired vaccines and children have died as a result.

The gamut of vaccinations include tetanus (TT) for both mother and child, measles mumps rubella (MMR), polio (OPV), diphtheria (DPT), vitamin A, deworming, and (BCG). CHIRAG and the government provide profile cards to mark the progress of each child's vaccinations, giving one copy to the parent and keeping their own identical record.

CHIRAG's immunization plans cover far more children than government plans. Most vaccines take two to three injections at specific time intervals, so consistency is imperative. Vaccination camps were the most effective and economical ways of distributing vaccines, but for distant places they would typically ride into a village and announce their arrival. The resident health workers would then spread the message that the vaccinations had arrived, and that the children who need them should be brought down along with any pregnant women for check-ups. Yet even when the health team travelled to villages consistently, women would often be busy working in the fields and unable to come. Other times the resident health worker was busy doing something else on that day, often she has overloaded herself with duties such as being the *balwadi* (pre-school) teacher or organizing a women's self-help group, and did not remind the village of the coming of the health team for vaccination. In remote villages there is too much dependency on the health worker and the extension team. There is a need to create a more sustainable immunization programme.

Health Problems of the Child

(a) Deworming

The findings of the survey also shows that 90 per cent of children have received no de-worming prevention. CHIRAG clinics supply de-worming pills, which are chewable and should be taken once every six months to prevent worms from developing, and can also be used at an increased dosage to expel worms from the body.

Ramsingh Bisht suggests even adults can use this pill to prevent worms. Many people of the hills complain of coughs, which is most likely attributed to worms in the lungs. Perhaps the reason so few people take de-worming prevention is that each pill costs 12 rupees, which is not unaffordable but may seem like an unnecessary expense when there is no education about its benefits, not even in assisted villages. The health education programme should focus on this aspect in their meetings.

Table 4.22 : Health Problems of the Child

Villages	De-worming		Any other Disease		Type of Disease			
	Yes	No	Yes	No	Diarrhoea	Premature baby	Mal nutrition	Pertussis
Almori	1	9	6	4	5	0	0	1
Kwedal	2	8	8	2	8	0	3	2
Kafli	1	9	6	4	4	0	0	3
Chataula	0	10	5	5	4	1	2	1
Simayal	0	10	5	5	5	1	0	0
Buribana	2	8	7	3	0	0	0	4
Total	6	54	37	23	26	2	5	11
Percentage	10.0	90.0	61.7	38.3	43.3	3.3	8.3	18.3

(b) Diarrhoea

Most women (61.7%) reported that their children experienced some kind of disease, the most common being diarrhoea, as reported by 43.3 per cent of the women. Most of the diarrhoea cases were reported by women from non-assisted villages and Kafli (17 out of 30). Diarrhoea is most common cause of child death in the developing world (Werner & Bower, 1995). Often caused by drinking contaminated water, the child dies of extreme dehydration and loss of electrolytes. Tragically, most cases of diarrhoea can be both prevented and cured in the home without the assistance of a trained medical professional, yet because mothers lack the knowledge, many children have died unnecessarily. Most cases of diarrhoea can be prevented by bringing drinking water to a boiling point. Sometimes health care professionals, such as the CHIRAG's current resident doctor, claim that drinking water must be boiled for a minimum of twelve minutes. Possibly because of the elevation and lower boiling point, water needs to be boiled a bit longer than at sea level, but even at sea level all organisms will be killed by simply bringing the water to a boiling point. It is the heat of the water as it prepares to boil, not the boiling water, that eliminates the contamination. Twelve minutes seems to be over and above the minimum requirement, and people may be discouraged from boiling their water if they think they must do it for such a long time, using so much precious fuel. Cases of diarrhoea can be cured by getting the child to drink an oral re-hydration solution (ORS), which is just a professional name for water with a spoonful of sugar and a pinch of salt. The very practical advice of Werner and Bower, authors of "Where there Is No Doctor", stress the immediacy of getting fluids into the child by suggesting that if no boiled water is available, the mother or health worker should go ahead and use water that has not been boiled instead of boiling water and waiting for it to cool. If a mother knows how to make her own ORS, then she need not even wait for a health professional and can cure her own child, possibly saving her life. (Huff E. : 2002)

When asked what the mother's did for the treatment of diarrhoea, some women (5) from village Simayal said that they had sought medical attention from a doctor in Nathuakhan, and others said that they administered the ORS solution provided by the CHIRAG extension staff. Women from village Kafli said that they use home remedies like salt and sugar solution and a local herb for the treatment of diarrhoea. One woman said she had a *'jagar'* ceremony to invoke the grace of the gods to cure her child. Unfortunately, the child died at six months. When I asked the HEW visiting this village why had this woman not administered the ORS solution, or used any traditional home remedies, she said that the woman's mother-in-law had great faith in the *'jagar'* ceremony and felt that it would cure the child. Perhaps a combination of the faith and replacing the lost liquids could have saved the child.

All these findings reiterate the importance of strengthening the promotive health care strategy which for its health education programmes can integrate folk forms like theatre, puppets, songs, etc. to give information on such vital issues.

(c) Common Diseases

Another common disease of children cough/pertussis was stated by 18.3 per cent of the women. One woman from village Buribana said, "when the child gets cough we make a garland of garlic and put it around its neck. Garlic has a lot of healing qualities. Along with garlic, we give hot water, ginger, honey and tulsi. All these help a lot in curing the cough."

Some (3) women from the same village also reported taking medicine for cough, from the local *vaid* or *Gunijan* (learned person).

Kunti Bisht from village Buribana said, "earlier when our children fell ill we had faith in traditional healing practices and home remedies, today the advent of new medicine has taken away our reliance on the traditional wisdom that we had. In fact sometimes we fear using our knowledge lest it upset the younger daughter-in-law in the family who does not have intrinsic faith in these remedies."

Kunti Devi's profound sharing links up to Ivan Illich's theory of Iatrogenesis, the medicalization of life wherein the control to cure/heal oneself with one's knowledge and wisdom is taken over by increasing dependence on modern medicine. A healthy way of life was a part of the total culture of this region.

Ritual Ceremony related to Child-Care – Annaprashan

The *Annaprashan ceremony* is performed at 8 months for girls and 6 months for boys. This disparity is because they feel the boy is weaker biologically and should be breast-fed a month longer than the baby girl before starting the cereals. Inadvertently this is beneficial to the girl child because she starts getting more nourishment a month earlier.

On this day the Pandit is called for a small *puja* and the mother, father and bhua (father's sister) feed the baby *kheer* with a silver coin. The child is dressed in new clothes. Some toys like bat, ball, bus, train, a pen and pencil and copy, a gun, a darati are kept in the courtyard and the child is left on the ground to crawl, whichever object the child touches first or moves towards it is believed that he/she will take interest in that when grown up.

According to Kunti, the HEW at CHIRAG clinic if a lactating mother gets her periods after 4 months then the mother-in-law cooks something sweet, feeds the child one tea-spoon first, then only they allow the mother to feed the baby. After being breast-fed the baby is brought out from the space where the mother is confined and purified by sprinkling cow's urine. They feel that the child is the embodiment of God, he is pure (*shudh*) until the day his mother gets per period, that is why they pre-pone the *Annaprashan*. If this is not done it is believed that the child will remain unhealthy and weak even after the *Annaprashan* ceremony. Most mothers continue to breast-feed only until one year. Some young mothers who are educated have started giving *dal*, water and boiled rice, they say they have learnt all this from the television!

SECTION-8

WOMEN AND HEALTH

Perceptions of Major Health Problems Faced by Women

Women are the source of life and the sustainers of health in the Kumaon Hills. In a place where traditions and social norms often treat women as inferior beings, to be responsible for the health and welfare of oneself, one's family, and one's village commands tremendous respect and authority.

Yet with the infiltration of outside medical knowledge and expertise, women's roles in the maintenance of health have begun to diminish. This is typical of rural areas in which development organizations have attempted to bring in improved health care and have inadvertently caused almost complete dependence on outside sources for health care. Developmental professionals are often guilty of ignoring the importance of indigenous knowledge. For the sustainability of developmental health care, it is essential to integrate modern practices with indigenous knowledge. Therefore, CHIRAG hopes to return the role of preventive health care into the women's hands by providing them with knowledge about health while empowering them to reduce their dependence on outside medical care.

Table 4.23 : Major Health Problems Faced by Women in general

Villages	Major Health Problems faced by Women					
	General Weak-ness	Back-pain	Leucorr hoea	White discharge	Burning sensation	Late Placenta
Almori	0	8	0	6	3	1
Kwedal	0	7	0	8	2	0
Kafli	4	4	0	7	1	0
Chataula	3	7	0	6	2	0
Simayal	4	9	1	7	6	0
Buribana	4	4	0	8	6	2
Total	15	39	1	42	20	3
Percentage	25.0	65.0	1.7	70.0	33.3	5.0

When asked what they perceived to be the greatest health problems women face, the top choices were white discharge and burning sensation (yeast infection or leucorrhoea), back pain, and general weakness.

A majority (70%) of the respondents said, white discharge, followed by backpain (65%); burning sensation in the hands and feet was considered a major health problem by 33.3 per cent of the women and general weakness by 25 per cent of the women. Some other problems cited by women were toothache, itching, swelling in the hands and feet, pigmentation (*chaiyaan*) and late placenta (5%). A respondent from village Almori said, "sometimes the placenta does not come for three days, the family waits eagerly and sometimes the woman dies."

The above problems were perceived by women as the major health concerns of women in the hills. In order to contextualize their sharing related to their own lives, women were asked what were the major health problems they faced personally.

What did they do, where did they go for help, if any, and did they try any traditional remedies?

Table 4.24 : Major Health Problems Faced as Respondent Women

Villages	General problems faced by the respondent women							
	Itching	Weakness	Back pain	W.discharge	Abortion	Burning	Irregular M.C.	Frequent PRE
Almori	2	0	9	7	0	0	2	5
Kwedal	0	0	8	5	0	0	3	0
Kafli	1	0	4	5	3	1	0	3
Chataula	0	0	7	8	2	0	0	0
Simayal	0	2	5	8	1	1	3	1
Buribana	0	0	7	8	3	1	4	5
Total	3	2	40	41	9	2	12	14
Percentage	5.0	3.3	66.7	68.3	15.0	3.3	20.0	23.3

A majority (68.3%) of the women stated that they suffered from white discharge, 66.7 per cent said that they had severe back pain, 23.3 per cent said that frequent pregnancies was a major problem for them, and 20 per cent of the women reported suffering from irregular menstrual cycle. The problems suffered by the respondent women are in a way similar to the health problems perceived by them that women suffer in the hills.

The second, and more crucial aspect of the question regarding what did they do and where they went for help, gives an insight into the health seeking behaviour of the women respondents, which was abysmally low. There is a self-efficacy theory of health seeking behaviour, which links women's notion of the self to seeking medical help.

Most of the women who suffered from white discharge said that they did nothing, only a very few (10 out of 60) said that they went to Nainital hospital, got an injection from Almora or got medicine from Nathuakhan. Four women from the villages of Buribana and Simayal reported that they had consulted the doctor at the CHIRAG clinic. None of them except one women from village Buribana reported using any home remedies even though there are known traditional remedies for these troubles. She said she bought some medicinal plants and herbal medicine from a vaid in Kwarab village. Perhaps women do not talk about their health problems in the family and white discharge is associated with the private parts, so they hardly speak about it.

Regarding back pain, only 15 per cent of the women reported using hot water for fomentation. A traditional method as reported earlier was heating a brick red hot, wrapping it in wet sack cloth and applying it to the back.

An equal number of women, five from village Almori (non-assisted) and five from village Buribana (CHIRAG assisted) reported frequent pregnancies as a major problem. The section on family planning has clearly shown how many women go in for contraceptive methods. However, more than seeing this as a numbers issue (which is the focus of health as a sector of development) it is important to understand the social fabric of the society that prevents women from having rights over her own body, and the number of children she would like to bear.

As regards the 20 per cent women who suffered from irregular menstruation none of them sought medical help for this issue, even though they came from assisted villages. While the community health workers and the HEWs are in touch with the women in the community, the absence of a gynaecologist or a lady-doctor to whom they can go for help is a major set back in the health care outreach strategy. This issue has already been referred to in the community health programme profile of CHIRAG. This aspect of course should be addressed by the primary health centre at Padampuri which has sixteen sub-centres and caters to a population of 20,000. A major recommendation should be a lady doctor at each PHC in a block, of the two MOI's.

The physical inaccessibility of the villages and the way the individual houses are located on the hill side (which is different from the Bakli system, houses in a row in one 'tok') makes it difficult for the healthcare providers to reach individual women in their homes. Added to this is the nature of the tasks the women perform, heavy-load heads resulting in severe back ache, lack of water to keep herself clean, inadequate rest and poor nutritional supplements.

What emerges from the major health problems of women in the Kumaon hills is that this issue has to be viewed holistically and not fragmented into compartments that further alienate women from their own wisdom and knowledge.

Lastly, the 60 women respondents from six villages were asked to share the changes they had perceived in the hill status of women in the last ten years. The perceptions of women from the assisted villages were distinctly different from those who had no access to healthcare.

Women from village Simayal in Ramgarh block said, "Earlier women were not aware, with the coming of NGOs (CHIRAG) there has been a great change, now women can also take their own decisions". Shanti Devi from the same village said, "There is a great difference in the status of women's health in our village, there is ante-natal and post-natal care of women, pregnancies are monitored, now we have complete immunization for children, growth monitoring....Now women go to meetings and speak out."

Kamla Devi also from Simayal added, "Earlier, we only relied on gods and goddesses, now women go to CHIRAG clinic, family planning methods are available, women are more aware than before and get operated after three children."

Women from village Chataula (also an assisted village) said, "A women is more aware and capable of looking after herself...earlier a women did not get enough to eat, she was anaemic, now everything is slowly changing."

Tara Devi from the same village said, "There is more knowledge now, laterines in the house, water in taps, ANC and PNC of pregnant women; immunization, all this has led to changes in women's health."

Women from village Buribana also expressed the same views, Kunti Bisht an active member of this village and the *Balwadi* teacher and CH worker of Chirag said, "The new generation has benefited greatly, they get supplementary iron tablets, have more health facilities and are better educated also. Because of the coming of electricity some work like grinding wheat at home has been replaced by electric mills, there is time to watch TV and get some information."

Women from Kafli (with a not so successful health programme) said, "only those in touch with CHIRAG have benefited, otherwise there is no change at all, women still suffer as they did except in some cases they fall ill less (like fevers, stomach problems, etc.)".

The women from the villages of Almori and Kwedal had a different story to share, a majority of them said, "Women face many problems, specially during pregnancy;......... there is no change, no facilities are available;......children are not immunized, no monitoring of pregnant women;.........we do not know, we are not aware of any changes". Only one woman said, "There have been some changes in women's awareness because of the presence of self-help groups".

Perhaps one cannot expect the women from these villages to say anything different, when they have no facilities. CHIRAG's community health programme really seems to have made a difference but they cannot go everywhere.

We have to rely on the government infrastructure, which needs to be made more accountable.

Traditional Health Care Practices – Indigenous Knowledge of Women – Promotive and Curative Aspects

(a) Bhagirathi Devi (CHW of village Kamola Sunkiya, Dhari Block), had a lot of wisdom and knowledge about healing and curing illness with locally available herbs and plants and cereals.

1. For cold and cough – basil leaves, piece of ginger, black pepper; this is boiled and lemon is added.
2. For stomach pain – vegetable prepared from nettles, 'bhichubuti'.
3. For stomach pain – make a paste of *gandhak*, put it on the navel of the child or adult. This can also be mixed with hing (aesophitida) for greater relief.

4. For fever – boil gahat and bhatt, two locally grown lentils and drink the water when it is hot.
5. For white discharge – Fry rice in pure ghee, boil in water and eat twice a day (this concoction helped Bhagirathi Devi herself in this condition in fact completely cured her).
6. There are many medicinal plants in this region if a child would swallow a small stone or a piece of wood or eat raw rice my mother-in-law would make a paste with a plant which grows near the river bed and give it to the child. In this way the swallowed object would pass out in the stool.
7. For cough – make a paste of the skin of *'darim'*, a type of pomegranate, and green turmeric and give a tea spoon to the child/adult. If a very young baby gets severe cough say on the day of the *'namkaran'*, 11th day, then green turmeric is boiled, made a paste of and while it is warm, applied on the head (*talu*), and some paste is put on the throat of the baby, the child will be totally cured.

When I asked Bhagirathi Devi how did people keep themselves healthy, she said by eating coarse grains (*mota khana kha kar*). They would eat grains like *mandua*, corn, jowar, *bhatt*, *gahat*. These were extremely nutritious and rich in protein and calcium. She said, "We would eat *gur* in the winter months, have pure *ghee* and cook all vegetables in an iron *karai* which would meet the iron requirements for the day. We always stored water in copper vessel as this water was brought from the natural springs located in the dense forest. Today a lot of the springs have got dried up because of extensive deforestation." When I asked her why copper vessels were used she could not give me the reason. But it was Kunti Bisht who said, "that all coliform bacteria present in the water get killed with copper. So drinking watered stored in copper vessels or filters is very good for preventing many water-borne diseases.".

Traditionally people had this wisdom and followed these practices at home, in fact during the rainy season they would boil the water and drink it.

Bhagirathi Devi said that health was linked to all aspects of living, the social situation at home, patterns of interaction all influence health. She said, "The mother-in-law is a woman and the daughter-in-law is also a woman, and therefore my mother-in-law did not discriminate against me in anyway, there was no tension between us and that made me healthy and happy. I too treat my daughter-in-law as a friend and help her with looking after the young children, the buffalo and cow, bringing water from the spring and sending the children to school."

Bhagirathi Devi is also involved with the Mahila Samakhya project in Dhari block. She said that in February this year, 2002, 150 women went in a procession to sit in a *dharna* at the DM's office in Nainital to protest against the presence of the liquor shops in Bhatelia. They reminded him that the chief minister had promised "an Uttaranchal free from the evil of liquor consumption." The women told him that if you want to give employment to people, why don't you open a factory of fruit jams, juices and jelly in Bhatelia; why does sit have to be a liquor shop? It is difficult for our daughters and daughter-in-laws to walk in this area, they said. Their protest was so genuine that the liquor shop was closed down at Bhatelia (however it has now shifted to Mukteshwar).

Bhagwati Devi's further sharing left me speechless, she said, "Educated women do not come together to protest for a cause, like women in the villages do for it effects their lives." How profound and true her words are, women in urban areas very rarely come together to protest for an issue, in fact the women of this region were largely responsible for the creation of this separate state of Uttaranchal. It is the urban-educated elite who have fragmented their lives into so many divisions that the interconnectedness is not visible to them. Our whole development process, initiatives and strategies are designed and directed towards providing services to people in the fragmented divisions.

Kishni Devi from Sargakhet village beautifully says, "*Swasthya aur Zindagi ek dusre se jure hain*" (Life and health are interconnected). Here, the word *zindagi*, encompasses one's whole life – physical, emotional, mental, and social. I wondered, how does this unlettered woman articulates the World Health Organization definition of health? The difference is perhaps that she lives the definition whereas we talk about it at meetings and seminars.

Interview with Radhika Devi – Village Kamola

From Bhagirathi Devi's house we walked through fields and orchards to the house of Radhika Devi who is also a member of the self-help group of this village which has been formed by *Chirag* for inter-loaning. According to Radhika Devi, there are many medicinal plants in this hill region which are used by the vaids to treat people.

One Vaid treated me for leucorrhoea with some medicinal plants. These grow abundantly in the oak forest where there is more water in the springs. The Kasturi found in the stomach of the Kasturi deer is also used for the treatment of several illnesses by the vaids in this region.

"Earlier people were very healthy", she said, "their digestive powers were strong. People stored water in copper vessels, cooked food in iron utensils and used only organic manure in their fields." The *mandua* that was grown in our fields which was highly nutritious and rich in calcium has been replaced by cash crops like cabbages, cauliflower and peas. The *Atta* that we get from the bazar in pre-packed polythene bags is not the same as the wheat flour ground in the *Panchakki*.

Radhika Devi's husband intervened and said, "Agriculture is the main occupation of the men in this region unlike Garhwal only 30 per cent of the men have migrated outside this region, as 70 per cent are farmers. ....earlier we never used *'sarkari khad'* (chemical fertilizers), we did organic farming and the production of cauliflower and cabbage as cash crops has only started from the last 7-8 years. In spite of this being predominantly an agriculture-based economy, there is no special focus on the farmer. We are completely dependent on nature. There is an organized *mandi samiti* meant for farmers, but the local farmer has no representation there and only *baniyas* handle the whole organization." Her husband's intervention in a way gave an insight into the patterns of traditional agriculture. Its linkage with health was already articulated by Radhika Devi herself.

Five women from neighbouring households gathered in Radhikabehn's house. They started discussing about the current programme of CHIRAG to vaccinate adolescent girls 12-19 years with the Rubella vaccine. The misconception floating in the village was that CHIRAG wants to reduce the population of the country that is why they are vaccinating young girls. Kunti (HEW) tried to dispel their fears regarding the above rumours. The women were eager to talk about themselves, they immediately included me in their inner space and said, "women's lives are so difficult, if a man had to bear the labour pain during child birth he would kill his wife with anger."

"Women undergo a lot of pain, the pain of ear-piercing, nose piercing, the pain of bearing a child, the trauma of being made to sit separately during menstruation, the pain of being considered impure, and if woman is considered to be manifestation of the divine goddess, then why all this suffering, pain!" said Pushpadevi from village Sunderkhal. She was wearing the traditional Kumaoni dress, a *lehnga*, men's shirt and a small waist coat. Her head was covered with a large *dupatta* and carried herself with a lot of dignity.

All this left me thinking deeply, and for a long time. Gender has now become integral to all discussions and programmes on development, yet do we have answers to their basic question.

Our whole model of interpreting the traditional wisdom of people and communities needs to be re-examined. We need to understand the health practices of women in the Kumaon Hills in a total context, rather than isolating them to arrive at inferences which relegates these practices as backward. The lived experiences of women related to their lifecycle events have to be viewed in the context of their world-view, and their integral relationship with the physical environment in which they live. For understanding the health practices of women one has to see their interconnectedness and inter-relatedness in a holistic manner – creating a rhythm and movement.

c. A women's initiative at the grassroots level was taken up in the Bhirapani area and in the Dhauladevi block by Adhar and Buniyad (community-based units of the NGO Sahayog). As a part of this initiative two workshops were held related to medicinal plants. Some elderly women from the community shared their knowledge regarding Dhatura oil which is tradionally used for back pain and joint pain. They also said that a powder made from *khaerwa* plant root and *dhol ka phool* was very good for the treatment of leucorrhoea, white discharge. On the second day of the workshop all the participants were demonstrated the entire processes of preparing the medicine and they actually prepared the same. At this workshop representatives from various women's groups were present, and the idea was that they would share this knowledge with other women in their community. On the last day of the workshop the women prepared a plan for the organization and management of this venture. Since the data has shown that most women suffer from back pain and white discharge the dissemination of these medicines would help in addressing a major health issue of the women of Kumaon.

As part of their management strategy women decided to use the money for the procurement of new materials for the medicine from the money they had collected in their SHG. At the same workshop they chalked out the guidelines to be used for the use of these two traditional medicines, e.g.,

- which patient should be given this medicine,
- how often, and
- how should the massage be done?

Women who were the carriers of this traditional knowledge demonstrated the correct method of the massage.

I. The constituents of the 'dhatura oil' are :

1. *Dhatura* root.
2. Mustard oil.
3. *Kacchi haldi*.

II. The constituents of the powder for the treatment of white discharge were

1. *Shatwari* root (*Kherwa* root).
2. Flower of *Dhaul*.

These are dried in the shade for six days and a powder is prepared, which when consumed three times a day with warm water is very effective in the treatment of Leucorrhoea.

One woman present at the workshop suggested that they would take these medicines when they travelled to their natal village and share this knowledge with their sisters. Initiatives and efforts like the above would go a long way in linking traditional knowledge and contemporary health needs of women.

By providing adolescent girls with knowledge about health care, stressing the importance of preventive care while integrating and encouraging indigenous knowledge, CHIRAG will stimulate greater empowerment for the women of Kumaon. During a meeting of local health workers and trained *Dais*, one woman described her definition of health to be having a disciplined and balanced life in harmony with the cycle of life. Many women expressed the desire to have their daughters educated about preventive health care, but also about major life events such as preparation for marriage and children. For this reason, it was envisaged that educating adolescent girls about health care will prompt discussions about the self in relation to her society and environment as aspects of good health, continuing to encourage the women of Kumaon to move beyond medical dependence to empowerment.

SECTION-9

TRADITIONAL HEALTH CARE PRACTICES

In traditional cultures, local health traditions have existed for centuries and have been catering to the requirements of people. The following section discusses some of the health care practises which are existing in the area of study.

Women as Keepers of Health and Healthcare Providers

Traditional health care systems are still alive in the watershed region, as women continue to practise their 'healing' knowledge and skills. These indigenous health practices have evolved out of people's needs and are closely interwoven with the day to day life of the villagers. These are not documented anywhere but are handed down to the generations orally, mostly through women, and hence are preserved.

Since women are the treasure houses of this knowledge, compared to the specialised knowledge possessed by 'Vaidyas', it is more frequently and regularly used. Most healers, recommend herbs for cure, a few women also specialize in the task of healing like men. At the household level, right from feeding the family to looking after the sick, it is the duty of women to take care of health. These indigenous health traditions besides taking care of common ailments, may also promote health practices at the promotive and preventive levels. Vaidyas are largely the guardians of the curative aspect of this ancient wisdom.

To emphasize, traditional health care systems, governed by food items as well as medicinal plants are still very prevalent in the watershed region. Besides Vaidyas, who commonly treat adult and children's ailments, the animal or *'pashu'* Vaidyas are also tremendously popularly in the area. Interestingly, in many of the villages in the Almora district holders of this specialised knowledge happen to be women. Though women are undoubtedly very knowledgeable and skilled in local health traditions, they do not value their expertise. This devaluation, has resulted in the erosion of the wealth of knowledge and has made an impact on the faith of people in traditional knowledge.

Changes

In recent times, the prestige and role of 'vaidyas' in communities of the area has suffered a lot and is increasingly becoming weaker because of various factors. With traditions crumbling all around us, these age old practices have also come under the threat of extinction, specially in the wake of increasing popularity of Western health care systems. Many 'allopathic' centres have come up in this region too. Western medicine, which provides immediate relief to the patient, has had an adverse impact on the popularity of the traditional system of medicine.

The profession is not highly popular amongst the new generation. Ever since the clearance of the medical examination, held by the Board of Indian Medicine, Lucknow, became an essential prerequisite for registration and thereafter medicinal practice, people feel discouraged to adopt the traditional knowledge systems. There are still quite a few people who practise it but they do it surreptiously, due to the fear of being caught. The formality of registration existed in the past too but the procedure was much simpler. Unlike today, a written recommendation, forwarded by 10-15 Gram Pradhans of the respective area in favour of the practitioner, was considered sufficient for initiating practice.

Another important factor behind the lack of interest of the new generation towards the tradition of their fathers and forefathers is the fact that, it does not provide enough income for a decent livelihood. Earlier also people used to refrain from asking for anything in return of their services/knowledge. They still do so as it is popularly believed that even the desire of anything in return of these services adversely affects the potency of the treatment and the knowledge. Therefore they accept whatever is offered to them in return for cash or kind. There are many people in the area, who are skilled in the art but do not practise it. Nandballabh is a well known Vaid in Almora district. So, to a great extent, it is the faith in the practitioners and not in the system, which has been eroded. This has in turn proved detrimental to people's pride for all traditional knowledge.

Earlier cash was strictly avoided as a medium of payment for services. Exchange was essentially done in kind, as ghee, grain, lentils, vegetables, clothes and sometimes animals too. Like other sectors (crafts, agriculture), here also cash has made its inroads into the system. Now-a-days, the services are mostly offered in exchange of money, and the quantum of services exchanged for kind has gone down substantially. Though people who have survived with their indigenous health knowledge still have strong faith in the traditional techniques of health care, the presence of very few knowledgeable practitioners around has forced them to turn towards modern medicine.

In order to overcome this, it is important to document the knowledge and preserve it as a legacy for the future generation, especially the 'promotive' and 'preventive' aspects of local health traditions.

The community normally resorts to various herbal treatments to cure ailments and diseases. Women, particularly the aged ones, know what and how to use for health promotion and disease prevention. Some of the diseases which were more prevalent in the yesteryears are as follows (local terms) : *Bai prasut* (complex set of symtoms relating to coldness), *Sansari* (fever with seizure), *Chaupara* (breathing difficulty) (locally called *'happa tappa'*), *Bukhar* (fever), *Piliya* (jaundice) and *Dadura* (measles) etc. Now Piliya, Pneumonia and Typhoid (these are also locally used terms and may bear no resemblence to the medical entity) occur more commonly and frequently.

Surprisingly a dearth of herbs or medicinal plants has not been an important reason behind the erosion of this system. A great number of these plants are growing in abundance in the forests, (mostly in *van* panchayats and occasionally in reserved and civil also), in fields, on the banks of river and within and outside the village. Nevertheless there are certain herbs which are much sought after. They are being sold to famous companies like Dabur. Some of them are roots of Hisalu, Kilmura, Hiva and Silver. Therefore, these plants are disappearing very fast and in the circumstances it becomes imperative to explore the possibilities to nurture and restore them. Besides, tapping the local sources, it is a common practice to buy some of the herbs from the market as well. Even earlier they were available in the open market of Almora.

Impact

The indigenous methods are claimed to be highly effective in keeping good health as well as in curing common ailments. The traditional knowledge regarding the preparation and usage of different herbs, despite being rich and invaluable has started diminishing, as fewer and fewer people are willing to take it up as their main profession. This has, unknowingly, affected the quality and richness of the knowledge and expertise. These methods have an edge health-wise over other systems of medicine. They are also easily affordable and are within the reach of the poor.

Healthcare Practices

Food and Promotive Health Care

Some of the popular practices prevalent in the area to maintain good health are associated with food habits. Like traditional knowledge in other sectors, in the field of indigenous health traditions too, women are the main carriers of this knowledge system. The health practices vary with different seasons.

Winter foods

- Gahat and Bhatt (traditional black legumes) are considered to be the hottest of all the legumes. These are eaten in winters.
- A very popular and spicy preparation of Gahat is called 'Thithani'. The legumes are boiled and then cooked with Asfoetida (*heeng*), cloves (*long*), chilly, ginger and salt.
- Ginger, Black pepper (also common to many other preparations) and cloves are ground and added to tea. This concoction helps in keeping the body warm, and also provides relief in cold and cough.
- *Bicchu ghas* (nettle) is believed to be particularly very effective in keeping the body warm during the winters. Normally not eaten very often these days, it was popular as a vegetable earlier. It is prepared after being chopped and boiled, lots of spices such as chillies, cloves, cardamom and asfoetida, etc. are added very liberally, along with a good amount of oil. It is prepared only after the rains in the winters and is more popular these days amongst the poor families. *Bicchu* plant is of two types : one with

and the other with fewer spikes. People prefer the one with more spikes, as it is supposed to be richer in vitamins. This preparation is also very popular in the Garhwal hills.

- *Methi* (Fenugreek seed) *laddu* is a very popular seasonal preparation. These days it is even available in the shops. It helps in keeping warm during the cold winter season. The seeds of this vegetable are fried, ground and after adding jaggery to it, the mixture is compressed into balls (*laddus*).
- Earlier instead of tea leaves, 'Banar' (cassia species) fruits, which is available in the wild, were added to boiling water and taken as tea.
- Its pods are plucked off when ripe, and the seeds are scooped out and roasted. They are then ground and added to the boiling water just like tea leaves. This practice does not exist anymore, because not only has tea become common but this preparation requires a lot of labor. Earlier *dalchini* (cinnamon) was also added to tea commonly.
- *Mandua* grain (a coarse millet) is considered extremely heating and nutritious. Its *rotis* with dollops of ghee are eaten in winters to keep the body warm and is a great source of energy. In earlier days when the *roti* was eaten by women during their forest and field trips, it kept them healthy and full of energy. It is also very high in calcium content, so that with its intake people seldom faced tooth problems. Today *Mandua chapattis* are mixed with wheat and given to pregnant women because of its high nutritive value.
- *Jaggery* is still popularly eaten after meals in this season. *Jaggery* tea, till today is preferred to ordinary sugar tea.
- Intake of *ghee* and milk was definitely much higher earlier in comparison to the present times. This helped in keeping good health and in improving body resistance.
- *Beru* (local fig) fruits when unripe and raw were popularly eaten as a vegetable, earlier, and the preparation involved the usual boiling and then addition of spices.
- *Chua* (amaranth) is also a traditional grain and its preparations are very fondly eaten in winters as it is considered heating. Seeds are roasted, followed by addition of *ghee*, water and sugar to taste. The preparation is popularly called *'chua halwa'*. (It is a popular dish of families in Maichun, Kharkoli and Balia (Almora district) as it grows in good amount here as compared to other places in the watershed.

- A nutritious preparation eaten during the winter months are *chappatis* of a mixed dough of *maans* (*urad dal*), soybean, *madira* (coarse millet) and *gahat*, which was popular in years gone by. The grains are soaked overnight and then crushed to fine paste. They are then mixed with *Mandua* flour and kneaded. Salt and red chilli powder are also added to the mixture and made into bread.
- A commonly eaten vegetable in the past was *Varmala* (*gethi*). People in remote areas of Almora district used to prepare it very often. It is a wildly grown grass which is found mostly in the *gadheras*. After being boiled, salt and chilly are added to taste. It is prepared in *ghee*.
- Palak continues to be a very important vegetable consumed during winter months. It is boiled for sometime in water then salt, chilly powder and other spices are added to it and the mixture is finally added to *Mandua* flour. This preparation is called *'dhapran'*. It is also considered to have a lot of heating effect.
- *Palak* (spinach) and *Mandua* flour are mixed to prepare another dish called *'kaba'*.
- *Madira* (coarse millet), *bhat, gahat dal,* and *gahat 'dubka'* are also eaten in winters. *Madira halwa* is commonly made also.
- Earlier 'tair' was also a very popular vegetable. It grew profusely near the homesteads and in the forests. The fruits are first boiled and then fried in oil, after removing the skin. Finally spices are added to the vegetable. It has been replace by potatoes now.
- Boiled pumpkin is still commonly eaten in the villages.
- *'Koni jyola'* is still eaten in far off villages in the remote areas of Kumoan hills. From here Koni was taken by people of the nearby villages, specially when somebody suffered with measles. This was taken in exchange of *manduwa, madira* and other traditional pulses. Koni is a millet and grows profusely in *Maichun* (Almora district) too. To prepare *jyola,* the grains are boiled either in buttermilk (if available in good amount, specially in economically well off families) or in water (more often in poor families) and then cooked in small amount of buttermilk. Finally, salt is added to the taste.
- Cannabis (*bhang*) seeds are added in vegetables particularly in *pinalu, arabi* and *jholi* (yoghurt) curry etc. It provides warmth as well taste and flavour to the preparation.

Summer food

- In summers buttermilk and curd are taken in large amounts as they are supposed to help in keeping the body cool and the stomach well.
- *Pudina* (mint) leaves are ground with salt, onion and green chillies to form a fine paste. This preparation is commonly called *'pudina chatni'*. It also gives relief in vomitings and diarrhoea.
- Rice *jyola* is a very popular preparation, wherein rice is boiled and then buttermilk or curd is added to it.
- Buttermilk and sour curd is added to wheat flour or gram flour and cooked till it becomes a viscous paste. The preparation is known as *'jholi'* locally. It is eaten mostly with rice.
- Cucumber is eaten raw in this season, in a good amount. It is usually eaten with 'cannabis *chatni*'. It quenches thirst as it contains water. *Raita* of finely grated cucumber with seasoning of *rai* seeds, keeping the body well hyderated in the hot season.
- A plant which was commonly used as a vegetable in summers is *'ugal'*. It was prepared by boiling water, followed by adding spices and *madira* to it. This preparation was popularly called *'rabra'*.
- Timil (a kind of fig) fruits also constituted an important vegetable consumed in this region many decades ago.
- Wildly growing grass called *'saujal'* and *'chormani'* were used as vegetable . They were boiled and eaten after adding spices.
- Cannabis *chutney* or *'bhang khate'* is a very famous preparation of the summers. Roasted cannabis seeds are ground with salt and chillies and then freshly squeezed lime/jamir juice is added, until the mixture becomes soft like sauce.

Rainy Season

- The young leaves of *Bethuwa* (A green leafy vegetable) plant are considered extremely rich in vitamins and were popularly used as vegetable. It is not in much use these days.
- Small fruits of *'beru'* plant are used in preparing vegetables, but this practice is also not as much prevalent as it was before.
- The young tender leaves of *'lingura'* (wild fern) plant make a very tasty preparation in this season. But again it is not as popular as it was in the past. *Lingura* and soybean (prepared separately) *jyola* are also eaten in summers.

- *Madira jyola* is also a much liked preparation in the area. It is prepared in the same way as rice *jyola*. Grains are boiled and then curd or buttermilk are added to the boiling mixture.
- People also used to eat potato leaves as vegetable, during the rainy season.

Food and Preventive Healthcare

Certain food items are normally avoided in winters because they produce cooling effect. The popular ones are *maans* lentils, *dubke* of *maans*, *bhatt* and *riyans*. *Bhat* is not eaten at night in the cold weather. Not much caution is needed in this season with regards to the diet, as digestion doesn't pose much problem.

In summer strict prohibition is to be observed to maintain good digestion. Egg and meat being hot are generally avoided. Likewise, *'gahat'* (black legume) is strictly avoided for the same reason. It is believed that its consumption can even induce nose bleeding. *Urad* pulses are also not preferred in this season as it is difficult to digest, and proper digestion also requires a fair intake of water. Also, *bicchu* grass (nettles), *gur* and food kept overnight are also avoided during summers.

Food items which are considered to be hot, are not recommended to the person suffering with red eyes.

Curative Practices

Winter

- When people suffer with throat pain, then the popular household remedy is to heat the salt slightly and wrap it around the throat to give relief in the pain.
- *Mandua* flour mixed properly in hot water and *jaggery* (coarse brown sugar commonly known as *'gur'*) is considered a very effective remedy in cold and cough. This preparation is locally known as *'bara'*.
- Gravy of fish curry is believed to be a good remedy for cold and coughs.
- Oil seeds, which were expressed at home earlier, are now taken to expressing machines installed at Barechina (Almora district). These are then used as a massage oil to relieve muscular pains and coughs specially in children.

- Wood ash is also very effective in coughs, specially for children. It is rubbed on their chest to give them relief.
- *Mandua halwa* is a highly potent preparation to treat cold, specially when jaggery is added to it.
- Warm water to which *Methi* (Fenugreek) seeds and ginger have been added, provide relief and effective cure to throat pain.
- *Gahat* legumes as mentioned earlier are considered to be hottest of all the pulses. People suffering with cold are generally given this dal.
- Banar (thyme) tea was preferred earlier by people suffering with cold.
- Juice of *Jamir* fruit helps in stopping vomitting.
- Juice extracted from *hisalu* leaves is very helpful in stopping vomittings and diarrhoea.
- Pine resin is applied on cuts and wounds as it helps to heal them.

Summer

- *Pudina chatni* helps in arresting vomittings, as well as in stopping diarrhoea. *Pudina* juice is also an effective remedy in this problem.
- *Jyola* is given to people suffering with diarrhoea and vomittings, and also for controlling fevers.
- It is believed that, *pinalu* (Coloccacia – *arabi*) leaves dipped in water if used to sprinkle water on doors and on the face of the patients, helps those suffering with malaria.
- Juice of *kirmaula* bark if dropped in the infected eye, helps in controlling infection.

Rainy season

- Radish leaves when tender, make a highly potent medicine for jaundice. 'Dubke' of black bhatt are equally effective in this disease.

General

- *Gahat* lentils are very effective in treating kidney stone problems. It is believed to exude heat, sufficient to melt stones.

- *Mandua rotis* are recommended to women after the delivery, as they are highly nutritious and energy giving.
- Turmeric paste is applied on the injured portion of the foot. Turmeric or *haldi*, is being used for a long time as an antiseptic on wounds. It is also boiled with milk to relieve throat irritation and for improving resistance against germs and diseases.
- Raw garlic is also very effective in stopping vomitting and in providing relief in gastric problems. For gastric trouble, one piece of garlic is given on the first day, followed by two on the second, three on the third and so on until the fortieth day . Then the reduction starts from the forty-first day with thirty-nine pods, thirty eight on forty-second day and so on till it comes back to one.
- For soft tissue injury Cannabis seeds are roasted in an iron utensil. Sand, turmeric powder and wood ash are added to it and it is turned into a paste. A knot of this paste is tied around the hurt portion.

The information given above in this section was shared by Reetu Sogani from Aadhar who has been documenting the traditional knowledge of women regarding these aspects.

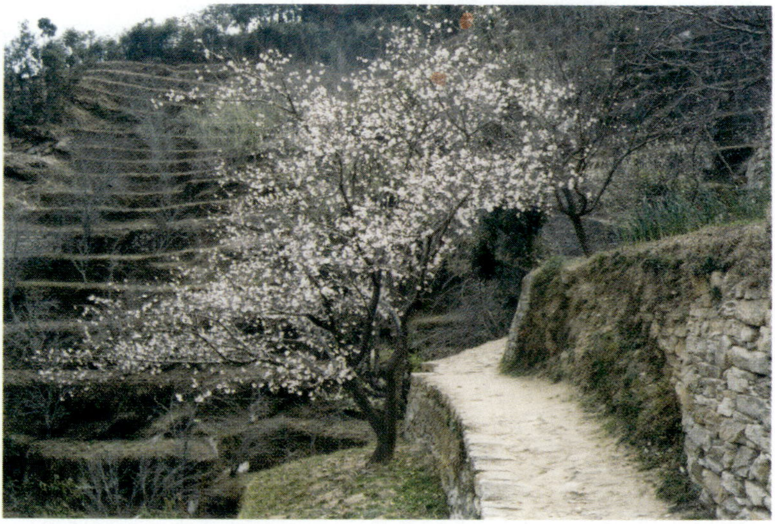

Plate 1 : Terraced hill-sides and orchards —A Village in Nainital District

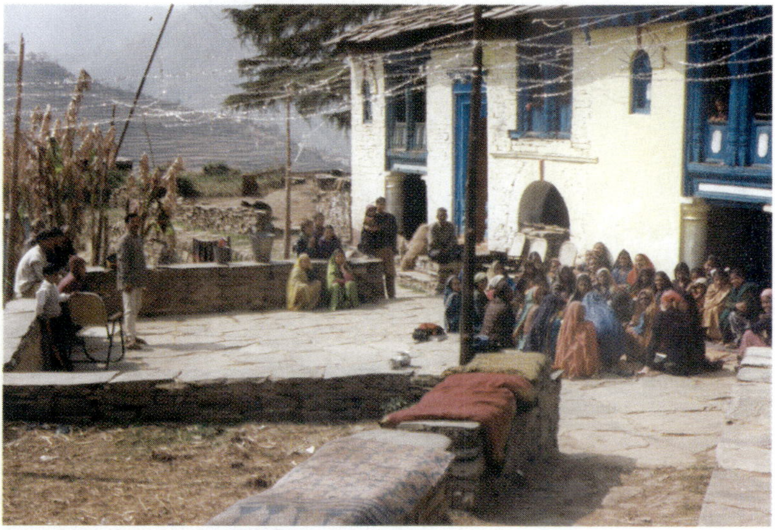

Plate 2 : A traditional Kumaoni house courtyard village Supitalla

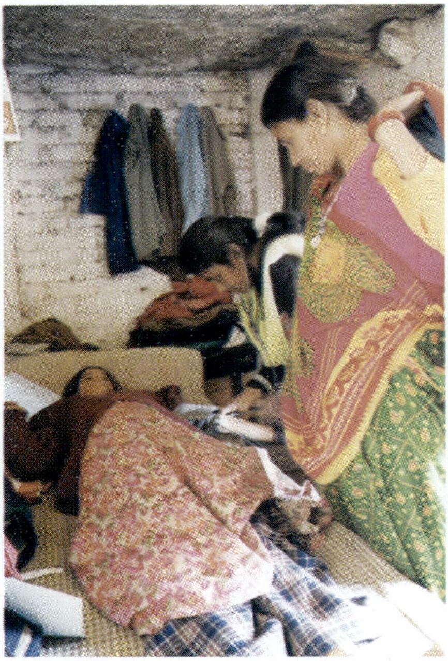

Plate 3 : Ante-natal check-up with community health worker Ganga, Village Supitalla

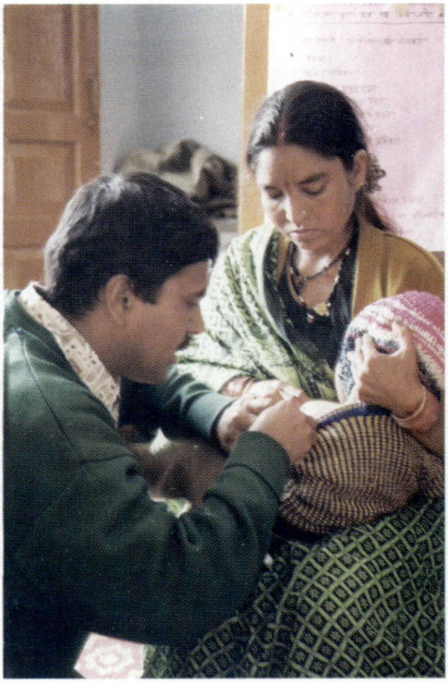

Plate 4 : Gangu, Development Assistant Health team CHIRAG— Giving BCG injections at an Immunization Camp in Kasialekh (Dhari Block)

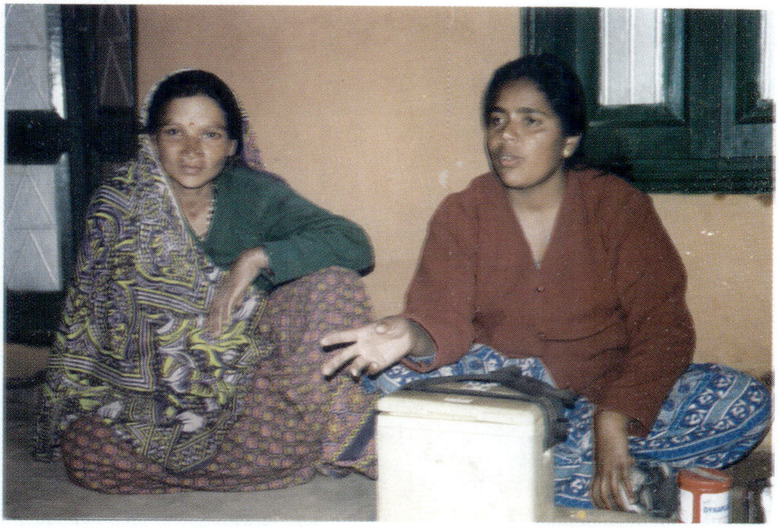

Plate 5 : Neomi, Health Extension Worker—CHIRAG talking to an anaemic woman in village Pokhrar (Dhari Block).

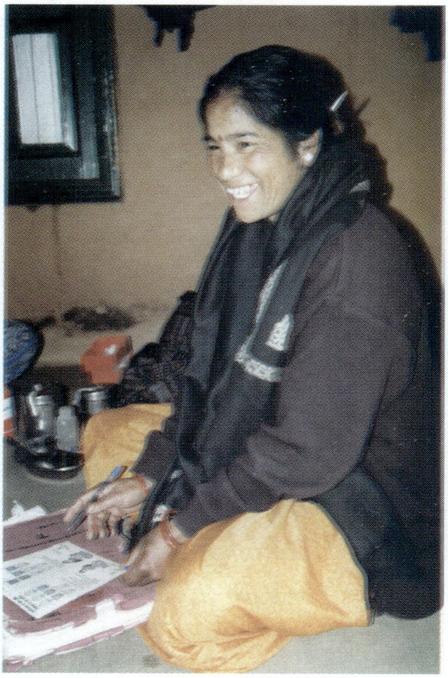

Plate 6 : Kunti, Health Extension Worker—CHIRAG growth monitoring records (0-5 years) village Pokhrar (Dhari Block)

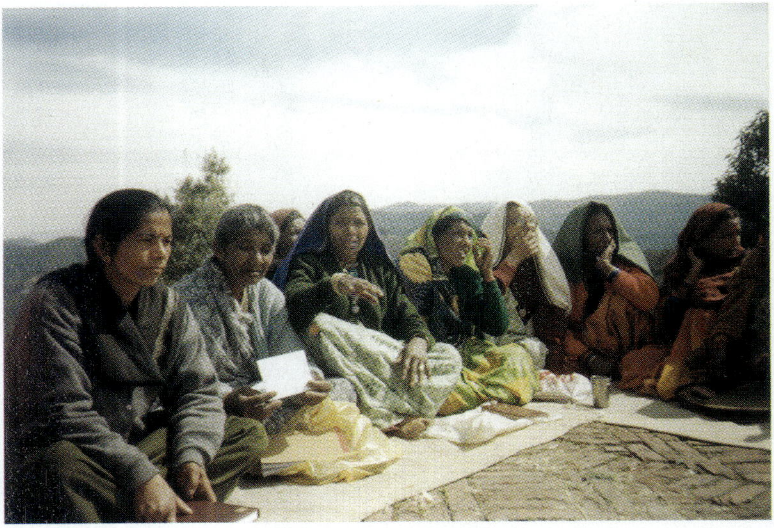

Plate 7 : Community Health Workers and *Dais* at monthly meeting Sargakhet Clinic

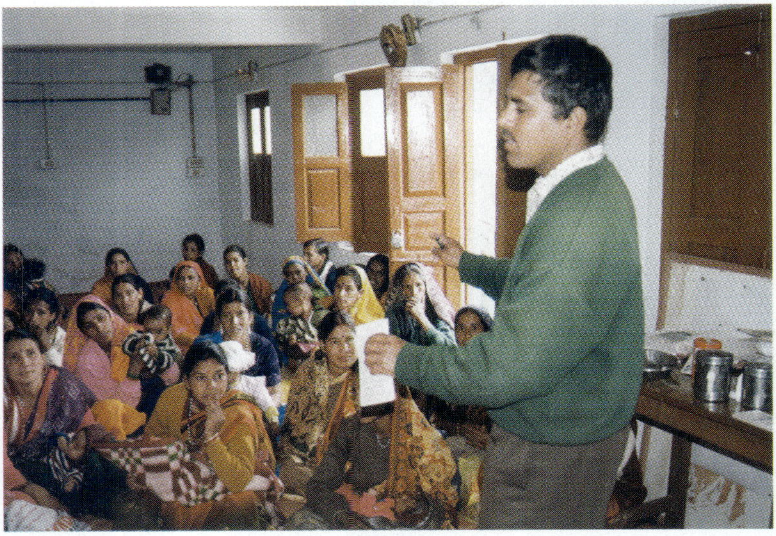

Plate 8 : Gangu giving a talk on 'nutrition education' to village women—Kasialekh

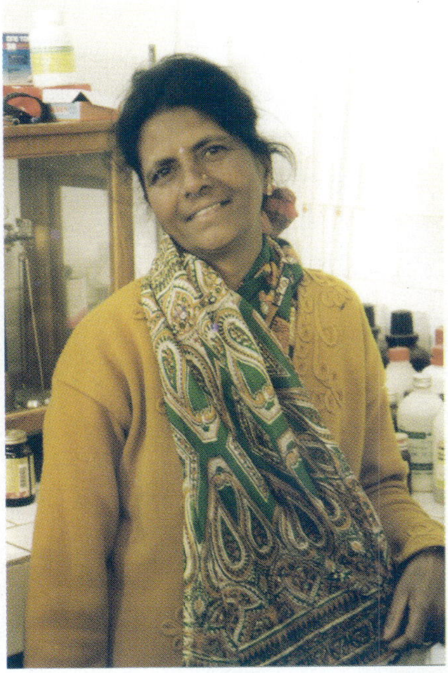

Plate 9 : Zarina —The trained *Dai* of CHIRAG at Sargakhet

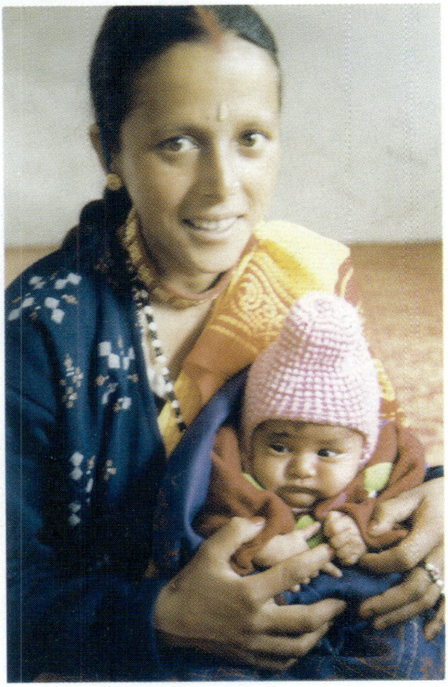

Plate 10 : A young Kumaoni Woman with her child at Kasialekh for an immunization camp

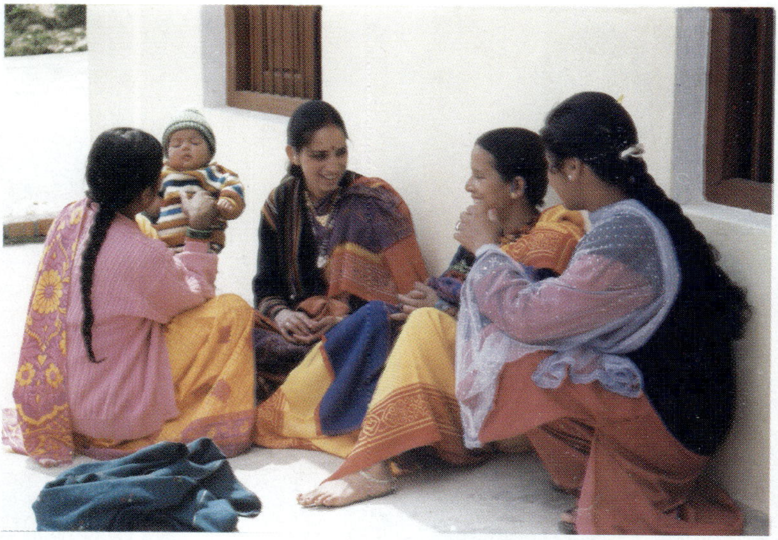

Plate 11 : Colourfully dressed Kumaoni Women with their children at an immunization camp at Kasialekh

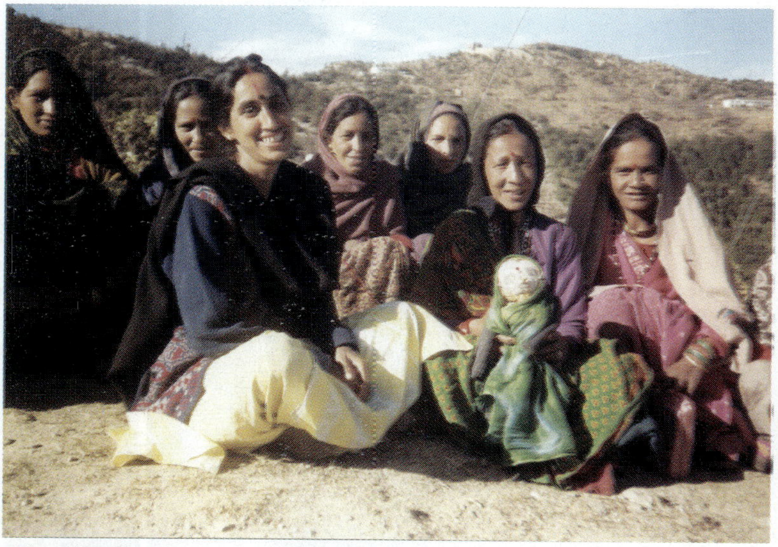

Plate 12 : Lata Harbola—CHIRAG, with a Self-Help Group (Dhari Block)

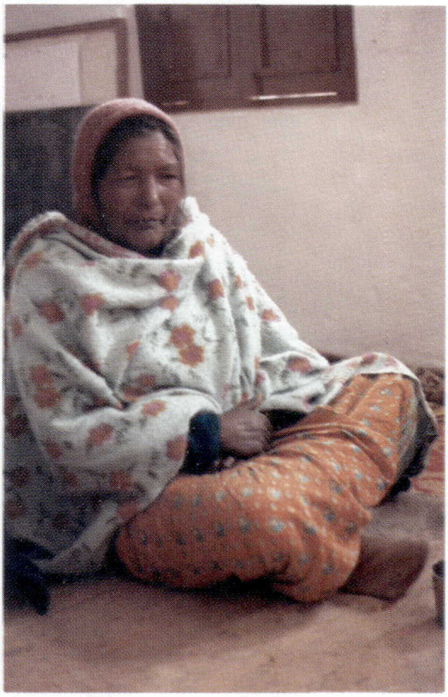

Plate 13 : Bachuli Devi —The *Dai* of village Navin Sunkhiya

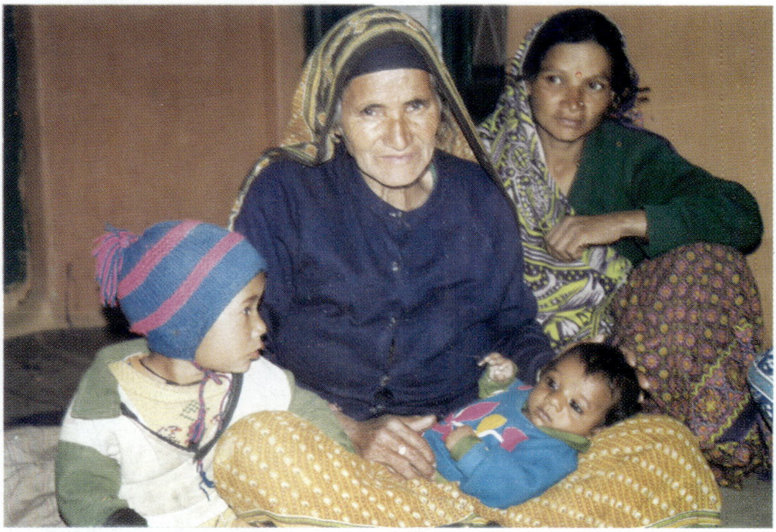

Plate 14 : Beena Devi—CHW and *Dai* of village Pokhrar with her grand-children.

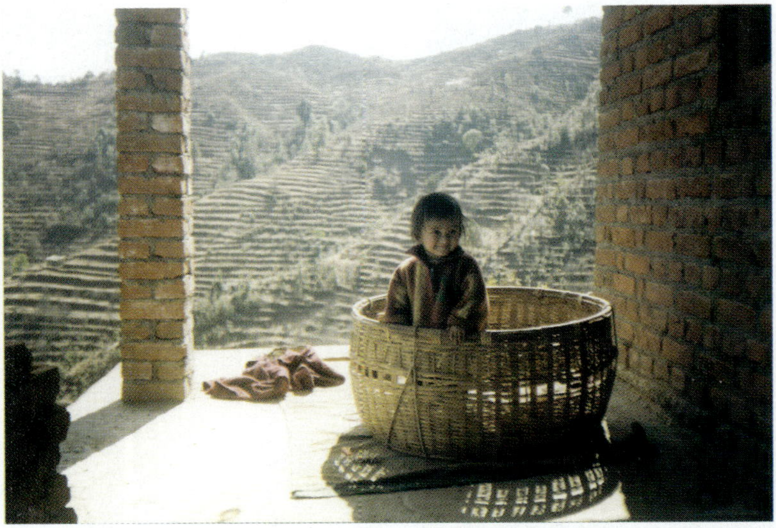

Plate 15 : A three year old Kumaoni child in basket—village Sunderkhal. (Dhari Block).

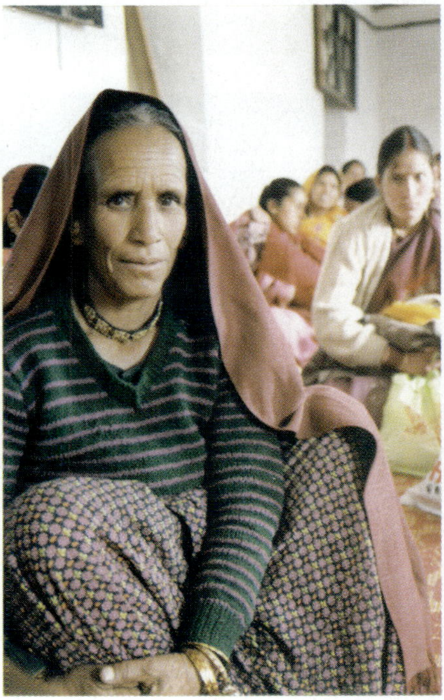

Plate 16 : Bhagirathi Devi—The Community Health Worker of village Kamola Sunkhiya (Dhari Block).

5

EMERGING TRENDS
A Holistic Perspective

While the quantitative and qualitative data, the various interviews and women's voices and experiences have been discussed in great depth in the preceding chapters some emerging trends and insights are viewed in a holistic manner and contextualized in this chapter, as follows :

1. Traditional Systems.
2. Traditional Practices.
3. Gender.
4. Male Participation.
5. Sustainability of Health Care Interventions and Initiatives.

    (a) Government
    (b) NGOs.
    (c) Traditional Health Service Providers.

Some Issues related to Community Health Programmes.

What Next ?

    (a) Salient Findings.
    (b) Some Recommendations.

Traditional Systems

Traditionally, living in the villages in Kumaon, including today in inaccessible areas, is characterized by a community oriented approach (sahbagita). This way of life not only reduced the hardships of women in terms of the management of human resources and natural resources, but this act of sharing also has a great bearing on the emotional well being of the community.

The earlier chapters have highlighted the theoretical-conceptual framework of health, being a function of a whole way of life, wherein the

Health ↔ culture ↔ environment ↔ work roles, inter-connectedness and linkages could be seen.

In remote areas, even today, the 'palta system' is operative in the community. In this system women go together to collect grass for each other's family. This enables the family to have access to grass in the winter months during which the availability is greatly reduced. Women who did not have help at home were benefited by this; and they said, *'mil jul kar kam karna chahiye'*, i.e., let us work together in a joyous manner.

During the sowing of rice or at the time of weeding of the *'mandua'* grain in the field a traditional group of singers called *'Hurkiyas'* came and performed in the fields. This was called *'bol lagana'*, by calling out or by singing it out. In this manner, during the winter months, the whole community participated irrespective of caste, class, age and gender. During these occasions women experienced a great sense of relaxation. The songs were often about old stories depicting acts of bravery, or were linked to the social problems of the community. This gave women an opportunity to express the creativity inherent in them. All this would fill them with enthusiasm and energy and also take off their mind from the hard task at hand.

Music played a very important role in the well being of the people. When women went to the 'gharat' the community water mill to grind the grain, they would sing together and then cook, eat and enjoy all night, near the river. This provided them an occasion to relax and share their concerns. (Capila: 2002)

Concept of Health

The integration and interconnectedness of health as a way of life emerged from the women's perception of 'good health', with Kishni Devi's sharing *"zindagi aur swasthya jure hue hain"*, i.e. health and life are linked, or are one and the same thing, not separate. She put the understanding of this issue into a clear holistic perspective. However, when we look at health as a sector development, it is just providing services and curing the disease which is the focus.

Environmental Factors

Another important resource which is linked to women's health is water.

Water ⟵⟶ Women's health.

There are two important aspects here of water, one is the availability and the other is the quality of water. Earlier water was fetched from natural sources, called *'naulas'*. The community managed the *naulas*, they maintained the cleanliness, keeping animals away. These were community resource management systems related to the effective use of water. Traditionally, 'naulas' were considered sacred. After marriage, for example, the bride and groom would go to the '*naula*' before going to the house and wash each other's face with the sacred water. In recent times pipelines have been introduced which have brought water to the door step of the house, unfortunately this process has isolated women from one another. In the mean time the '*naulas*' have also been neglected and when water is depleted in the '*naulas*' women go to the '*ghadera*' which is the deep gorge located at the base of the valley. This has increased the work load of women and it has effected their health adversely. Also related to water availability are the reproductive tract infections that women suffer from, because they do not have enough water to clean themselves.

In most societies, women are traditionally responsible for managing water resources. Experience shows that modernization often forces them out of their field of responsibility. It is thus all the more important to involve women actively in the planning and implementation of water projects. Special efforts must be made, since participatory methods do not automatically ensure that the interests of women are represented. Women should not only be seen as water users in the household sector, their role as producers must be taken into account.

Other aspects of community participation which affected the health of women were, for example, when a child was born in a family, if for some reason the woman was unable to breast-feed the baby, she would never know from where the cow's milk to feed the child was coming, it could be from a neighbour's house or any other household in the village. There was a great sense of sharing which produced a feeling of well being. The housing structures also contributed to this aspect. In the *'bakli'* system the houses of four brothers were in a row, and the women of the four households supported each other in the work roles as well as in taking care of the children, which reduced the pressure on the individual woman. This system has now broken down to individual houses on the hill side represented by the *'bagicha'* system. (Fig. 5.1).

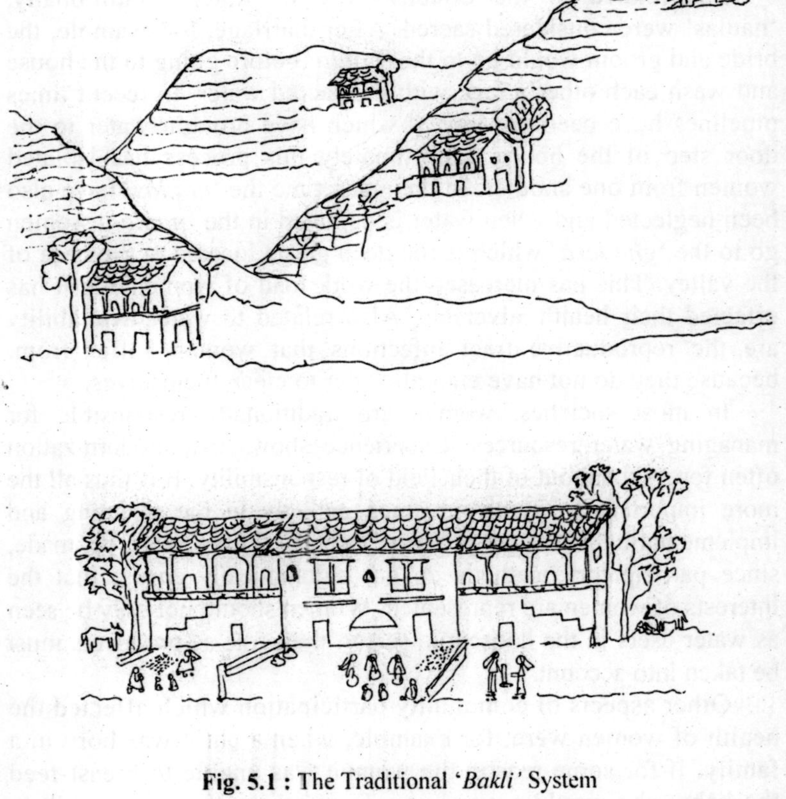

Fig. 5.1 : The Traditional '*Bakli*' System

Another aspect of traditional agriculture which indirectly has a bearing on women's health is that grass for animal feed was available from traditional grains like *'mandua'* and *'madira'* which was very beneficial for the animal's health. When vegetables like peas and cabbage are grown one does not get any grass for animal feed and women have to work harder to procure it, as the animals are crucial to their sustenance in the hill region.

Food Consumption Patterns and Globalization

The chemical composition of grains like *mandua* and *madira* shows that these varieties are extremely rich in calcium, protein and minerals. Lentils like *'gahat'* (which incidently also helps in dissolving kidney stones) *bhatt*, soybean, *rajmah*, are also a rich source of protein. As discussed in the section on concept of health, the consumption of these has been greatly reduced effecting the nutritional status of the women who are buying ground wheat (*atta*) or fine grain from a central ration shop. The woman who is the holder or practitioner of knowledge related to all aspects of traditional agriculture, today finds her knowledge or *jankari*, sidelined or considered quite useless and this has affected her self-esteem and indirectly her health.

Globalization → Traditional agriculture → Women's self-esteem → Health.

Earlier on, it seems, women were the originators of traditional knowledge and had great confidence in their knowledge system which they utilized for their livelihood.

Traditional Practices

The shift from traditional agriculture to the market economy has reduced women's confidence in their own knowledge system not because they do not value it or do not know the usefulness of that practice, but because of other influences like globalization, consumerism and the market economy forces which have to be taken into account. Even school curriculum does not give value to this knowledge, instead it imposes a pre-determined colonial framework on the people.

The Fourth World Conference on Women held in Beijing in 1995 stressed the gender approach as a crosscutting task affecting every policy field. The chapter on "Women and the Environment" of the Beijing Declaration and Platform for Action point to the extreme disequilibrium between the rights and responsibilities of women. Some specific issues raised were :

- Women should be involved in environmentally-relevant planning and decision-making processes.
- Traditional knowledge and female skills in the sustainable use of biological diversity should be preserved.
- The rights of women to the natural resources they manage and their powers of disposal over such resources should be recognized.
- National strategies and legal standards should be elaborated to protect women's rights and give them a share of the benefits arising out of the utilization of biological diversity.

For a long time "farmers" were in general defined as male. This approach overlooks the work of women, women's knowledge and role in agriculture and environmental protection. The UN Convention on Biological Diversity (CBD) highlights the special role of women in the conservation and sustainable utilization of biological diversity, because the experience and practices of women, in their capacity as managers of natural resources and holders of knowledge, differ as a rule from that of men.

Today as interviews with women and other resource persons have revealed, the forces of market economy and cash crop agriculture have reduced community participation. "We would rather spend four hours extra on our field and earn more money than spend time on a neighbour's field," said a farmer in village Simayal, Ramgarh block.

A study conducted in Almora district by the field staff of the NGO Sahyog, looked at some other aspects of the decision-making process. In the area of agriculture, they found through PRA techniques that men were the handlers of all the processes of the 'cash crop economy'. They decided on what crops to grow, in which field they are to be grown, how to sow the seed, the spacing, amount of water to be given, how the cash was to be spent, which animal to buy or sell and women were reduced to unskilled labourers in their own field. The decisions women made related to bangles, bindis, gift items for a wedding, or some utensils for household use.

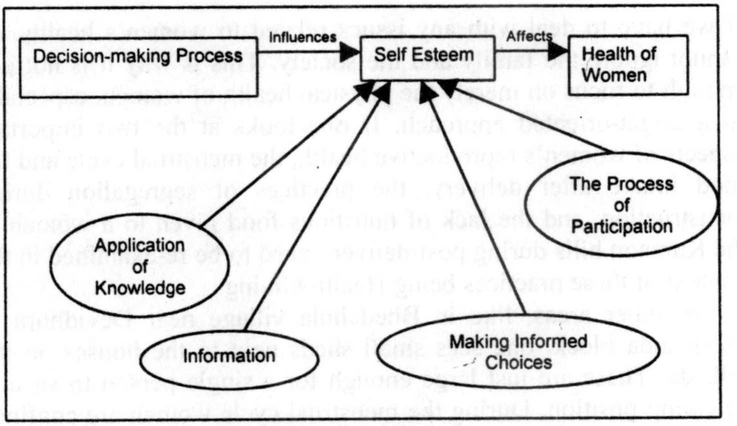

Fig. 5.2 : Decision-making Process

The manner of utilizing the knowledge that women have in the context of the socio-cultural environment and the needs of the community is of great significance to their health and well-being. We need therefore to give value to women's knowledge and develop a system of integration of the traditional and new forms of agriculture so that the correct balance is achieved.

Women's Health – The Family and Society

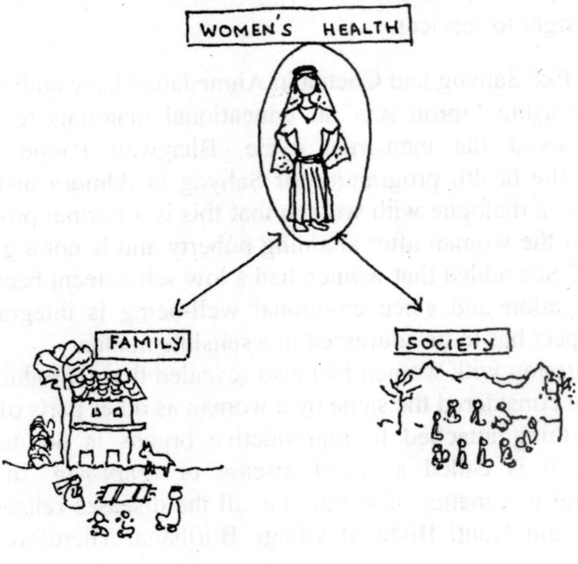

Fig. 5.3 : Women's Health —The Family and Society

If we have to deal with any issues related to women's health, we cannot ignore the family and the society. This is why it is not just enough to focus on merely the physical health of women, especially as a target-oriented approach. If one looks at the two important aspects of women's reproductive health, the menstrual cycle and the food intake after delivery, the practices of segregation during menstruation, and the lack of nutritious food given to a woman in the Kumaon hills during post-delivery need to be re-examined in the context of these practices being Health-Giving.

In other areas, like in Bhedchula village near Devidhura in Okalkanda block, one sees small sheds next to the houses on the hillside. These are just large enough for a single person to sit in a squatting position. During the menstrual cycle women are confined to these sheds for 3-5 days. At a meeting in this village some of the women expressed that "we start hating our own body; we are impure and because we do not have access to water, for which we have to walk for miles to the *'ghadera'* deep down in the gorge, we cannot keep ourselves clean.

Even though I did not see the same practice in the villages in the Dhari and the Ramgarh block, the above sharing raised some important issues about reproductive right of women.

- The right to information.
- The right to cleanliness.
- The right to services.

Some NGOs like Sahyog and Chetna in Ahmedabad have addressed this issue by using 'apron sets' as educational materials to give information about the menstrual cycle. Bhagwati Pande who worked with the health programme of Sahyog in Almora district, said, "we have a dialogue with women that this is a normal process in the body of the woman after attaining puberty and is not a god's gift or curse." She added that women had a low self-esteem because of this segregation and since emotional well-being is integral to health this aspect has to be addressed in a sensible manner.

The discussion with women had also revealed that reproductive organs are not considered the same by a woman as other parts of her body. "Everything attached to reproductive organs is not to be talked about, it is called a secret disease or *'gupt-rog'* in the vernacular, and is a matter of shame, i.e. all the diseases related to these parts", said Kunti Bisht of village Buribana. Therefore the terminology and language has a great impact on the way something is perceived by the people.

Towards this end, i.e. linking women's health to family and society, a "reproductive health *shivir* (meeting)" was held at the Dhaula Devi block PHC in Almora district where about 100 women from various villages in the age group of 20-60, and 50 men had gathered to have a dialogue on the impact of the values, beliefs, ritual and taboos of the family and society on women's health.

During this meeting younger women of the family posed certain questions to the elderly women present, in the presence of the men. These questions were: why are there so many restrictions related to food intake? why are we considered unique and unclean during menstruation? why can we not keep ourselves clean (restrictions related to availability and use of water)?

They also focused their questions on the access to health services, these questions were addressed to the doctor-in-charge of the PHC and the ANM, but unfortunately none of them were present to answer these questions. Based on this meeting a resolution was sent to the CMO of Nainital district for action.

Another issue of significance in the context of women's health and the role of family and society is that the entire emphasis is on child health and not on the health of the mother. This is evident from all the rituals, ceremonies starting from the first menstrual cycle after marriage which is a celebration of the possibility of motherhood, to dietary restrictions during pregnancy and post-delivery, all of which are centred around the idea that the baby will get sick; it is difficult for the baby's delicate digestion; and, so on. After delivery the women is considered impure for 22 days and is not allowed to touch food and water, while the baby is carried around the house and loved and cared for by one and all.

At the level of health services also 'child health', in terms of immunization, breast feeding, supplementary feeding, growth monitoring gets more attention than maternal health services. While the mandate of all the PHC's is to reach maternal health services, it is clear from the analysis of the data that this is not the case. The focus of the ANM, if at all she does visit a village, is immunization and family planning (both are target-oriented activities). Added to all this is the physical inaccessibility from interior villages to health clinic/centres, both in terms of distance and non-availability of transport for women. Three significant factors that are emerging from this study are that women have a lack of :

- Awareness of health problems.
- Access to health services.
- Control over their own health.

Thus, women's health concerns have to be addressed at three levels :

1. Promotive, 2. Preventive, and 3. Curative.

	Promotive	Preventive	Curative
The individual Women (*mahila*)	"	"	"
The family (*parivar*)	"	"	"
Society (*samaj*)	"	"	"

Fig. 5.4 : Traditional Health Practices related to the Reproductive Phase of Women

The focus of this research has been to examine the traditional practices related to the promotive, preventive, and curative aspects of health care at the level of the woman, the family and the society; the values, beliefs and rituals related to the reproductive phase of women, what is being done to address these aspects, and how this is being operationally carried out in the field. The above important perspective has to be kept in mind while understanding the various issues related to women and health. Since these are not mere biological events in the life of a woman, the way the family and the society perceives these events and celebrates them, represents the essence of this culture. Culture is therefore a very important determinant for understanding the health of the community.

Perhaps the sectoral approach to health does not address the above framework. Since women are stake-holders in this process, therefore, in order to enable women to analyze these health-care practices they need to develop their critical abilities. For this purpose a whole process has to be initiated, a dialogue has to be started. If one believes in the people, and has faith in their knowledge and skills one has to enable them to walk through a process. In this process the role of the facilitator/CHW at a meeting becomes very crucial.

Those who are more vocal get heard, but the 'voices' of women (like the *akal mahila*) who are single, widowed, destitute, who do not participate actively remain unheard. Listening to women's voices, creating awareness about their rights related to health care and access to health services empowers them. After the recent panchayat elections in Uttaranchal representatives of women's groups at the village participated in the meetings at the gram sabha level to decide which issues have to be raised at the gram panchayat meeting. At a meeting I attended in Dhari block women representatives had raised the issue of the ANM not visiting their village. This led to immediate action as the issue was taken up with the medical officer in charge at the PHC. It is thus clear that women's meetings can become an important entry point for health issues. They felt that only when one builds the capacity of people and makes them aware of their rights with special reference to health services can one talk about a "people-oriented sustainable health programme". People should know why being healthy by themselves is important, instead of being dependent on an outside agency.

In the context of traditional health practices one can say that a critical analysis of any practice can lead to a healthy development. Flexibility and openness are very important. If a practice has to have sustainable implications it is not just the management of the resources but also the utilization that is important. For example, if oak leaves have to be used, the pruning has to be done in such a way that the stem remains healthy and produces a richer bio-mass. The way it is pruned is also important. If one is looking at sustainability, one has to take care of the needs of the people as well as the needs of the future generation. This involves moral responsibility. Thus, when one talks about traditions one has to be inclusive and not just focus on the needs of those who already have access and control to the means and materials. The age of specialisation has fragmented the individual and alienated him or her from that integration and interconnectedness which was the hallmark of societies that lived in close proximity to nature and environment.

It would be more important here for the community to develop a critical approach to understand that all traditional practices may not be health-giving. The question arises, how does one decide whether a practice is useful ?

- If a practice is not based on discrimination.

- If it does not violate a right.
- If it does not lower the self-esteem of an individual.
- If it does not promote violence on not just woman but also other marginalied sections of the society.

The points are not exhaustive and there may be so many others that need to be considered.

Gender

Health needs to be seen in a holistic way. It is not only an economic, or social issue but it is also deeply connected with gender.

Gender ⟷ health.

Since the focus of this research has been on the reproductive health aspect of women's lives, what emerges is that the adolescent girls health concerns need to be addressed, since she is going to be the future mother. (In Part II of this book on Action research these aspects have been applied to the new generation.)

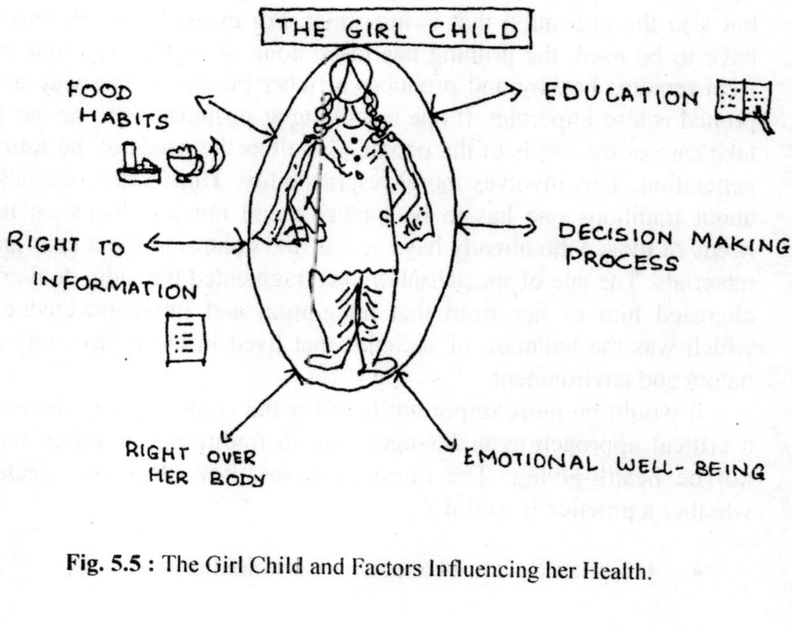

Fig. 5.5 : The Girl Child and Factors Influencing her Health.

- Education
- Emotional well being
- Decision-making process
- Food habits
- Right over her body
- Right to information

The above diagram illustrates that the health of the girl-child (adolescent) is linked to all these parameters. Based on the insights from the major health problems faced by women in Kumaon hills, there emerges the need for the education and training of adolescent girls in Uttaranchal on 'reproductive and child health issues, reproductive rights and gender' which is the trinity for human dignity. (According to Farah Francois, 2002, at the III National Raushni Deshpande Memorial Lecture.)

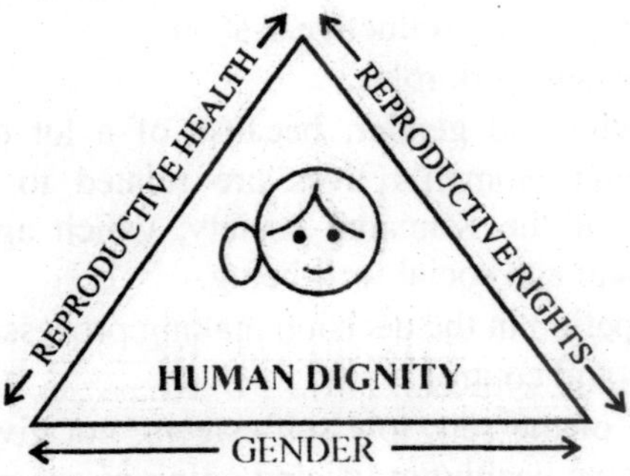

Fig. 5.6 : The Trinity for Human Dignity

According to Bhagwati Pande who now works with Pragati Sahyog in Almora, a dialogue on health issues was initiated at the grassroots level. Here, at this meeting, they took up one issue related to the reproductive phase, e.g. delivery, and asked the following questions:

- Where will the delivery take place?
- Who takes the decision?
- During an emergency what is to be done?
- Where will the finances come from?

The answers to all the above were that a woman does not participate or have any role in the critical decisions related to the important phases of her life which affect her HEALTH. All the decisions are taken by the elderly women of the family, who have a lot of lived experience related to delivery and the men in the family. In village 'Kanyager' in Dhari block Hema, a thirty year old Kumaoni woman, after delivery of a girl-child, had developed jaundice. The Chirag HEW informed the family that she was severely anaemic and needed hospitalization urgently. But the men and elderly women opposed this and Hema died when she could have been saved, her voice was unheard.

The issue of gender in the context of women's health needs to be addressed at multiple levels:

- Discrimination right at foetal stage/food intake.
- Lack of access to education/information about services available and reproductive system.
- Gender and work roles.
- Patriarchy and gender, because of a lot of the practices governing women's lives are related to the patriarchal system of the Kumaoni society, which again effects her emotional and social well-being.
- Participation in the decision making process.
- Access and control.
- Notion of the self, low self-esteem, not giving importance to her own health/not voicing opinions/not being heard.
- Social and familial pressure to produce a male child.

Male Participation

Linked to the issue of gender is the emerging importance of male participation which plays a very significant role in determining the health of a woman during her reproductive phase. Male participation in the pregnancy, pre-delivery, and post-delivery phase definitely effects the health of a woman. For example, if the husband is sensitive to what she eats and the amount of work she does during pregnancy and post-delivery; and if he is able to influence or have a say in the matter in the family then his participation would have a direct bearing on her health. Male participation in the reproductive phase related to contraception is also of critical importance. Our data has shown that women undergo tubectomy after giving birth to four children, here too her health suffers as she is not able to get adequate rest. The percentage of men going in for vasectomy is only 3 per cent. The two child norm of the government also adversely effects the health of the woman in traditional societies. If she has produced two sons and goes in for an operation, the family is very supportive, but if she has had two girls the pressure on her is so strong that the 'taunting' and sarcasm takes a toll on her emotional well being. The pressure of aborting the foetus is very strong if it is a girl-child and multiple abortions are carried out until she produces a male child. All this effects her health, quite obviously, but is seldom taken into account. Perhaps male participation in the reproductive phases of a woman's life is a concept which is not in line with the culture of this society, however significant it may be.

Sustainability of Health Care Interventions and Initiatives

(a) Government.
(b) NGOs.
(c) Traditional Health Service Providers.

Access to Health Services

Our survey of sixty women has clearly indicated that access to health services in areas where NGOs are not working is very low, (e.g., villages Almori and Kwedal) and there is still great dependence on *Dais'* for delivery. Traditional untrained *Dais* are still preferred by families because of their rich experience in delivery. In remote areas where there are no facilities for immunization, ante-natal and post-natal check ups and growth monitoring, the role of the *Dai* as a care giver and service provider assumes a critical role. NGOs like CHIRAG have developed a system of building a close interaction between the CHW and the *Dai* in the village. In fact the HEWs keep meeting the family of the pregnant woman so that they can educate the family on important issues like food intake during pregnancy and post-delivery.

Perhaps this important aspect should form an integral aspect of the CHWs and *Dai's* six monthly training programme.

From the whole process of owning responsibility for one's health and the health of the family and community, emerges the concept of sustainability. That which is viewed from the outside can never be sustainable. Traditional knowledge is sustainable because people are the repositories of that knowledge, it belongs to them, they utilize it for the benefit of the individual, the family and the community.

Outreach

CHIRAG's outreach programmes with reference to maternal and child health services extend to 15 villages in the Sargakhet area and 8 villages around the Sitla area in Ramgarh block. Access to health care for ante-natal and post-natal check up, growth monitoring, immunization, family planning and other referral services have been in place in these 23 villages for a period of 15 years. The health extension workers (HEWs) are responsible for the promotive, preventive and curative aspects of maternal and child healthcare under the able guidance of a qualified doctor.

Many discussions around the issue of sustainability of the health programmes of CHIRAG at the village level were held with the Community Health Workers, the *Dais* and the HEWs at their monthly meeting held on the 28th of every month at Kasialekh/Sargakhet clinic. Based on their experiences some of the ideas that the HEWs came up with were that the 15 villages where health interventions had been going on for the last 15 years could be put on a grid as follows:

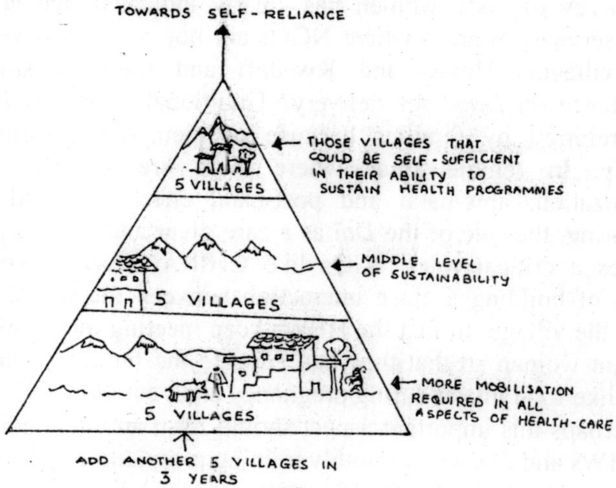

Fig. 5.7 : Moving towards Greater Sustainability

When the CHWs were asked at the same meeting, how they would sustain the programme at the village level, some of the suggestions they gave were :

1. The creation of a *'Swasthya Ghar'*,

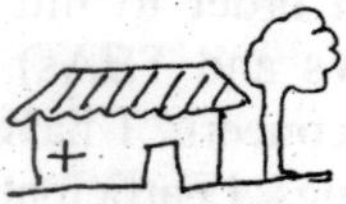

2. CSM – Contraceptive Social Marketing – i.e. they would make a list of all the eligible couples in the village and supply them with condoms/oral pills for a nominal price.

One of the CHWs said, "We will do all this for the development of our village, we will attend every meeting and raise health issues of significance at these meetings". Their major concern was the stipend that they received from CHIRAG (Rs. 200 per month), but they were convinced that when they started disbursing medicines at the community level and charged a nominal fee for their services they would be able to make more than the stipend.

Another significant issue for sustainability is how does the community perceive the CHWs role. A comment of one of the CHWs was that "*Dais* have no problem of sustainability as they are highly respected because of their special skills in the community, but we have to make our own place". This initiated a lively discussion. The CHW is chosen democratically by the community, she is one of them, they have faith in her, so there is no reason why she should feel diffident about her role in the community. If people become stake holders in the process of health care they will ensure that the health programme is sustainable.

Some problems voiced by the CHWs were the need for health education :

> "We can only give those medicines in the community that we have knowledge of", said one CHW.
>
> "We need to understand the relationship between height, weight and arm circumference, e.g. what supplementary nutrition should be provided to a child who comes in the yellow/red band" said another CHW.
>
> "Our health intervention in the village level meetings needs to be strengthened, at every meeting we should have a health issue to discuss, educational materials should be made available at a common centre" said Kunti Bisht the CHW from village Buribana.

These concerns voiced by the CHWs reiterate the importance of the promotive aspects of health care which need more attention than has been given hitherto.

In order to illustrate the role of the health service providers (CHWs and TBAs) at the grassroots level, and address issues of their concern, I have shared the discussions of one of the several meetings, I participated in, to listen to their 'voices'.

Community Health Workers and Trained Birth Attendants (TBAs) meeting at Kasialekh 9th May, 2002.

Agenda (1) : To understand the major problems faced by CHWs and TBAs at the field level.

Agenda (2) : To discuss 'methodologies' for strengthening the 'promotive' and 'preventive' aspects of health care delivery with special reference to the performance appraisal and monitoring systems of CHWs at the village level.

Agenda (3) : To elicit responses regarding the job responsibilities of CHWs and TBAs from them.

Discussion

Major problems encountered by CHWS and TBAs at the village level were as follows :

(i) Opposition of elderly family members, particularly the mother-in-law for ANC and immunization.
(ii) No interaction with the *Dai* of the village.
(iii) Some women in the village say that they are shy to have a check-up.
(iv) No materials available for health education.
(v) Low salary.
(vi) How do the CHWs and TBAs become self-sufficient and independent in their work roles, if Chirag was to move to other villages.
(vii) No training for CHWs for the last 5 or 6 years. There should be a training every six months, to strengthen their knowledge level.

(viii) To create a *'swasthaya ghar'* in each village where the *'swasthya sevika'* is available (could be her house or any other place mutually chosen by the village people) :

- medicines
- bandages
- contraceptives

should be available here.

(ix) Receipt book to be printed by CHIRAG so that people know that the money they are giving for services rendered are properly utilized properly.

(x) Many villages do not have *Dais* (15 CHWs + 9TBAs in 15 villages. Every *Dai* and Health Worker should train one another woman who is interested in this work to learn their skills, so that these services are strengthened. The *Dai* of Kafli village Radhika Devi however opposed this saying, "it is very difficult to give your inherent skills to anyone else – this is god's gift".

(xi) To strengthen the component of health education. Towards this all CHWs agreed to hold two sessions every month at a women's meeting held in their village. The theme for these would be decided at the health workers meeting held on the 28th of every month.

The Community Health Workers requested the HEWs to provide educational materials related to the selected themes for that particular month to the health workers at the meeting. A system for recording these sessions was developed :

1. Topic:
2. Date:
3. Venue:
4. Materials used:
5. Number of women present:
6. Issues raised:

Each health worker would record these sessions in her diary.

The job responsibilities of the CHWs were enumerated with their participation, as follows:

1. Health education.
2. Counselling.
3. Growth Monitoring (0-5 weight)
4. Contraceptive Social Marketing.
5. Record keeping.
6. Dissemination of simple medicines.
7. Linking patients to clinic/hospitals for specialised care.

The HEWs were also asked to keep a record of the two meetings held with the CHWs and TBAs every month. These minutes/records would go a long way in strengthening the systems and methodologies being used.

Since the area concerned around Sargakhet is 15 villages, each HEW (Neomi, Kunti, Gangu) would look after or be responsible for the monitoring and record keeping system of 5 CHWs. This would ensure greater interaction between the two groups.

SOME ISSUES RELATED TO COMMUNITY HEALTH PROGRAMMES

The chapters before have shown that during the last 20 or 25 years, a great many attempts have been made to bring basic health care to communities by the government and the NGOs. A great deal of financial help has been allocated and given to various programmes planned by highly trained experts at many levels. It is clear that for many reasons, like bureaucratic indifference, delay and corruption, the results have been disappointing, often since suffering due to disease, sickness etc. has not been mitigated. However, community health programmes in villages, especially by NGOs has in many ways helped people to meet their health-related needs. Programmes which are considered successful are those which have the following important areas in common :

1. Importance of decentralization growth which has focused on local levels, while showing slow beginnings these have gradually developed and evolved in response to the needs of the particular communities, which means that these programmes have remained decentralized at the planning and decision-making levels which take place at the village level.

2. Involvement of local people – especially the poor – in each phase of the programme emphasizing that the disadvantaged members of society, apart from local leaders, also play a leading role in determining priorities. This allows consciously to help and strengthen the position and bargaining power of the people.
3. The planning 'blue print' in this approach does not follow a predetermined course, as programme content and health workers training is flexible, a continuous process where participants at every level are invited to help shape, change, and criticize the plans. Implying thereby that instructors, students, health workers and members of the communities are constantly evolving and adapting according to local needs.
4. Those programmes work well where committed leaders whose aim is both not only for a just society but where the first responsibility is towards the people, so that even when the programmes are successful they continue to focus on the critical needs of the people with whom their contact continues to be in terms of a close relationship. (Werner & Bower: 1982)
5. A recognition and vision of good health that is contextualised within a framework of improving the entire social and cultural situation, i.e. health activities considered as state of wholeness and well-being are linked to social development. It means emphasizing the role of relationship between one's self and the other and a clear understanding that the influence of all people's well-being is essential. As it has been emphasized throughout earlier chapters, it is this critical awareness that has become a key part of training and community work.

When many of the above highlighted points are not followed in many health programmes, their failure is not surprising since these objectives and approaches remain at the top planners level without a follow up of implementation especially because community participation has come to generally mean "getting people to do what we decide". In doing so these communities are seldom self-governing and self-sustaining, and become instead increasingly dependent on the 'government, *sarkar*', to give aid and services. This is where corruption also enters strongly, this dependency on authority is a continuation of colonial manner of administration which continues to haunt us even after so many years of freedom. The growth of vested interest is helped in this manner, as is the case with many programmes in India that is too well known to narrate here. (Bower &Werner:1982).

In short, the biggest obstacle is the unwillingness of experts, professionals, and health authorities to let go of their control, so that the responsibility is first to the people rather than to the health system. This seldom allows the people from the village community to grow and become leaders, take initiative in health programmes, instead they become servants or auxiliaries to visiting doctors, nurses, learning to fill forms, etc. In this way such health workers win little respect and have no influence on the community. Seeing this manner of operation, it discourages many young workers who become either corrupt or quit, especially the government sponsored programmes which many feel then is only a pipe dream that has been tried yet has failed.

However, despite the centrally controlled programmes (Government) the NGOs with effective community participation are outstanding examples of success where the goal is a "community-strengthening approach" to health care. These programmes have a wealth of variety in terms of innovation and adaptation to local conditions, where the health worker speaks out for the 'voiceless' poor, where human dignity, loving care, and fairer distribution of land, wealth, and power is kept upper most in their mind. These are movements beyond any dogmas either religious or political doctrines, invoking greater faith in small, self-directed programmes that allow for searching questions, criticism and allowing communities to form their own conclusions for factors that shape their health and their lives. (Bower, et. al : *ibid.*)

Thus, it is this approach to the training, role, and responsibilities of community health workers, ideas and methods and a practical human vision, that is being shared around the world through a series of informal networks.

Innovative Methods of Health Education

Health education is an important component of the 'promotive' health care strategy. The preceding chapters and the analysis have clearly brought to focus that women's health has to be addressed at three significant levels :

- Promotive
- Preventive
- Curative.

While the second and the third aspects are being addressed in some form by the formal/informal health care interventions, it is the promotive aspect of health care that has to be strengthened. The aim of a health worker is to be people-centred, to help those who are the weakest, and to make them self-reliant. Thus community health education is appropriate to the extent that the poor and powerless gain greater control over their health and their lives. Effective health workers need to develop approaches very different from what most of us have experienced in schools everywhere in the world, i.e. to critically examine different ways of teaching in order to adapt to people's ways of traditional learning, ways they are already used to enjoy.

In this context, it is significant to examine the methods that are to be used and the way we relate to the trainees, beyond stating that we are to be people-centred. A culture-centred approach, say, by using stories (especially true stories told from personal experience), puppet shows for children, games so that discovering things for themselves and learning becomes exciting. Learning could perhaps be useful by doing, is how workers will be more able to help others, by relating to the student and trainee. This is to encourage them to question authority and to think for themselves, then they will gain attitudes and skills useful for helping people meet their biggest needs. This involves a sense of equality, inviting cooperation, welcoming criticism, questioning, initiative and trust say, by living and dressing modestly and while working in the community.

Instructors and trainers need to have discussions about sharing and self-reliance because essentially even health development growth depends on this idea, even when food, water, cleanliness knowledge, resources, opportunities need to be shared. Self-reliance is a measure of health, since a sick person needs to be cared for completely and can do almost nothing for him/her self. Health is closely related to people's ability to care for themselves and each other – as equals. To illustrate, in order to start discussions certain questions like the following may be asked :

1. How are persons who are sick different from persons who are healthy?

2. Who are better able to care for themselves? Who needs to be taken care of?
3. Who have more problems, the rich or the poor? Why?
4. What do health and well-being have to do with self-reliance? Of a person? Of a family? Of a nation?
5. Can you give examples from your own experience?

After discussing these question, one may ask:

1. What should be the main goal of health education?
2. What should be your responsibilities as a health worker?
3. What new approaches to health care require new approaches to teaching and learning?

In other words, health workers not only need to know how to break down and teach or build up people's self-confidence and community strength, they also need to understand why such methods are important, by experiencing and practicing appropriate teaching methods during their training. It has to be constantly kept in mind that health education is to enable a person to gain the knowledge, skills, and awareness necessary to meet life's needs. The health worker's training itself must set an example, is very important, if he/she is to be a 'leader for change'. In the context of the latter there are a few suggestions which may be useful for the group leader or the facilitator :

1. To sit in a circle so that everyone can see each other's faces.
2. To teach the same way as learnt one's self, by drawing information out of the people from their own experience.
3. To use words the people understand and check often if this is happening by asking them.
4. To develop thinking capacity, ask a lot of questions which allows for critical thinking for themselves.
5. Emphasize the most useful ideas and information in their community, say hygiene, importance of ante-natal and post-natal checkups, immunization, etc. In this way encourage women to relate what they have seen and learned to real needs and problems in their own communities, and to discuss what action they might take.

6. Encourage women to relate what they have seen and learned to real needs and problems in their own communities, and to discuss what action they might take.

To reiterate, those trainings give best results which keep the language simple, focus on what is most important, and use learning methods people are used to and enjoy. This is to be done within the framework of an 'open-ended dialogue' in which many answers come from peoples' experience and helps people in finding ways to gain more control over their health and their lives so that true social transformation takes place where social equality is the basis, and where oppression, exploitation, and corruption is actively opposed. In stating all this, ultimately the health worker is accountable to the community, especially the marginalized sections of the community whose interests she/he defends. (Bower, *et.al.* : *ibid.*)

Briefly, the important concepts that need to be focused on and strengthened in training Community Health Workers are as follows:

1. Critical analysis
2. Social awareness
3. Communication skills
4. Teaching skills
5. Organization skills
6. Innovation
7. Self-reliance
8. Use of local resources
9. Local customs
10. Confidence building
11. Abilities of women and children
12. Human dignity
13. Methods that help the people to grow stronger.

What Next ?

Salient Findings

Before proceeding to decide on the next steps it would be significant here to refocus on the salient findings of the research on traditional health practices of women in the Kumaon Hills emerging from our discussion in Chapter 4.

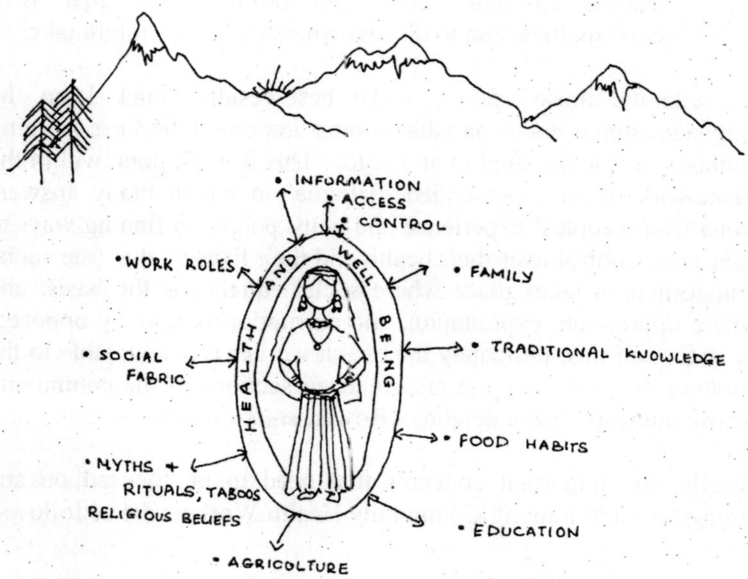

Fig. 5.8 : Women's Health has to be viewed 'Holistically'

What has emerged from this research on traditional health practices, continuity and change, is that we need to build a matrix wherein these practices intersect with the modern medicine system in order to provide a more holistic health care strategy for women and children in this community.

From our detailed analysis of the traditional health practices it is apparent that culture is an important determinant for understanding the health of any community. The conceptual framework outlined in Chapter 1, becomes very clear as one proceeded to understand these issues with reference to women in the Kumaon Hills. In fact Kishni Devi's articulation that life and health are one, not separate, is very clearly illustrated in the voices of the women and in their sharing of their health concerns.....

1. What comes across from the perception of women about 'good health' is that they are aware of the fact that not only the body, but the environment, village, family – society in general – are all inter-linked in the creation of good health. Their ideas in a way reflect the WHO definition of health

which takes into account the physical, emotional and spiritual well-being of people.

2. The shift from traditional agriculture to 'cash crop economy' wherein there is more emphasis on growing potatoes and cabbage and vegetables has changed the food consumption patterns greatly in this region, thus affecting the nutritional quality of the food consumed.

3. While health professionals encourage women to increase their normal food intake during each trimester of pregnancy, for many women in Uttaranchal, social and cultural constraints make this an unlikely option.

   It was interesting to note that access to extension health programmes caused no differentiation in the proportion of women eating normal, more, or less amounts of food in all of the six villages. The beliefs that permeate the post-delivery food intake practices have to be seen in a context, wherein individual lived experiences find expression into a practice. It is critical that this aspect of maternal and child health is addressed by integrating the traditional practices with promotive health care strategies.

   Nutrition education should therefore form an important aspect of the promotive health care strategy. Here emphasis should be given to the value behind the practice and then initiate a 'dialogue' to discuss the merits and demerits of existing food restriction practices during menstruation, delivery and post-delivery. This would be very beneficial for the village women. This task could be performed by the HEW/CHW/TBA and the ANM within the government health infrastructure. The importance of giving the first milk to the new born baby should also form an integral part of maternal and child-health education.

4.a. Fruit bearing trees, plants, the cow, cow's milk, *naulas* (water springs) are all considered sacred in this culture, therefore a menstruating women who is considered impure cannot come in contact with all these items.

4.b. Not only are there restrictions for movement within the house, a menstruating woman is not welcome or allowed in community spaces, the village temple, neighbouring households and her presence is absolutely forbidden on social or religious occasions like marriages, prayer meetings, *jagar* ceremonies and other religious festivals. This social isolation effects her emotional health.

4.c. Health Service Providers at the grass roots level like the CHWs/TBAs can play an important role in disseminating information about how to prepare sanitary pads which women can use during the menstrual cycle. They can reinforce the importance of menstrual hygiene which will protect women from the severe RTIs they suffer from. Promotive health care has to include these aspects so that women can move about freely during their menstrual cycle. This would have a significant bearing on their emotional well-being. Women also need to be given knowledge about their reproductive system. Awareness generation is a prerequisite for action.

5. Promotive health education and interventions should focus on patterns of work distribution in the family, especially during the reproductive phase of a woman's life. This is particularly important in the context of women in the hill communities who continue to perform back breaking tasks during their menstrual cycle, delivery and post-delivery. Decreasing women's workload needs to be coupled with education about resting for at least one month after delivery. This can be done by educating the community about sharing the workload during a woman's pregnancy. If it is unlikely that men will participate in "women's work" then local women's groups can organize to assist one another.

6. As regards ante-natal and post-natal services the survey reveals that while accessibility is a strong factor in determining whether the women will receive care, increased awareness of its benefits and availability is also a key factor. Familial opposition from elderly women of the family to receiving ante-natal and post-natal services needs to be addressed by awareness generation and continuous reinforcement of the benefit. A 'family-oriented' approach to maternal and child health care which takes the whole family along (including the men) needs to be strengthened and developed. This should become an integral aspect of any pro-active health care strategy. Since family bonds are so strong in this culture and the family is a sacred unit, such an approach would go a long way in creating and sustaining health care systems which are 'health giving'.

7. Traditional *Dais* are the repositories of the indigenous body and health knowledge. Their good practices are culturally appropriate since these maximise the use of locally available resources, thereby providing a palpable life force energy, and assume the naturalness of birth. In this way these practices work at bodily, emotional, social and sacred levels. Any health care system must give value to their wisdom and support their work with appropriate training and new methods which can be integrated with their knowledge. The *Dai* belongs to the community and owns responsibility for the well-being and health of the women in the community. She is seen as a care-giver and supporter by people, a role that is often ignored.

   The research about the beliefs and practices of the Dai in Kumaon reveals that while a great many of the practices are appropriate and she is the key health resource person in the village, any training programme will have to take into account these various socio-cultural aspects of the *Dais* themselves, so that areas of conflict can be explored. Such a training programme can be rewarding for both the *Dai* and the trainer, as each can benefit from the other's experience.

   It is interesting to note here that the ANM who is the representative of the government primary health care infrastructure at the village level has very little role in ensuring safe delivery. In the villages of effective CHIRAG assistance the role of the ANM seems to be almost negligible in ante-natal care and in directing women to have their deliveries from trained *Dais*. Wherever the NGO outreach programme is effective the govt. infrastructure in providing health care seems to recede. However, a more effective interface between the two would go a long way in changing the status of mother and child health in the country.

8. When the mother is able to cut the cord of her own child, she retains ownership over the health of herself and her family. Often when development organizations begin to educate about new practices, they put less emphasis on reinforcing beneficial traditional practices that allow the people whom they are assisting to remain in control of their own health. A partnership can be developed between the development organization and the local people by synthesizing local and scientific knowledge of health. Rather than stealing control of

health knowledge, they should create a participatory atmosphere, which will lead to greater sustainability. Teaching the mothers as well as the *Dais* how to sterilize and bind off the umbilical cord allows the mother to participate in sustaining the health of her child. The example of *Dais* rather than mothers cutting the cord is just a shadow of the underlying problem this survey intended to uncover – that assisted villages have begun to shift from sustaining their own preventative health care to increasing dependence on curative health services.

Many health workers and *Dais* are intelligent and well-respected within their communities. Yet there are those who are skeptical of new health practices. However, when another woman of equal standing explains to the other that she has tried the new method and discovered its benefits, even the skeptics must think twice. Thus, increasing awareness through health education is very important.

The need to have training for *Dais* of all villages and not only NGO assisted villages is very important. Many women who experienced problems shared that they did not seek any medical or professional help but only consulted the *Dai*, who is very wise and has years of experience to support her knowledge and wisdom. This total reliance on the village *Dai* is a pointer again to the crucial role they play in the traditional as well as modern health-care scenario.

9. Social familial pressures to produce a son has a great bearing on the mental and social health of the woman. A woman who has given birth to a baby girl is under a lot of mental tension because of the socio-cultural pattern of life in this region. She sees her own life reflected in a way in this new born girl, overburdened with workload, repeated pregnancies, frequent abortions, lack of access to health care, lack of decision-making in using contraceptives, and lack of freedom in mobility. All these factors pose a constraint on her mind and this tension manifest in a number of health related problems in women. A supportive and caring environment, attitudinal change and health education sessions giving value to the girl-child would help in creating a healthy environment.

10. One of the objectives of the PHCs is to provide immunization to the children in the population covered by them. This role is performed by the ANM. However, the absence of these

services in areas where the NGOs health outreach programs are effective, and who provide these services with great consistency makes the government PHCs unaccountable in a way. In remote villages there is too much dependency on the health worker and the extension team. There is a need to create a more sustainable immunization program. A greater interface between the NGOs and the PHCs would go a long way in creating this sustainability. It is only recently that this is happening in the villages where CHIRAG is working, and they are now coordinating with the PHC doctor and ANM for providing immunization. If this happens the NGOs can concentrate on capacity building and training of their CHWs and TBAs for greater sustainability of their health care programs.

11. A focus on women's health seeking behaviour makes it apparent (ref. for details Chapter 4) that since most of the problems women experience are connected with their private parts, they neither speak about them nor seek help unless it becomes a critical situation. In this context the social fabric of the society and the women's notion of the self-play an important role. The presence of a lady doctor at each PHC in a block would help in this regard. It is not at all easy to find a doctor to provide sustained health services to a community as has been the experience of CHIRAG. Most medical professionals prefer to be in towns and metropolitan cities, rather than serve a community that critically needs care.

12. Local communication networks and performance genres like puppets, folksongs, folk theatre and folk tales can be used effectively for giving information on vital issues related to the health of women and children in the community. These would strengthen the promotive and preventive aspects of health care.

13.a. The major health problems experienced by women in this region are pelvic inflammatory disorders (PID), which includes severe back pain, white discharge, frequent headaches, excessive bleeding, repeated pregnancies, burning sensation in hands and feet, anemia and general weakness. There is a direct correlation between the work roles performed by women, the dietary restrictions during important reproductive phases of a woman's life and the health problems experienced by her.

13.b. What emerges from the major health problems of women in the Kumaon hills is that this issue has to be viewed holistically and not fragmented into compartments that further alienate women from their own wisdom and knowledge.

13.c. Women are the source of life and the sustainers of health in the Kumaon hills. In a place where traditions and social norms often treat women as inferior beings, to be responsible for the health and welfare of oneself, one's family, and one's village commands tremendous respect and authority.

Yet with the infiltration of outside medical knowledge and expertise, women's roles in the maintenance of health have begun to diminish. This is typical of rural areas in which development organizations have attempted to bring in improved health care and have inadvertently caused almost complete dependence on outside sources for health care. Developmental professionals are often guilty of ignoring the importance of indigenous knowledge. For the sustainability of developmental health care, it is essential to integrate modern practices with indigenous knowledge. Therefore, NGOS working with health care need to return the role of preventive health care into the women's hands by providing them with knowledge about health while empowering them to reduce their dependence on outside medical care.

14. People's faith in traditional knowledge systems and the healing powers of the local vaids is diminishing. Herbs and medicinal plants grow abundantly in the forests of this region. They are still available, but the younger generation does not have as much faith in this system. Documentation, and cataloguing of these herbs and medicinal plants for all aspects of health care and giving value to the knowledge of 'gunijan' and vaids as well as the wisdom of the women would give an impetus to this valuable source of knowledge. When people's knowledge is recognized and given value they see themselves as stake holders in a process and not merely as a statistical beneficiary.

15. Providing adolescent girls with knowledge about health care, stressing the importance of preventive care while integrating and encouraging indigenous knowledge, will stimulate greater empowerment for the women of Kumaon. Many women expressed the desire to have their daughters educated

about not only preventive health care, but also about major life events such as preparation for marriage and children. For this reason, we hope that teaching teaching adolescent girls about health care will prompt discussions about the 'self' in relation to the society and environment continuing to encourage the women of Kumaon to move beyond medical dependence to empowerment.

Some Recommendations

Briefly, to reiterate, the following are some of the recommendations that have emerged from the study in the context of women's health :

- The social system which marginalises women from access to adequate resources, from decision-making processes; which determines early marriage, immediate proof of fertility, "son-preference", heavy workload requires deep-rooted changes in patriarchal attitudes. It follows that men need to be targeted (rather addressed) and sensitized. In fact reproductive health cannot be improved without involving men. Since they hold the reins of decision making in their hands, they need to be mad aware of contraception, STD, AIDS, importance of woman's access to ante-natal care, safe-delivery systems, etc.
- Social taboos and rituals, belief systems, etc. which have been perpetuated by religious/cultural institutions can be mobilized in a constructive manner to carry the message of 'safe motherhood'.
- CHWs and TBAs, or Mahila Mangal *Dais*, in the absence of any other alternative, are repositories of strength and knowledge for the village women, and a good medium of change. The logic of this is proven when village women were asked how they gained health awareness.
- New opportunities, through the involvement of women in panchayats, other statutory bodies like JRY, Indira Avas Yojana, NGOs, etc., can introduce 'social' development at grassroots level. Women pradhans, and women panchayat members, etc., can become effective pressure groups for ensuring better health care systems and practices. (Srivastava : 2001)

- Ensuring better outreach to health care systems can counter socio-cultural and economic limitations that are barriers to women's access to health. More lady doctors, better medical staff, adequate medical supplies and other strategies need to taken into account especially in mountain terrains where regular refresher programmes need to be undertaken by the staff, keeping in mind the strategic link of the *Dais*.
- Extremely heavy load work for women, in the procurement of food, fuel and water requires greater attention and perhaps we need to look at alternatives, such as the installation of pumps, fuel efficient stoves, introduction of proper natural resource management techniques to increase the production of fodder (introducing traditional techniques also), and locally available food (such as berries, leafy vegetables, nuts etc.). Introduction of appropriate technologies to increase fuel and heat consumption in winter months.
- Use of media to spread the message of Reproductive Health, such as radio, pamphlets, puppet shows, local *haats*, market centres, fairs, festivals for dissemination of information.
- Infrastructure in the form of roads and transports systems to ensure timely health services.
- All these suggestions and recommendations will work if the basic aim for sustainable improvement in reproductive health status of women is kept in mind. The larger problems of women's status in the social fabric of Kumaon Hills has to be addressed, so that they live with dignity.
- The adolescent girl-child who is systematically ignored by policy makers, needs to be made aware of Reproductive Health and related issues. A good place for intervention would be creating Kishori Samooh's or 'Kishori Sanghs' at the village level, or organising systematic Trainings in Reproductive Health Issues for groups of adolescent girls so that specific socio-cultural needs can be addressed. This would contextualise their learning in an environment where they live and grow and to which they relate.

PART II

TRAINING OF RURAL ADOLESCENT GIRLS IN UTTARANCHAL ON REPRODUCTIVE AND CHILD HEALTH ISSUES

An Action Research

6

ADOLESCENTS – A PROFILE

A. INTRODUCTION

Adolescence represents a cognitive and social transformation from dependent childhood to relatively independent adulthood, marked by intense psychological, physical and intellectual turbulence and change. The term adolescence means "to emerge" or "to achieve identity". It is a complex change of status that is influenced by the individual's personal endowment and experience as well as the individual's culture. It is also considered to be one of the most critical periods for learning and receptivity of learning. Psychologically, individuals become more capable of abstract thinking, foresight and internal control; and acquire greater awareness of the environment, capacity for empathy and idealism.

"Adolescence is a period of physical, psychological and social maturity from childhood to adulthood extending from the onset of puberty to the attainment of full reproductive maturity". (WHO 2000) It is a time when puberty is experienced. Physically, adolescents begins to reach their adult size, their bodies become sexually defined and reproductive capability is established.

Adolescence is a tumultuous period that many people find difficult to cope with. Society, as if taking a cue from the physical changes, often imposes regulations and codes of conduct on adolescents that adolescents find difficult to observe. "During this phase of transition, the adolescents have to straddle the ambiguous terrain between childhood and adulthood. Like adults, adolescents move into larger world and respond proactively to their environment. However like younger children, their present settings and their access to future resources like economic and marital opportunities are controlled by adults" (Schegal, 1995).

Adolescents also include a whole gamut of categories – school going and non-school going, drop-outs, sexually exploited, working adolescents (both paid and unpaid), unmarried adolescents as also married males and females with experience of motherhood and fatherhood (Ministry of Health and Family Welfare, Country Paper, 1998).

Adolescence is complicated by non-simultaneous nature of the changes, i.e. different aspects of behaviour or physical appearance occur at various stages. This suggests a need to move beyond an overall emphasis on adolescents towards different interventions at different stages of adolescence.

The three main stages of adolescence may be discerned as :

1. Early Adolescence (9-13 years) – This stage is characterised by a spurt of growth the development of secondary sexual characteristics.
2. Mid-Adolescence (14-15 years) – This is distinguished by the development of a separate identity from parents, of new relationship with peer group and the opposite sex and of experimentation.
3. Late Adolescence (16-19 years) – At this stage, adolescents have fully developed physical characteristics (similar to adults), and have well informed opinions and ideas (NCERT, 1999).

Demographic Profile of Adolescents

A pre-requisite for planning of any intervention is the comprehensive situational analysis of adolescents.

* In India, adolescents account for 21.4 per cent of the population.
* According to Central Statistical Organization (CSO) in India, this percentage of adolescents is decreasing gradually year after year.

Population Distribution of Adolescents in the Total Population

Population Distribution of Adolescents in the Total Population

Year	Age Group 10-14 Years		Age Group 15-19 Years	
1981	13.2	12.6	9.9	9.4
2001	12.1	12.1	11.0	10.5
2016	8.7	8.7	8.3	8.3

Source : Population Council of India, 1998.

- The sex ratio for adolescents in the 13-19 years age group declined from 897.7 in 1981 to 884.2 in 1991, although it rose to 890.4 in 1996, (Office of Registrar General, 1996)
- According to CSO (1999) in India among the older adolescents age group, female mortality is significantly greater than the male mortality as female adolescents begins to experience problems of early pregnancy, the effects of malnutrition and anaemia.

Mortality Rates of Adolescents

Year	Age Group 10-14 Years		Age Group 15-19 Years	
1995	1.3	1.4	1.7	2.0

Source : Population Council of India, 1998.

- According to National Family and Health Survey (1998-99), though the legal ages of marriage are 18 years for females and 21 years for males, nonetheless, early marriages continue to be the norm. In India, 50 per cent of women aged 20-24 years are married before 18 years. Out of this, in rural areas the percentage of women who are married before 18 years is 58.6 per cent, which is in sharp contrast to urban percentage of 27.9 per cent.
- According to Indian Institute of Population Sciences (1992), There is a sharp contrast between the fertility rate of rural and urban population, in the age of 15-19 years old adolescents – in rural are 23.3 per cent and in urban-42.4 per cent.
- Adolescents are vulnerable to contracting STDs due to early onset of sexual activity, low contraceptive use and likelihood of partner change. Young people between the ages of 10-25 years make upto 50 per cent of all new infections. In India, the epidemic continues to shift towards women and young people (India Responds to HIV/AIDS, UNAIDS, 1999). In addition to this, studies across South Asia (Mehta, 1998; Jeejebhoy, 1996) on sexual activities and knowledge indicate the following :
- The magnitude of adolescent girl's sexual activity is lower than that of boys due to fears of social disapproval.
- Parents and teachers play a minor role in both giving information as well as being reluctant to impart such information. The majority of the information on sexual and

reproductive issues is obtained from peers, which can be sometimes being misleading and inaccurate, thereby resulting in negative perceptions throughout the reproductive years of adolescents.

- Knowledge about sexual and reproductive issues, safe sex and preventive behaviour is extremely poor.
- The education system doesn't adequately meet the needs for imparting sex education.
- Sexual and reproductive decision-making by adolescents is constrained by age and gender factors.
- There is a huge unmet demand for adolescent health facilities, information and counselling services.

All the data indicate that the RH (Reproductive Health) needs of the vast number remain ill served. Until recently, the special needs of this group have not been sufficiently addressed. There is increasing recognition now, that reproductive health needs of the adolescent girls have to be articulated in terms of information and services so that they can make informed choices leading to improvement in their health status. Access to reproductive health services to unmarried adolescents seems to be an emerging issue for this group. Helping adolescents develop into healthy, productive adults requires a safe and supportive environment, accurate information, counselling and training to build their life skills.

Why Focus on Adolescents

"In India, adolescents account for one-fifth of the population with an estimated 190 million adolescents, constitute a significance group meriting separate attention". (UNFPA, 1998)

Adolescents represent a major potential human resource for the overall development of a nation. Actions taken during adolescence can affect a person's life opportunities, behavioural patterns and health. For physical, socio-cultural, economic and psychological reasons, young people are typically poorly informed about how to protect themselves sexually and are thus particularly susceptible to unwanted pregnancies and STDs including HIV/AIDS.

As studied by Jeejebhoy and Rama Rao in 1990, reproductive health in general and adolescent reproductive health needs in particular, are poorly understood and served in India. In many societies, despite recognition that there is an increase in adolescent sexual activity outside marriage, there is often considerable reluctance among influential bodies that provide education to young people about sex, reproductive health and contraceptive methods that might prevent these consequences.

Adolescents in India : Issues at a glance

There is a growing awareness and concern about the fact that the sexual and reproductive health in India is characterised by high rates of unwanted pregnancies, unsafe abortions and STD and HIV infections. This can be interpreted as a result of social change in response to economic development, rapid urbanisation, transitional flow of media messages and a loosening of traditional gender roles. Many people are unable to attain optimal reproductive health because of incomplete knowledge about health and sexuality, high-risk sexual behaviour, the unavailability of poor quality of reproductive health services; existing gender bias and limited power of many women over their sexual and reproductive lives.

In the absence of systematic and correct information on matters related to sex and sexuality, the youth are facing a dilemma between traditional Indian norms and modern Western influences. Ignorance is what adolescents face regarding their own sexuality and physical well being, their body and their health. What is urgently required for both adolescent girls are programmes, which will help them to understand and deal with issues of sexuality.

"Providing access to accurate information to the adolescent group should be seriously considered." Some NGOs have considerable experience and potential in organising such activities, which could be tapped. The "gate keeper" of information for adolescents should be taken into confidence for imparting service (UNFPA : 2000). Issues that are of grave concern regarding adolescent reproductive health are discussed below. These are :

- Marriage age and fertility behaviour of adolescent girls.
- Sexual activity in adolescent girls.
- Teenage pregnancy in adolescent girls.
- STD and RTIs in adolescents.
- HIV/AIDS.
- Contraception in adolescent girls.
- Female Genital Mutilation (FGM) in adolescent girls.

Marriage Age and Fertility Behaviour of Adolescent Girls

Marriage is as yet a generally accepted norm in India, unlike perhaps in the advanced West. Among the major problems of adolescent reproductive health are those resulting from the traditional early marriage of girls that still prevail in many, especially rural, parts of the developing world. (WHO, 1989)

Nationally, about 39 per cent of women aged 15-19 years are married out of which 26 per cent get married by 15 years of age, and by 20 years of age about 71 per cent women are married. Although the minimum legal age of marriage for girls is 18 years (according to Child Marriage Restraint Act, 1978), still a majority of women and their parents are not aware of this legality and child marriages continue to take place in large numbers, especially in rural India. (UNFPA, 2000)

Adolescent marriage is synonymous with adolescent fertility. The Total Fertility Rate in India is 3.5 (children per women), while the age specific fertility rate of women aged 15-19 years is 116 births as compared to 243 for women aged 9-24 years, per 1000 wome.n (India, 2002) Mothers aged 15-29 years contribute more than three-fourth of the total fertility and out of these, adolescent girls, in the age group of 15-18 years, contribute 23 per cent. Thus child bearing is concentrated among younger women. Increasingly, early parenthood means lost education with lifelong loss of earnings as well. (UNFPA, 2000)

A more universal consequence of early and more frequent child bearing is the increase in population size and growth rate. It also leads to chances of anaemia during pregnancy, retarded foetal growth, premature birth and complications during labour and also increase in maternal and infant mortality and morbidity rate.

Teenage Pregnancy in Adolescent Girls

Pregnancy and childbearing in girls during early adolescence constitute increased health risks as compared to fully developed women particularly if the girl does not receive adequate prenatal care. More than 15 million adolescent girls give birth every year, but there are great regional differences in adolescent fertility levels. For girls ages 10 to 14, maternal mortality rates may be 5 times higher than for women in their early twenties, and their children are also more likely to fall sick or die in infancy. An increase in the age of marriage, a fall in the age of menarche and no decrease in sexual activity is a greater risk of adolescent girls becoming pregnant outside of marriage, which involves social stigma that might prevent pregnant adolescent girls from obtaining prenatal care.

Women who become mothers during their teens generally end up with less education and fewer job opportunities. This, in turn, exposes them to a greater risk of poverty. Many studies have shown that in the case of adolescent pregnancies, partners are by and large friends. Significant proportion of adolescents becomes pregnant as result of rape or non-consensual sexual activity, suggesting the prevalence of violence against adolescent girls. This is further supported by the fact that – "8 per cent of India's 26-27 million annual births are to mother under 19 years of age" (NIPCCD, 1998)

Abortions in Adolescents Girls

As per service statistics, compiled by Government of India, about 1 million abortions are performed annually under MTP Act. In addition, around 6 million illegal abortions are performed by a variety of medical and non-medical practitioners, most of whom are unqualified, untrained and induce pregnancy termination at unqualified places using dubious methods. Adolescent girls constitute about 25 per cent of these abortions (UNFPA, 2000).

According to UNICEF (1991), it is estimated that roughly 5 million abortions occur annually in India, of these, about half a million are performed under the health services network, while another 4.5 million occur illegally. Adolescents largely unmarried constitute a relatively large proportion of abortion seekers.

"Adolescent girls constitute a disproportionate (25%) portion of the 5 million abortions performed annually" (NIPCCD, 1998). Studies have shown that lack of information on contraception, the cost of health, lack of confidentiality, limited access to safe services and delay in realising or admitting to the pregnancy among adolescent girls, are some of the main causes of abortions in adolescent girls.

STD And RTIS in Adolescents

Adolescents also constitute the group most susceptible to STDs due to physiological and social factors. Yearly, 5 per cent of all adolescents contract STD. RTIs including STDs, are now being recognised as a serious health problem especially with the recognition of the role that RTIs play in the transmission of HIV/AIDS. All community based prevalence studies of women's health that have been conducted in India indicate that the rates of RTIs are very high.

Young people are at a greater risk of contracting STDs due to early onset of sexual activity, frequency of partner change and reluctance to use barrier methods. Every year, 1 out of 20 adolescents contracts a curable STD, not including viral infections. Also, of the estimated 333 million new STDs that occur globally every year, at least 111 million occur in younger people aged 10-24 years (UNFPA, 1998). Although, most of these are treatable and curable if caught early, young people are likely to be ashamed and guilty about contracting it, likely to delay or avoid diagnosis and more prone to self-treatment, which can prove very dangerous (NIPCCD, 1997).

When young people lack guidance and information, and measures to prevent exposure are inadequate, they will be less likely to seek timely professional medical help and more likely to undertake dangerous self-treatment. The consequences of this may be permanent impairment of health, infertility, psychological damage and even death, with long-term affects not only on their immediate families but also on society as a whole.

Contraception in Adolescent Girls

Adolescents have little, inadequate and incorrect information about fertility and contraception. Even if they come to know of contraceptives, few use them, which may be because of ignorance or difficulty in obtaining them (FPAI, 1998). Further, a study done by UNFPA has shown that knowledge of family planning in India is far from being universal. Although knowledge of one contraceptive method, usually sterilisation is nearly universal, general knowledge of four or more methods is still low. Lack of knowledge breeds and perpetuates myths and misconceptions. In India, 44 per cent of currently married women aged 15-45 years practice family planning. Male participation in accepting the responsibility for contraception is also low; only 1.9 per cent of total sterilisation's were vasectomies in 1997, according to a national level survey finding. (UNFPA, 2000)

Statistics show that the age of women and the level of contraceptive use are closely linked, i.e. age increases, the use of contraceptives also increases. Besides this, illiteracy is another factor that contributes to low contraception usage.

Another development aspect that may influence the use of contraception involves the fact that adolescents are usually still influenced by the values of their parents and other adults. As a result, they are less likely to obtain contraceptives beforehand.

Adolescents and Reproductive Health

The health of adolescents is a concern that has gained prominence during the last decade both in developed and developing countries. Reproduction related health matters are of vital importance to young people as they take on their adult roles. As stated above, while adolescence is a time of growing sexual awakening and interest, there is tremendous curiosity but little authentic information on sexuality.

Adolescent sexual and reproductive health refers to the physical, mental and emotional well-being of adolescents, and includes freedom from unwanted pregnancy, unsafe abortion, sexually transmitted infections (STIs), including HIV/AIDS, and all forms of sexual violence of coercion. In the past, adolescents were largely neglected in both health and family planning programmes. This is partly explained by the fact that in many societies adolescent are not considered sexual beings until their marriage. Another factor in this systematic neglect is the unfounded fear that providing information and services would encourage premarital sexual activity.

Since the subject of adolescence sexuality remains taboo in most societies, there is widespread ignorance among young people of the risk associated with unprotected sexual activity. When young people lack guidance and information, they are less likely to seek timely professional medical help and more likely to undertake dangerous self-treatment. The consequences of this may be permanent impairment of health, infertility, psychological damage and even death.

A further problem of uninformed and unprotected adolescent's sexual activity is the increased exposure to STDs. A major set of problems of reproductive health in adolescents results from the profound socio-economic change- taking place in most developing countries. The average age of menarche has fallen, there is a trend towards later marriage and young people and often less, directly supervised than was the case in the past – all of which have the effect of increasing the opportunities for sexual encounter.

These above illustrated studies, highlight the need for education to address mistaken attitudes and help these young people realise their greatest potential.

Reproductive Health : Its meaning and importance

Reproductive health is a state of complete physical, mental and social well-being are not merely absence of disease and infinity in all matters related to the reproductive system and to its functions and processes. (Programme of Action adopted at International Conference on Population and Development, Cairo, September 1994).

Reproductive health, therefore, implies that people are able to have a satisfying safe sex life and that they have the capacity to reproduce and the freedom to decide if, when and how often to do so. Implicit in this last condition is the right of men and women to be informed and to have access to safe, effective and affordable and acceptable methods of family planning of their choice, as well as other methods of choice for regulation of the fertility which are not against the law, and the right to access the appropriate health care services that will enable women to go safely through pregnancy and child birth and provide couples with the best chance of having a healthy infant.

It also includes sexual health, the purpose of which is the enhancement of personal life and relations, and not mere counselling and care related to reproductive and sexually transmitted diseases.

Reproductive Rights

There are certain Reproductive Rights recognised with reproductive health. These have been endorsed and strengthened at the fourth world conference at Beijing in1995.

The reproductive rights are :

1. Right to reproductive and sexual health.
2. Right to reproductive decision-making.
3. Right to equality for men and women.

4. Right to sexual and reproductive security, including freedom from sexual violence and coercion and the right to privacy.

The UNFPA, the WHO and the International Planned Parenthood Federation make the protection of reproductive rights a central focus of their work. These rights entail –

1. Right to life.
2. Right to liberty and security of the person.
3. Right to equality, and to be free from all forms of discrimination.
4. Right to privacy.
5. Right to freedom of thought.
6. Right to information and education.
7. Right to choose whether to marry or not to marry and to find a life partner and plan a family.
8. Right to decide whether to have or not to have children.
9. Right to health care and protection.
10. Right to the benefit of scientific progress.
11. Right to freedom of assembly and political participation.
12. Right to be free from torture and ill treatment.

(*Source* : Parivar Seva Sanstha, Newsletter; *Sampark,* Reproductive Rights – Increased Choices For Women; July-September 2001)

Reproductive Health Approach

Reproductive health approach links demographic concerns including fertility reduction with a range of other objectives like improving the health and socio-economic status of women. The 1994 ICPD report established a growing international consensus on a new approach to policies to achieve population stabilisation.

Reproductive Health programmes should focus on the needs of the actual and potential clients, not only for limiting births but also for healthy sexuality and child bearing. In India, the implications of the reproductive health approach would be to shift the focus from the use of family planning as tool intended essentially for population stabilisation to using family planning as long as one among a constellation of interventions that would enable women and men to achieve their personal reproductive goals without being subject to the additional burdens of disease and death associated with their reproduction. Such a shift in emphasis is more likely to address the needs of women who are at risk of unwanted birth and in doing so assist the country to accelerate fertility decline.

Reproductive health interventions would enable clients to make informed choice, to receive counselling and education for responsible and healthy sexual behaviour; to access user-friendly service for preventing unwanted pregnancy and safe abortion; maternity care and child survival and management of reproductive tract infections.

Adolescent Reproductive Health Needs

The need to promote culturally sensitive family life education to reach adolescents in and outside of school settings :

- The need to provide a full range of accessible, acceptable and affordable ARH services;
- The need to train services providers about the special needs of ARH programmes;
- The need for advocacy in support of the development of ARH policies;
- The need for more data and research on ARH;
- The need to promote gender equality in adolescents in the design of programmes affecting ARH;
- The need for management information on special needs of adolescents for policy and programme development;
- The need to train youth on "leadership skills"; and
- The need to study the socio-cultural issues and utilise the relevant materials to support programme promotion and implementation.

Role of Mass Media

In the process of discovering their sexuality, adolescents rely heavily on mass-media entertainment – radio, T.V., films, magazines, books and more. What young people see and read about sex in popular entertainment is often what they do. However, it has been observed that T.V. being a family entertainment channel does not cover sexual aspects explicitly and have little importance for acquiring information about sexual development and reproductive health. It has been observed that information and knowledge gained through media is usually inadequate, improper, unrealistic and titillating. Doubts are seldom clarified, emotional relationships remain unexplained and responsibility never taught. On the contrary, they spread increased sexual and gender stereotypes.

Influence of Peer Group

Friends and peers play an important and predominant role for girls in providing emotional support in issues related to sexual development and reproductive health. Adolescent girls get the majority of their insight about reproductive health by discussing with each other. However, what they learn from each other is probably very little, as far as accurate information is concerned.

In the absence of proper guidance from the adults, adolescents obtain information from media and their friends who are equally ill informed. As a result, they usually succumb to bear pressure and develop social myths related to sexual behaviour." (*India Today*, 1998)

"Peer groups are acknowledged as a credible source of information. Project interventions should therefore focus on strengthening information delivery through peer group mechanisms, wherever possible." (UNFPA, 2000)

Role of Schools

(School-based interventions through "Family Life Education" Programmes – A recent phenomena in India)

With more children than ever before receiving education, schools are an efficient way to reach school aged children in an organised way. School also holds potential to have positive effect on health and learning of students.

Since most parents are reluctant to impart Reproductive Health Education due to lack of knowledge and fear of consequences, this leaves the school authorities and teachers to take up the responsibility. Among all the agencies, which touch the lives of children, school is the only institution, which leaves the opportunity to have children over a prolonged period.

In India, population education has been integrated into the school curriculum since 1980.

However, this has concentrated mainly on micro-demographic issues. Currently, the AIDS pan-epidemic has given fresh impetus to school reproductive health programmes. The Ministry of Health and Family Welfare has joined hands with Ministry of Education and Department of Youth Affairs to impart AIDS education among school children. Family Life Education (FLE) is the only widespread programme for youth adults all over the world. These brief programmes, held mostly in schools, may encourage abstinence, teach reproductive health and physiology, build skills in problem solving, decision-making, and life planning, and in a few cases, discuss contraception. Many now cover HIV/AIDS as well, while other in school and outreach programme focus exclusively on AIDS prevention. Impact has been modest. FLE programmes can increase knowledge and improve attitude toward health sexual behaviour.

However, it is equally important that unless teacher has a positive attitude towards imparting instructions on sexual development and related facts to youth in schools, any programmes of introducing Reproductive Health Education in curriculum may not be successful.

"The school has the potential to provide an excellent base for large-scale programming and high coverage of adolescents in countries but lacks adequate staff, space, materials and time for training and adapting prototype curricula to reproductive health needs of adolescents". (WHO, 1999)

Parent-Child Communication

It is generally agreed that home should be the best source of child's first exposure to the information about sexual matters, to gain standards of acceptable behaviour, self-control and the realisation of the role of its sex in adult life.

"Parents do not inform their children about sexual development and other issues deliberately since they fear that sexual enlightened and educated youth will want to implement and act out this sex knowledge directly in his behaviour. In other words, it might dispel irrational anxieties about sex and lead to sexual experimentation." (Powers and Baskin, 1969)

"Studies indicate that parents do not talk to their children about sexual development and reproductive health since they feel themselves to be ill equipped and uncomfortable to dose. They are embarrassed to initiate or participate in discussions about these matters with their children" (UNFPA, 1993).

B. GOVERNMENT APPROACH, POLICIES AND PLANS*

Introduction

While worldwide one-fifth of the population is that of the adolescents (March 2000), in India they account for 22.8 per cent, i.e., 230 million between the age groups of 10 to 19 years. As they are the future of the country, bearing in mind their population numbers and special needs, it might be one of the ways to also contribute to the socio-economic development of the country. This includes gender justice, population stabilisation and through harmonious living, improving the quality of life, and moving towards positive stimulation through providing a congenial environment. This, in order that they recognise themselves as productive and participating citizens of the country and their respective sub-societies, by imbibing them with idealism.

Several working groups have debated at length on policies and programmes to define the parameters for the group of adolescents. For example, in the Draft Youth Policy they have been defined as the age group between 13-19 years for boys and from 11-18 years for girls; constitutional and labour laws consider those of the 14 age groups as children, whereas the Reproductive and Child Health Programmes mention adolescents between the age 10-19 years, the same as is done by UN agencies. Considering all this, the Planning Commission Report states that it would be most appropriate to consider the 10-19 age group as a definition in many contexts.

The Approach

The complex and inter-sectoral nature of adolescents implies that no one sector is more crucial than the others to influence the entire range of factors are that impact on the situation of adolescents in India. To reiterate, any policy-framework therefore must acknowledge the importance of a multidimensional approach and that of a holistic perspective. The analysis of the current situation is

---

* Based on the *Report of the Planning Commission working group for 10th Plan, 2000-2001.*

this; the government can play a positive interventionist role by focusing on key areas that have wide ramifications.

Adolescents are important since they will be equal citizens as adults who are expected to participate in democratic processes. They have an inalienable right to good education, training and information on a range of issues, including health and reproductive rights so that they can make informed choices free from influence and coercion. Here it is important to differentiate between the socio-cultural expectation and economic pressures working on adolescent girls and boys so that the policy and programmes need to be designed keeping in view these gender differences and avoid stereotypes currently prevalent in the society. Consequently, all programmes need to bear the inclusion of both boys and girls and there is evidence for this that by the exclusion one group from the other, many self-developmental programmes have suffered. It may be noted that those programmes that have simultaneously worked with boys and girls in the same community have recorded positive changes in the larger social milieu.

In this context, the Report says that the needs and aspirations of poor children in the rural and urban areas have to be kept in mind also, as these are different from those of the middle classes, i.e., the situation needs to be prioritised in favour of the most disadvantaged of the urban and the rural poor. Further, it says, the following programmes are the critical areas of national concern which will attract adolescents, sustain their motivation by their full involvement in the developmental objectives :

- Education levels that prepare the ground for social, cultural and economic advance.
- Health and nutrition that effects inter-generational impact.
- Delayed girls marriage age that is correlated to education delayed childbirth and lower mortality and morbidity among the new borns.
- Environment and sanitation.
- Entrepreneurship through development skills in economic activities.
- Empowering new strategies for increasing livelihood possibilities so that poverty is eradicated.
- Creation of a new culture of compassion genders equity, and so on.

- Education of adolescents is important because it is obviously a special period, physically, emotionally and cognitively so that ideally it should be so designed that it helps in their development. This is being emphasised because at present school curriculum are far from being relevant for the majority of this group, despite the recommendations of the National Policy on Education. The subject and activity taught seldom matches their identity and specific problems, which have a lot to do with motivation, interests, personal inclination, etc. These groups' own intuitive constructions and theories need to be kept in mind.
- An important area is that of health education, which is often neglected since formal school curriculum seldom looks at health in a holistic manner in terms of the human body, its normal functioning, disease and prevention to causes of malnourishment, social deprivation and even social beliefs and indigenous knowledge about health and disease.

Situational Analysis

Taking the above into account, given that literature is sketchy in this regard, a situational analysis may be attempted if planning as to be based on a realistic and reliable assessment of the situation. The following headings may be prove useful.

Population distribution in age groups.

Because of high fertility during the last two decades, the share of the population of adolescents has risen sharply and this requires special attention by the fact of sheer numbers and will determine the size and growth pattern of India's population.

Sex Ratio

According to 2001 Census, the female to male ratio is 933 : 1000, indicating perhaps gender discrimination and other factors. It varies from state to state, of course, viz. 1058 in Kerala, 990 are Chattisgarh, and 861 are Haryana and 874 in Punjab. There is obviously the son-preference syndrome in India, so that girls are most often neglected social and physical, so that 25 per cent or 3 million girls never get to see the age of 15, and even high mother mortality between 15-19 years of age. Hence it is crucial to consider this gender discrimination in any planning process.

Education and Literacy

The positive influence of the above factors is well known, such as education of girls and lower fertility, child mortality and other social development indicators. While gender gaps in terms of literacy has been increasing and is less than 10 per cent as against 20 per cent before the 1990s female literacy rose by 24 per cent between 1981 and 1991.

For girls between the age of 10-14, and by 22.5 per cent between the age of 15-19 years. The corresponding figures for boys are 10.2 per cent and 9.2 per cent respectively.

It is thus notable that only 49.6 per cent of boys and 30.6 per cent of girls in the 15-19 age group have ventured beyond middle class school in rural India. Corresponding figures for urban areas are 67.4 per cent for boys and 63.8 per cent for girls. There is a wide range in terms of regional variations, e.g., in Kerala it is 93.24 per cent for boys and 97.15 per cent for girls all between the 11-14 age group; while for Rajasthan female enrolment is 33.5 per cent and male enrolment is 78.57 per cent; and so on. There are similar variations and some inexplicable declines in various states, and some of the causes are poor attendance, high dropout rates, and inaccessibility of schools, unimaginative and dysfunctional schools, disinterestedness of teachers, social attitudes and expectations. Girls are especially burdened because of taking care of siblings, domestic responsibilities, and absence of female teachers and low parental educational levels.

Drop-out rates are high such as between class I to X it is 70 per cent and even then only 40-60 per cent get through class X and XII examinations. Many people feel that schools don't teach dignity of labour, so that adolescents tend to aspire for white-collar jobs and in this sense 90 per cent of the youth are considered to be unemployed, instead of being an asset to the country.

Psychological Concerns

Given the sensitivities involved at this age, when habits and behavioural patterns are formed in addition to skills, developed exposure to social and cultural values is important, especially at this times of exposure to different media and other global influences. A pilot study by Urivi Vikram Charitable Trust indicated for example the following :

- 73 per cent of students could not communicate with their parents and 56 per cent even with their friends.
- 31 per cent did not understand much in class and 28.5 per cent students were not able to study effectively.
- 40 per cent student found difficult to concentrate and 37% examination fear and fear of failure.

Career Options

As a consequence of all these factors there are little career options and adolescents are driven into vocations and careers unrelated to their aptitude and suitability. Choices are made out of parental and social pressures, and there is almost a complete lack of career guidance.

There thus arises the possibility of deviant behaviour, especially drug abuse, pre-marital sex, anti-social behaviour; 4.54 per cent were drug-users in the age group 12-17, and 13.86 per cent in the age group of 18-23 years.

One may say that no knowledge of sexuality, menstruation and reproduction is provided in a healthy manner so that distorted notions are perpetuated among adolescents and this is the case in rural India also where even knowledge of contraception, STDs and AIDs is not known. All this has led to anti-social behaviour and high crime rates in many regions. Adolescents counselling, information and health services are therefore a must for planning purposes.

Nutrition

Nutrition is very important at this stage of life in terms of weight gain, height and skeletal mass gain. There are hardly any programmes for this purpose as the focus is on lactating mothers or pre-school children. If malnutrition at this stage is not recognised it leads to other malfunctions obviously. For instance, rapid growth of already malnutritioned children increases the severity of under-nutrition, iron deficiency leading to anaemia that is harmful for adolescent girls that later leads to the risk of miscarriages, maternal mortality, birth of still born and poor academic performance and low productivity, etc. To Illustrate, in Rajasthan 93.3 per cent girls suffered from 1-3 degree of chronic energy deficiencies, and the caloric intake was deficient by 26 to 36 per cent along with a 23-32 per cent deficiency in proteins.

Age at Marriage

There is high correlation between the age at marriage, fertility management and family health with educational levels. While the marriage for illiterate girls is 15 years, it is 22 years for women who have completed school. 30 per cent of adolescents (age group 15-19) are married and those between 25-29 years 94 per cent were married (NFHS-1998-99). In rural areas the age is about two and a half years less compared to the urban areas. The median age at first birth for women (20-49 years) is 19.6, and the 68.3 per cent for adolescents married before they are 18 in Rajasthan, 76 per cent in Bihar, 17 per cent in Kerala and 11.6 per cent in Punjab.

Fertility Rates

Most fertility occurs within marriage, so that this institution is of paramount importance for knowing about fertility rates. NFHS 1 report of 1992-93 states that 36 per cent of married adolescents (age group 13-16 years) are already mothers or pregnant with their first child, those in the 17-19 age group are 64 per cent. These fertility rates differ from state to state, e.g. adolescent fertility is 153 births (per 1000) in Madhya Pradesh, 143 in Haryana, 141 in Maharashtra, and as low as 38 is Kerala. Thus, it seems that while knowledge about family planning is becoming widespread, availability of services is lacking especially for the age group between 15-19.

Age-specific Mortality

While adolescents are generally healthy compared to old age groups, the male-female differentials in mortality is very noticeable, probably because of the low nutritional diet of the girls and early marriage that often leads to maternal morality.

Crimes against Adolescents

Violence is a global phenomenon and India with its growing urban and semi-urban areas at effect of the new technological changes, life-style patterns, etc. is no exception to this specially against women and girls. Adolescents are both perpetuated and perpetrators of crimes. This is a growing phenomena both at home and outside which has taken many shapes and forms, ranging from eve-teasing and abduction to rape, incest, battering and so on; along with it the social stigma that is attached to the females which prevents registration with the police and very few, therefore, convictions.

Policies and Major Programmes Concerning Adolescents

Ninth Five Year Plan (1997-2002)

This document mentions adolescents mainly in the sections on women and children, health and youth. This includes commitments towards the child, to universalise supplementary feeding with a special emphasis on adolescent girls, to expand girl's scheme and to assess the health needs of adolescents in the RCH programme. However, adolescents are not treated as a separate category, and considered to be as human capital for productive development, less than a commitment to their recognition as human beings, people.

Draft National Youth Policy (2001)

This document provides a comprehensive overview of youth issues and concerns which come closest to a policy on adolescents. Nevertheless there is no official policy about it. It does however state "that working with youth and not merely for youth" does suggest the importance of their participation; and in this manner providing space for the contribution of you to communities and to social development. The thrust areas of empowerment gender equity and an inter-sectoral approach hints at a move towards a right approach and a people-centred approach to development. It also gives a special focus to adolescent health, their education including non-formal education and their nutritional requirements as 'they are the most important segment of the population'.

National Policy on Education (1986 modified in 1992)

It emphasises the eradication of illiteracy especially for the 15-35 age group and universalisation of primary education. However, it too fails to recognise adolescents as a separate group *per se,* even though it talks about meeting the vocational needs at the high secondary level.

National Population Policy (2000)

It has recognised the earlier invisibility of adolescent's views them as a section, which needs to be addressed, and that they will play a crucial role in the context of replacement level of fertility when hopefully the population of India will stabilise. There is a special mention about developing a health package for adolescents and enforcing the legal age at marriage.

Draft Health Policy (1999)

It fails also to follow a life-cycle approach to the health needs of women, and it is in this wider context of women that the health of adolescents is mentioned with regard to their nutritional needs, not treated as a separate group.

Draft National Aids Policy (2000)

In this context too specific mentions of adolescents is neglected even though they are crucially relevant in terms of the strategy of the national health policy, as unprotected sex is a major source of AIDS, and STDs because of lack of sex educational, experimentation, peer pressure, etc. that makes adolescents a especially vulnerable segment.

National Nutrition Policy (1983)

This too does not focus on the youth as a separate category, in fact boys are not even mentioned, it is only girls within the role as mothers and housewives that there is any mention of adolescents as a group.

National Policy for the Empowerment of Women (2001)

This document recognises the girl-child as a separate category and adolescent girls seem to be covered thereunder, for purposes of nutrition, education, violence against them, sexual abuse, their rights and a holistic approach to health.

In general one may thus conclude that though adolescents are mentioned in the various documents mentioned above, none of them address themselves to a holistic view of adolescents as such. It is high time then that a nodal department is needed to co-ordinate and monitor policies and interventions for adolescents and needs clear visibility in terms of their perceptions and participation in all of the areas of nutrition, health, education, health, family welfare, AIDS/STD and other diseases, sports, etc. This approach even in the States is being followed in terms of the Centre's thrust areas.

Programmes for Adolescents

Without specific mention of adolescent needs in any comprehensive schemes, a number of government departments have interventions that impact the lives of adolescents, nevertheless these are vertical programmes that do not take an integrated view. Some of these are as follows :

(i) Kishori Shakti Yojana, earlier called Adolescent Girls Scheme, in the department of women and child development, for improving the nutritional and health status of girls (11-18 years), through non-formal system, providing vocational and home-based skills, etc. In this the Balika Smridhi Yojana aims at delaying the age of marriage and finally eliminating child marriages.

(ii) The Nehru Yuvak Kendras have health awareness programmes through various activities, to provide a forum for increasing awareness of many of the issues mentioned all along.

(iii) The implementation by a central ministry to provide educational facilities including scholarships and hostels for tribal girls.

(iv) The Mahila Samakhya programmes which aims at ensuring, equal access to educational facilities for adolescent girls and young women. It runs the Mahila Shikshan Kendra in project areas in Karnatak, Gujarat, Uttar Pradesh, Andhra Pradesh, Bihar, Madhya Pradesh and Assam. Kishori Melas and other activities are organized to create educational opportunities for self-development. Sarva Shikha Abhiyan as part of the

National Literacy Mission provides quality elementary education to children between the age of 6-14 years.

(v) Department of Family Welfare has its Reproductive and Child Health Programmes to provide for maternal care, including safe motherhood and nutrition facilities, etc. that are subsumed under the general target group of women. There being no mention of boys in these schemes.

(vi) The Department of Health has programmes that cover school Aids education, which includes radio and TV talks, and running de-addiction, centres and the NGOs do the same.

(vii) Rajiv Gandhi Drinking Water Mission that provides safe drinking water and sanitation facilities in all schools in India.

(viii) The Directorate General of Employment and Training provides facilities of registration in employment exchanges, and vocational training to adolescents after class VIII or X.

(ix) The Swarn Jayanti Swarozgar Yojana (SGYS) provides vocational and skill training to youth and adolescents and also Training of Rural Youth for Self-Employment; both run by the Ministry of Rural Development.

(x) Lok Jumbish, Rajasthan organises since 1992 residential Adolescents' Girls Camps of about 6 months duration for providing primary education and various empowerment activities, and reproductive health other relevant issues for adolescents.

(xi) In Haryana, the Department of Women and Child Development provides information and generates awareness regarding basic health, sanitation and reproductive health. They also implement life skills for adolescents for personal, physical and mental development.

(xii) There are a fairly large number of NGOs, which address adolescent issues either in an integrated manner or sectorally, especially the involvement of adolescents and the community from the project formulation stage itself.

Areas of Focus on Adolescent Girls

Young girls are drawn into adulthood rather soon, with no time to explore their own person hood, because of taking care of young siblings, even rearing their own children, responsibilities of household thrust upon them. In this way they are confined within closing boundaries that are defined by social norms that have to be carried out even if it means subservience, sacrifice, uncritical obedience, etc. Consequently, they are inhibited, dependent, insecure, and other psychological complexes within this vast socio-cultural scenario.

Thus, there is an urgent need to have a structure that provides broad educational opportunities and strategies to discover for the girls their potential and become empowered citizens. This is a challenge that requires interventions, some of which have started already by many agencies, in the areas of health and nutrition issues, economic activities and educational programmes. Wherever such schemes have functioned they have provided role models not only for the younger siblings but even the older sisters and women in the larger community question of gender discrimination and greater resistance of violence towards them.

It is in this context that residential education camps have been an extremely effective mechanism for providing support for a learning environment. When such education is available the girls can be weaned away from household responsibilities, towards becoming trained leaders for other girls in specific programmes, such as female literacy which is very low generally speaking. Here the aim is to integrate education with life skills, vocational, and social awareness for developing holistic models of education.

This approach requires the creation of a learner-friendly environment with a flexible curriculum, as also involving the girls in decision-making process and management of camps and centres. The teachers in these camps have to be carefully chosen so that the girls who come there after fighting great odds in both the home and the social set up imbibe these values. This is why it is crucial in these interventions, to have women facilitators and workers who continue to garner family support and are able to mobilise the community so that newly trained girls are influential for others to aspire for the same results. It is here that the role of the mother is crucial, especially in getting support from the peer groups during and after the camp. This is helpful in the long run since follow-up activities are required for the girls need to be absorbed in a subsequent developmental programme, say, as teacher or health workers, etc.

For instance, the "Educating Adolescent Girls; Opening Windows, Janshala Program, 2001" has shown visible benefits. The girls became very attentive, hard working, and exceptionally keen to learn, had exhilarating experience, their personalities changed into one of self-esteem, confidence and having the ability to communicate with others. For some parents it was a matter of pride to seem them like this and some even managed to postpone their *'gauna'* or early marriage. All this was possible because of the absence of an authoritarian-bureaucratic set-up, which is always judgemental and even discriminative having no sensitivity for the girls who are already coming from a state of being marginalised. This scheme goes beyond textbooks and their potential is discovered through song, dance, theatre, craft as well as games.

In short, the aim is to design such an interesting and meaningful curriculum that can compensate for the early years of social and educational neglect, so that it motivates the girls to continue with enhanced zeal and confidence; that is, it empowers them to change their own situation in life and the community around them.

New Strategies and Opportunities

For purposes of providing the above stated meaningful and empowering learning environment, the plans have to be very innovative, truly relevant and life-oriented. Some voluntary groups and government programmes are currently carrying these out but more concerted effort is required all over the country, each state on a sustained basis. The following is a suggestive list of possible activities that provide diverse educational opportunities to adolescents :

- Residential Camps and Institutions.
- Village Melas on Health and various issues.
- Community Action Projects managed by the young, e.g. watershed management, afforestation, etc.
- Village/mobile libraries run by youth.
- Kalajathas and Travelling Theatres based on performing arts.
- Open Learning Courses.

Summing Up

In India, adolescents account for one-fifth of the population with an estimated 200 million adolescents. Adolescents are very vulnerable group of society, and especially adolescent girls. All these girls are going to be mothers of near future. Any lacunae in their reproductive health can have harmful effects in the long run and short term. This age group (14-19 years) was specifically chosen for Action Research in the Kumaon Hills, as this is the period of rapid physical growth in adolescents, with development of primary and secondary sexual characteristics along with maturing of reproductive functioning. At this stage, needs and urges of adolescent are sexually oriented and they may indulge in wrong behaviour. Also the knowledge of sexual and reproductive health is extremely poor amongst adolescent girls and especially of slum and rural areas. This is why it becomes very important to impart training to the adolescent girls, living in remote areas of the Kumaon Hills, regarding their own reproductive functioning and related issues at this crucial age.

Adolescence is the age where school drop out rate is high among adolescent girls, thus preventing them from pursuing higher studies. Also as long as the problem of maternal mortality, teenage pregnancy, unsafe abortions, STDs and HIV/AIDS are allowed to persist much of the energy, creativity and idealism of youth will be lost to society. These problems are preventable provided the young girls themselves are involved in the elimination of these risks. These girls must be given every opportunity to develop to their full potential as healthy individual, after getting the correct information on the subject instead of hearsay sources of information. This study thus recognises and addresses the diversity of reproductive health needs effectively, and hopefully will help to further develop a holistic approach in order to address the problems of adolescent girls in the hill regions, so as to result in healthy and responsible behaviour.

All the above reasons make it essential to focus on adolescent girls of the Kumaon Hills, and address their informational needs regarding reproductive health issues. The focus on adolescent girls of this area is an attempt to build the knowledge base and create awareness regarding reproductive health issues.

ADDRESSING THE NEEDS OF ADOLESCENTS – CHIRAG CONCEPT

CHIRAG, as stated in Chapter 3 has been working at the grass roots level for nearly 15 years in the Kumaon Hills. Not withstanding the usefulness and importance of all its interventions, it is amply clear that something vital remained lacking at this juncture. Instead of reacting to repair the damage that has already taken place, the focus of development work in the region has to shift to pro-active, preventive and promotional activities, i.e. what the community does for itself to remain healthy and keep its environment healthy. This is imperative to make the process self-sustaining and sustainable.

This pro-active approach can only be achieved through education, training and motivation in a systematic and sustained manner. Only thus will villagers accept and participate in new approaches, attitudes, and appropriate technology. Women are potentially the most effective community based agents to bring about this awareness as they occupy a crucial role in the subsistence economy of these isolated communities. Not only do the women of these mountain villages fulfil household duties, but also they have the additional responsibility of taking care of the cattle, collecting firewood and fodder from forests, and fetching water from springs.

Of primary importance is the need to create a sense of self-confidence among women in their ability to improve the quality of their lives with the minimum of external assistance. With this objective, CHIRAG has been able to form over sixty women's groups with a membership of over 750 women. Highly successful women's empowerment (*Mahila Shakti*) programme helped provide technological alternatives that greatly reduced the drudgery of women of many mountain villages. Income generation programmes have assisted many women gain financial independence. While such programmes are very useful, the need has been felt for a programme to empower young adolescent women of the area. Typically, women aged 25-60 are associated with the women's programmes currently coordinated by Chirag. Younger girls, or those newly married, are often unable to participate either because they are in school, or as new *'bahus'* (daughter-in-law) they are expected to do housework. A need has been expressed for initiating a programme aimed at these young women. This is particularly important as young women, typically get married and relocate outside CHIRAG's project areas. Many of these women have been to primary schools or *balwadi's* administered by CHIRAG, or have seen their mothers attend CHIRAG's women's groups meetings or benefit from biogas plants built by CHIRAG. Yet once they marry and move away, they are on their own and lack the self-confidence to play an effective role in their new community.

To fulfil this need, CHIRAG established a Learning Centre for adolescent girls, *Kishori Shikshan Kendra*, for young women in the age group 13 to 20 years. Unmarried girls, who had studied to at least class-V, would be the target group. There are hardly any girls in the region that have not completed primary schooling. However, many girls do dropout by the time they get to class VIII. The target group, therefore, covered mostly girls who had dropped out from mainstream education. Newly married young girls who had migrated into villages of the area were also included.

Objectives

The objective was to provide the future generation of rural women in Uttaranchal with a broad based educational programme which takes them beyond literacy and enhances their knowledge base, skills and abilities to deal with real life situations that they will face as adults. The idea was to empower them to play a more effective role in building a better future for themselves, their families and the community as a whole. Most importantly, this would help seed villages in areas where Chirag does not as yet work, with women who are self confident, knowledgeable about a range of issues, and able to act as catalysts for change in their new homes.

To achieve this goal it was intended to integrate the gender perspective in all the content areas as this would emphasize the significance of social and cultural change to overcome gender biases and discrimination. The fundamental principle guiding the selection of content, teaching methodology and curriculum would be to ensure that the overall approach is learner-centred, gender-sensitive, multi-sectoral and holistic. This is not to say that adolescent girls are being viewed merely as assets whose productive and reproductive potentialities need to be enhanced and regulated respectively. Chirag does not see them primarily as development objects. Such an approach automatically determines that only that which is useful is relevant. And usefulness is generally defined as that which directly betters their daily lives. While Chirag would ensure that the curriculum is relevant in the above context, the criteria for relevance and usefulness would be more holistic. It was envisaged that appropriate content and methodology would develop the Adolescent Girls' capacity for critical reflection and questioning.

The real challenge facing CHIRAG was to create a gender sensitive curriculum for Adolescent Girls to cover the whole gamut of interlinked "content" areas (to suit these mountain villages) and develop a teaching methodology which motivates attitudinal and behavioural changes. In addition, the future use of distance education would be kept in mind in developing the curriculum, which, in any case, will keep evolving and changing as the years go by. The principal content areas, which would be addressed at learning centre, are shown in the Figure 6.1 below :

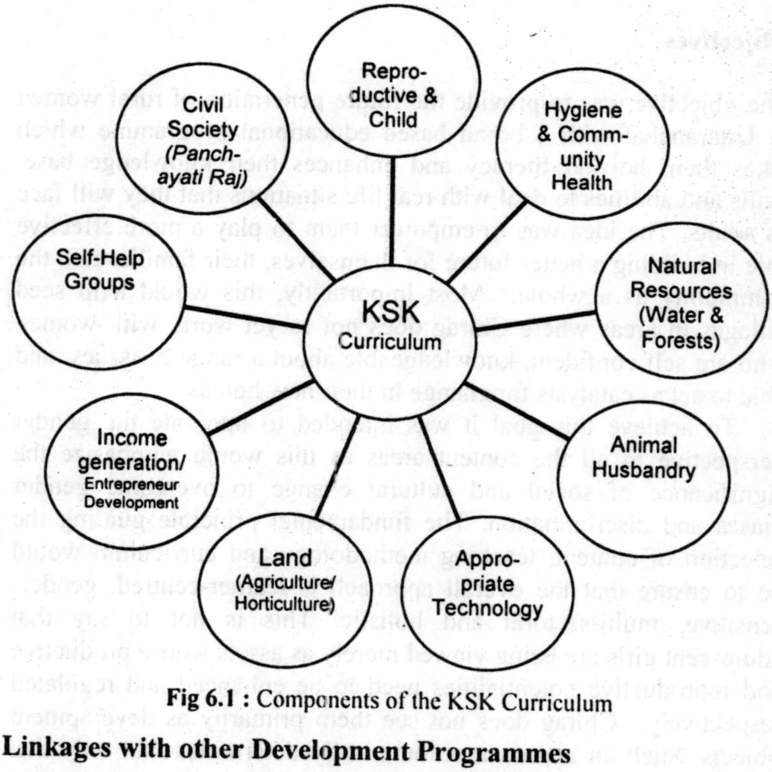

Fig 6.1 : Components of the KSK Curriculum

Linkages with other Development Programmes

It is important to recognize that such a programme for adolescents cannot exist in isolation and its success would naturally depend on the extent to which it is integrated with other interventions. As mentioned earlier, the concept of the Learning Centre evolved as a result of CHIRAG working in this area for more than a decade and the plan was to integrate it into the overall development process. Thus members of CHIRAG's health team would be involved in helping design and implement the RCH and community health modules, the in-house agricultural graduates will provide inputs for the land-care module, and so on.

Involving parents and encouraging community participation was to be important elements of this project. The focus was, firstly, on improvement of the status of adolescent girls and secondly, investment in them as the key to future development in the rural areas of Uttaranchal with a sensitive understanding of the fragile mountain ecosystem. CHIRAG does not underrate the importance of addressing the needs and concerns of adolescent boys in their own right but, given the dominant role that women play in the rural economy of Uttaranchal combined with the widespread gender discrimination, CHIRAG would like to give priority to adolescent girls. Once this project is well established, CHIRAG would formulate a similar and parallel programme for adolescent boys.

C. NEED ASSESSMENT FOR ADOLESCENT GIRL'S TRAINING CENTRE, CHIRAG

CHIRAG in its 15 years of development work in the Hill State of Uttaranchal has experienced that despite the implementation of development programmes at the village and community level there has not been any significant change in the status of youth in the region. One reason for this could be that the programmes so far have not focused on the interests and needs of this section of the population and in fact have laid no emphasis on creating awareness amongst the youth and involving them in the development process.

Keeping the above rationale in mind, CHIRAG felt the need for a training centre for adolescents in this region. Adolescent girls were chosen as the focus initially, because women are the backbone of the hill economy. The adolescent girls training centre would give training on skills related to issues and concerns that are paramount in the lives of the young girls who live in this region. Natural Resource Management, Income Generation, Health, Panchyati Raj, and all other areas dealing with the political, social and economic life in the community would be addressed.

Strategy

Phase 1 : Before establishing this centre it was deemed imperative to find out the perceptions of women and young adolescent girls about the creation of such a training centre.

For this purpose a questionnaire was developed in order to seek the responses primarily in the area covered by CHIRAG, namely, Sitla, Kasialekh, and Suyalbari. This was to elicit responses in the context of health, education, agriculture, environment and panchayati raj, etc. This individual and collective group contact was carried out in 32 villages with women and adolescent girls. The figures of this report are attached herewith.

Phase 2 : A detailed module would be prepared, based on the assessment of the existing knowledge and awareness of every subject, and would be tested at an informal level.

Objectives

- To elicit opinions with regard to the establishment of an adolescent training centre for girls.
- Establish rapport with the community.
- To find out in which areas or subjects the girls are interested in.
- On the basis of the above to develop a training strategy.

Method : Group and individual discussion on the basis of the questionnaire at an informal level.

Area : Sitla, Kasialekh, Suyalbari.

Age : 13 to 20 years

Findings of the Survey

Q. 1 What are the desires/aspirations of adolescent girls?

Table 6.1 : Desires/aspirations of adolescent girls

	Education	Female Progress	Employment	Right of decision making	Self-sufficient	Communication	Learning skills	Do something	Happy family	Contentment
Numbers	23	42	9	10	20	5	6	7	6	4
%age	16.3	29.8	6.4	7.1	14.2	3.5	4.3	5	4.3	2.8

From the 32 respondents, 141 multiple answers were received. 30 per cent of the respondents stated that there should be focus on women's development, 16 per cent said that they valued education and 14 per cent said that they would aspire to build self-confidence in themselves.

Q.2. What are the problems that a girl generally faces after marriage?

Table 6.2 : Problems faced by girls after marriage

	Harmony	Desire supp. By in-laws	Dowry Menstruation barren	Knowing.	Excess workload	Fear	No career.	Husband no support	Dual role
Numbers	23	20	14	9	17	8	4	6	4
%age	21.2	18.5	12.9	8.3	15.7	7.4	3.7	5.5	3.7

A majority of the respondents stated that the greatest problem they face after marriage is to create a place for themselves in their new household, and maintain a harmonious balance with all the family members. 18 per cent stated that they have to suppress their desires because of pressure from in-laws. 12 per cent of the respondents stated that segregation during menstruation; barriers and the emphasis on dowry are some of the other constraints they would face after marriage.

The other problems stated by them; dual role of women, no support from the husband and not being able to make a career for themselves. The responses clearly show that the adolescent girls were very aware of what happens after marriage.

Q. 3. What is the information that your daughter has about health? How aware is your daughter about the health issues?

Table 6.3 : Information about health issues

Personal hygiene	Food-drink	Vaccination	Home cleanliness	Home remedies	Protein	Environ sanitation	Covered food water	Primary first aid	Pregnancy problems	Problems	Lack of information
11	23	14	11	3	1	14	1	1	1	23	3
10.3	21.6	13.2	10.3	2.8	0.9	13.2	0.9	0.9	0.9	21.6	2.8

Only 21 per cent of the respondents had some knowledge about nutrition and a balanced diet, 21 per cent stated women face many health problems and only 13 per cent knew about personal hygiene, immunisation and household sanitation. In relation to health, 0.9 per cent had information about first aid or problems faced during pregnancy. Surprisingly only 2.8 per cent knew about home remedies to cure illness. During informal discussions with the adolescent girls while administering the above questionnaire, it came across that they did not know much about their own body, the reproductive system and how menstruation takes place.

Q.4. Do you think women/adolescent girls should be educated on life skills?

Table 6.4 : Adolescent girls' education about life-skills

How?	Yes	Know	Outside work	Computer	Social skills behaviour	Literacy/ signature	Accounts bank	Bus board
2	24	1	1	1	2	6	6	1
4.5	54 .5	2.2	2.2	2.2	4.5	13.6	13.6	2.2

54 per cent of the respondents stated that they would like to get information on how to deal with their life cycle events.

Q.5. Do you think your daughter should learn the art of managing the household at minimum expenditure?

Table 6.5 : Daughter should learn art of household managing

Yes	Very imp.	Budget/business.	Savings
29	10	6	2
61.7	21.2	12.7	4.2

61.7 per cent of the respondents said that it is very important for girls to learn the optimum utilisation of resources at the household level. Others stated that they would like to learn how to prepare a budget and plan their expenditure accordingly.

Q.6. Does your daughter know the appropriate use and maintenance of natural resources?

Table 6.6 : Knowledge about maintenance of natural resources

Traditional know-how.	Incomp. Information	Desire to know	Don't know	Little bit	No time
16	4	4	10	6	1
39	9-7	9-7	24-3	14-6	2-4

39 per cent of the respondents said that they knew traditional methods of utilising their natural resources for household consumption. 24 per cent said that they did not have any information about this, but would like to know more.

Q.7. Do you think your daughter should have information about agriculture and new technologies?

Table 6.7 : Information about agriculture and new technologies

Yes	Knowledge	Very important
30	1	2
71.4	2.3	4.7

71 per cent of the respondents said that if information about new technologies related to agriculture were given to them they would be extremely interested. Since women and adolescent girls work in the field this information or skill would be extremely useful to them.

Q.8. Do you think your daughter should know about the commercial aspect of animal breeding and their maintenance?

Table 6.8 : Knowledge about animal breeding and their maintenance

Yes	Very important
29	9
76.3	23.6

Almost all the respondents said that if they were given information about the breed of cattle and buffalo and how to take care of them, it would be very helpful to them. In Kumaon it is the women who take complete care of the animals.

Q.9. Do you think your daughter should have information about self-help groups?

Table 6.9 : Information about self-help groups

Yes.	Functional necessity	Know it
29	10	2
70.7	24.3	4.8

As regards the information about the formation of self-help groups nearly 94 per cent said that they would like to know about these self-help groups and their distinct features.

Q.10. Should your daughter know about the appropriate technology and micro-business?

Table6.10 : Knowledge about appropriate technology and micro-business

Yes	Very important	Unity of women/income generation
3	4	11
67	8-6	23-9

All the respondents both women and girls stated that they would like to get information on small-scale enterprises for income generation. They could see this as a pre-requisite to self-sufficiency and women's empowerment, as shown in the table below.

Q.11. Do you want your daughter to select a field of choice and use it for income generation to give and economic support to the family? If yes, which one?

Table 6.11 : Income generation and support to family

Yes	Jute	Embroi-ery	Sewing	Knitting	Crochet	Weaving	Dye	Food savouries	Computer
9	2	22	28	30	18	12	2	8	11
3.3	0.75	8.30	10.5	11.3	6.7	4.5	0.75	3	4.1

Papad	Soap	Candle	Card	Envelope	Chalk	Coaching map	Gardening	Screen printing	Animal husbandry
12	6	9	6	12	8	4	8	6	2
4.5	2.2	3.3	3.6	4.5	13	1.5	3	2.2	0.75

Block printing	Bindi	Tooth paste	Sofaset	Decoration things	Alpana	Wooden puppets	Krishi	Bee-keeping
2	9	8	1	15	6	4	4	1
0.75	3.3	3.1	0.37	5.6	2.2	1.5	1.5	0.37

A variety of responses were received to this question. The important aspect was that all the respondents felt that they need to learn some skill for income generation – weaving, knitting, embroidery and sewing were the more favoured skills for income generation.

Q.12. If you have to link your product to the market, what are your means and sources?

Table 6.12 : Means to link product to market

CHIRAG support	Outside support	Self-help	Women's coop	Society	Marketing facilities	Nearby shop
2	3	4	4	4	3	6
7.6	11.5	15.3	15.3	15.3	11.5	23

23 per cent of the respondents stated that they would market their produce in the nearby shop, as it would be easy to send their products there. 15 per cent women said that they would market their produce themselves through women's groups or societies.

Q.13. Do you feel to gain all this information a training institute should be established?

Table 6.13 : A training institution to be established for getting information.

Yes	Within the village	Nearest village	Very imp. Must	In winter also
23	2	2	2	1
76-6	6-6	6-6	6-6	3-3

All the respondents answered in the affirmative for the establishment of a training centre for adolescent girls. Some felt that it should be a residential training centre, while others stated that it should be located in their village or at the most the neighbouring village.

Q.14. If yes then what sort of training it should be? What are the resources and facilities it should have?

Table 6.14 : Type of training and its resources

Conducive environ no noise	Nearness	Safety factors	Roadside	Big centre	Vehicle	Good Arrangements	Latrines	Things; computer books	In village	Good trainers	Residential	Increase in income
19	5	4	3	3	7	3	2	14	5	7	6	11
21.3	5.6	4.4	3.3	3.3	7.8	3.3	2.2	15.7	5.6	7.8	6.7	12.3

21.3 per cent respondents said that it should have an environment conducive to learning, be in a quiet place and have infrastructure facilities like computers, be located on the roadside, have its own vehicle and should provide safety and security for the girls.

Q.15. Why do you want your daughter or yourself to get education?

Table 6.15 : Advantage of education

Yes	Will not be deceived	Decision-making	Good future	Self-sufficient	Will do more	For marriage	More knowledge	Difficulty in marriage
12	8	5	7	7	7	3	4	2
21.8	14.5	9.0	12.7	12.7	12.7	5.4	7.2	3.6

Women respondents stated that they would like to educate their adolescent girls so that they can be self-sufficient take their own decisions and have a good life in the future. 14.5 per cent also stated that she would not be deceived if she is educated.

Q.16. What are your expectations after the training?

Table 6.16 : Expectations from training

Increase in income	Decision for better life	Practical training	Increase knowledge	Recapitulation	Camaraderie	In winters	Health knowledge	Learn everything.	Successful housewife
17	6	2	11	4	2	1	1	7	1
32.6	11.5	3.8	21	7.6	3.8	1.9	1.9	13.4	1.9

32.6 per cent of the respondents said that after their training they would be able to increase their incomes, 21 per cent said that such a training would enhance their knowledge level, and some said it would give them skills to be a successful housewife!

Q.17. Will you send your daughter if CHIRAG establishes such a training centre?

Table 6.17 : To attend CHIRAG's training centre

Yes	Quickness in work	If in the village, then only	Safety and security
28	1	1	1
90.0	3.2	3.2	3.2

90 per cent of the respondents said yes to send their girls to such a centre, while 6.4 per cent said if it was held in their village and if the environment was safe and secure.

Highlights

From the Survey it became evident that women and adolescent girls were certain that a learning centre based on life-skills education and focusing on the major lifecycle events in a woman's life would be of great value for the future of women in this region. An integrated approach focusing on all aspects of the life of a woman in the hills was emphasised – much in line with CHIRAG's vision. Income generation, small business, self-sufficiency, skills in natural resource management, agricultural and animal husbandry and Reproductive Health information were seen as being useful.

On one of my visits to village Buribana in Dhari block, I learnt that Mahila Samakhya (head office Lucknow) had created Kishori Sanghs at the village level, to provide young girls a forum to speak about their concerns to each other. A Saheli who was in charge of the group had received training in Lucknow, and shared with me that a group of adolescent girls (13-19 years of age), met every Sunday near the village temple from 11 a.m. to 1 p.m.. (Fig. 6.2).

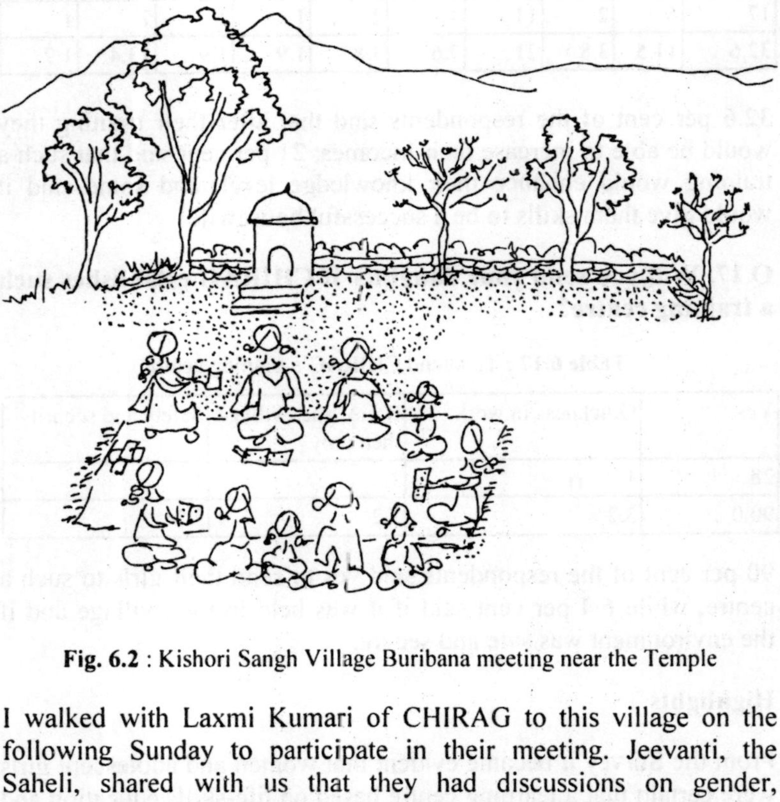

Fig. 6.2 : Kishori Sangh Village Buribana meeting near the Temple

I walked with Laxmi Kumari of CHIRAG to this village on the following Sunday to participate in their meeting. Jeevanti, the Saheli, shared with us that they had discussions on gender, patriarchy, social fabric of society, legal rights of women and so on at their meetings. When I asked them if they talked about health issues like segregation during menstruation, emotional and psychological changes experienced while growing up, marriage, reproduction, nutrition and health, self-development, they all said they would certainly like to know about all these issues but had not given much thought to it all.

When I shared CHIRAG's vision of a learning centre – they were all excited but expressed reservation about it being residential. So many ideas had come in, we had heard the voices of adolescent girls/mothers/young women, and it seemed very clear from their sharing that an adolescent training centre was a felt need.

D. A LEARNING CENTRE FOR ADOLESCENT GIRLS

Kishori Shikshan Kendra

Keeping the findings of the Need Assessment Survey in mind Chirag decided to establish a learning centre for the adolescents of the region. To reiterate, the adolescent girls were the main focus of this learning centre in the initial phase, as it is these girls who would grow up to be the future mothers. The training centre, aptly called the Kishori Shikshan Kendra (KSK) focused on a comprehensive training module that started with "understanding One-self" and went on to "Understanding the community" and "Local self-Governance and Legal Rights". It dealt with the personality development aspect of the adolescent girls and encompassed the technical training modules concerning all the vital life issues that women of these hill region come across in their lives. The entire training duration was that of six months with a number of vocational training sessions interspersed.

Objectives

The following were the major objectives of the training centre for the adolescent girls :

1. To provide the future generation of rural women in Uttaranchal with a broad based educational programme which takes them beyond literacy and enhances their knowledge base, skills, and abilities to deal with real life situations they will face as adults.
2. To empower them to play a more effective role in building a better future for themselves, their families, and the community as a whole.
3. To help seed villages in areas where CHIRAG does not as yet work, with women who are self-confident,

knowledgeable about a range of issues, and able to act as catalysts for change in their new homes.

4. To integrate the gender perspective in all the content areas so as to emphasize the significance of social and cultural change to overcome gender biases and discrimination.
5. To ensure that the overall approach to the training is learner-centered, gender-sensitive, multi-sectoral and holistic.
6. To create awareness, build capacity and sensitize these adolescents towards the existing components and forces of nature, the harmony in their equilibrium and appropriate management of the existing natural resources.

I have stated in the Prologue and Chapter 3 that CHIRAG's intervention at the grassroots level in the Kumaon Hills began with a focus on health. The role of women in the hill economy has been emphasized throughout the book and the detailed analysis of their health status has clearly reflected that these issues need to be addressed at multiple levels in a holistic manner.

From the integrated approach to life-skill education for adolescent girls, the component chosen for the first training was "Reproductive and Child Health Issues".

The Process

The first part of the book looked at the traditional health care practices of women in Kumaon Hills. It viewed this aspect in the following steps stated briefly:

- Secondary sources.
- Interviews with resource persons, *Dai's*, Community Health workers (CHWs) Health Extension workers (HEWs), NGO personnel staff, Chief Medical Officer (CMO), Primary Health Centre (PHC) staff.
- Study of 60 women in six villages of Ramgarh and Dhari Block of Nainital district with special reference to the reproductive phase
  - Menstruation
  - Pregnancy
  - Delivery

- Post Delivery
- Family Planning
- Child Health
- Major Health problems of women
- Food Intake
- Work roles

- Emerging Trends: A Holistic Perspective and Recommendations.

CHIRAG's Concept of a Learning Centre

- Need Assessment for Adolescent Girls' Training Centre, CHIRAG. Survey of 32 villages.
- A Learning Centre for Adolescent Girls – Kishori Shikshan Kendra. Detailed Focus on RCH for first training of Kishori Shikshan Kendra (KSK)

1.

Identification of modules Education materials on RCH For Adolescents	VHAI NIRANTAR JAGORI CEDPA UNFPA ASTHA	SUTRA CHETNA

2.

Desk Review of Modules/
Selection of choose a future
By CEDPA

3.

Based on analysis of Health Care practices of 60 women - developed A 5 day training module on RCH	Sharing Proposed module with resource person.

4.

Hiring Saheli's for mobilizing adolescent girls to join a training centre at two field centres
- Kasialekh
- Reetha.

5.

Admission Strategy :
Registration forms, nominal fees taken.

6.

a. Capacity building of CHIRAG staff:
'Training of trainers' (TOT) of Chirag field staff (23 participants) focus on Adolescent Health Issues. Methodology of use of 'choose a future' by the team from the NGO 'Prerna', Delhi. May 31st to June 4th, 2002. Dhokane Training Centre.

b. RCH training of Chirag field staff (the same participants as TOT in June 2002) 10th-11th August 2002.

7.

Formation of 2 groups of 20 adolescent girls each at Kasialekh and Reetha centre.

Mon. Tues. Wed. – Reetha	10-12 noon…vocational skill.
	12-2 p.m.… Life-skill education.
Thurs. Fri. Sat. - Kasialekh	10-12 noon…. Vocational skill.
	12-2 p.m.…Life-skill education.

8.

Strengthening attendance of adolescent girls at both field centres by:

- Home visits.
- Adopting an adolescent girl by CHIRAG field staff from the health team, the women's programme and MCC team.
- Inviting role models to address the group for sustaining their interest.

9.

The Course Components.

10.

a. First five day residential RCH training of adolescent girls from Reetha Centre (19 participants)
2nd-6th Sept. 2002 by *Prerna* team from New Delhi. Assisted by CHIRAG Staff at Dhokane Training Centre.

b. Second five-day residential RCH training workshop of Adolescent girls from Kasialekh (17 participants) by CHIRAG KSK staff and inputs by health Extension workers of CHIRAG.
11th-15th Nov. 2002 at Dhokane Training Centre.

11.

Innovation in the programme.

12.

Impact of Training.

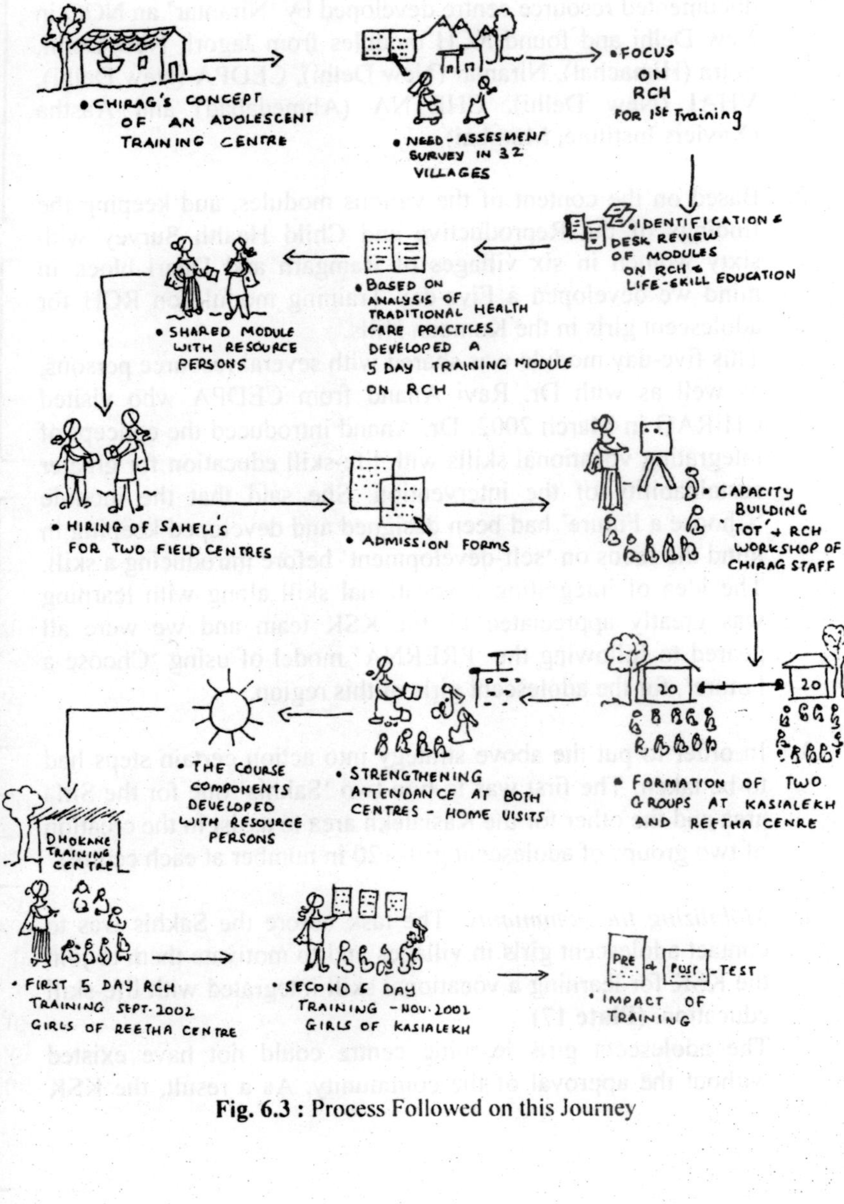

Fig. 6.3 : Process Followed on this Journey

Methodology

1. *Desk Review of Modules on RCH.* I visited various libraries and resource centres of NGOs and UN organizations working in the area of RCH. I met Mridula Seth from UNFPA, who shared with me several modules on RCH including the now published IWAG modules on life-skills education. I visited the well-documented resource centre developed by 'Nirantar' an NGO in New Delhi and found RCH modules from Jagori, New Delhi, Sutra (Himachal), Nirantar (New Delhi), CEDPA (New Delhi), VHAI (New Delhi), CHETNA (Ahmedabad) and Aastha (Xaviers Institute, Mumbai).

2. Based on the content of the various modules, and keeping the findings of the Reproductive and Child Health Survey with sixty women in six villages of Ramgarh and Dhari block in mind we developed a Five-day Training module on RCH for adolescent girls in the Kumaon Hills.
   This five-day module was shared with several resource persons, as well as with Dr. Ravi Anand from CEDPA who visited CHIRAG in March 2002. Dr. Anand introduced the concept of integrating vocational skills with life-skill education for greater sustainability of the intervention. She said that the module 'Choose a Future' had been designed and developed keeping in mind the focus on 'self-development' before introducing a skill. The idea of integrating a vocational skill along with learning was greatly appreciated by the KSK team and we were all geared to following the 'PRERNA' model of using 'Choose a Future', for the adolescent girls of this region.

3. In order to put the above strategy into action certain steps had to be taken. The first was to hire two 'Sakhis' one for the Sitla area and the other for the Kasialekh area to assist in the creation of two groups of adolescent girls (20 in number at each centre).

4. *Mobilizing the community.* The task before the Sakhis was to contact adolescent girls in villages and to motivate them to join the KSK for learning a vocational skill integrated with life-skill education. **(Plate 17)**
   The adolescent girls learning centre could not have existed without the approval of the community. As a result, the KSK

team conducted village level meetings and SHG meetings to make the community aware of the KSK's objectives. Further, the KSK team also conducted orientation meetings for CHIRAG Community Health Workers who play a major role in mobilizing the community towards women issues and have a deep understanding of the existing social dynamics and local problems. These health workers, in turn, spread the objectives of the program in their work areas where they have been working for over a decade and have a strong social standing and credibility.

Efforts were made to involve the parents, particularly the mothers, who were regularly visited by various members of the CHIRAG team. The mothers were also kept abreast of their daughter's progress. There were several meetings arranged specifically for the parents where the general progress of the girls was discussed and views/suggestions invited for specific problems that the team or the girls were facing. The objective of such meetings was to sensitize the parents towards the special needs of the adolescent girls and take them into confidence for smooth running of the training programme. Open discussions were held to gauge the expectations of the parents and their concerns (if any) from the programme.

In addition, CHIRAG staff not connected to the KSK programme directly but who formed an integral part of the community through various other CHIRAG projects took part in the KSK programme by becoming guardians ***'Kendra Abhibhavak'*** of certain adolescent girls. This was very beneficial, as these extension staff members of CHIRAG are from the community themselves and are also closely associated with people from the community. Their role was to regularly visit their wards during the residential trainings thereby helping reassure the parents of the girls and focusing attention on one-to-one basis.

Capacity building of associated staff

(a) A five-day residential Training of Trainers (TOT) was held at the CHIRAG training centre at Dhokane on *Bhavishya Ka Chunav* – a training manual by CEDPA/PRERNA. The external resource persons – Ms. Vineeta Nathani, Executive Director, PRERNA and Dr. Ashraf Ansari, Founder member PRERNA, conducted the training. 23 members of CHIRAG staff attended it.

The TOT conducted by PRERNA focused on initiating the CHIRAG outreach staff in the areas of health Women's empowerment and education to the innovative methodology of the manual 'Bhavishya ka Chunav' (Choose a Future). The first two days of the residential training focused on introducing the manual, the objectives of the entire training and the pedagogical issues related to learning. The trainers divided the participants into groups of two and gave each group a session from the manual to use from the third day. The presentations were structured in a way that all aspects involved in the use of the manual were delineated upon, in great details. There was flexibility to use innovative methods other than those listed, and to weave in the culture specifics to make it relevant to the needs of the adolescent girls, who would be trained in the future.

While one group made the presentations a few groups sat around as the 'audience' pretending to be adolescent girls and actively participated in creating a real life situation. The remaining groups were made observers and gave feed back along with the trainers. The feed back was based on

(i) Presentation of content.
(ii) Visuals made.
(iii) Methodology of involving the audience.
(iv) Innovative use of learning techniques (role play, quiz, etc.).
(v) Confidence in delivery.

The feed back sessions provided useful insights to all the groups about the use of the manual, and one could see that the presentations improved as the day went along. Trainings always generate an 'energy' that is difficult to define and put into words. The entire CHIRAG staff who participated in the five-day workshop seemed enthused, and for Pratima Singh and me it seemed like another step towards the fulfilment of 'The KSK dream' had been taken.

(b) This training was followed by a two-day residential Training of Trainers (TOT) at the Chirag training centre at

Dhokane on 'Reproductive Child Health' and other related issues, a component, which had not been covered in detail at the previous TOT.

While the five-day workshop in June 2002 had focussed on the use of the manual 'choose a future' the two-day workshop on RCH issues (for the same staff) touched on the following aspects:

(i) Definitions of Reproductive Health.
(ii) Myths and Conceptions related to Adolescent Health.
(iii) Aspirations/Anxieties during Adolescence.
(iv) Adolescent health services.
 (a) Health Officials.
 (b) Health Arrangements.
 (c) Health programme.
(v) Emotional, Physical and social changes during Adolescence.
(vi) Body Mapping, male/female.
(vii) Menstruation, myths and conceptions.
(viii) Family planning, various methods, advantages and limitations – breast-feeding as a method of contraception, other natural methods
(ix) HIV/AIDS–STDs.

This exercise in capacity building of the CHIRAG staff (other than those directly connected with the KSK) and the Health programme was an important step in the 'process' of the development of the KSK. As stated earlier the idea was to give trainings to adolescent girls on all aspects of life in the Hill Communities and the TOTs were envisaged to provide the necessary skills to the staff to make their trainings more participatory and experiential in nature. In fact I observed a remarkable difference in the way the Health outreach staff were structuring their health education sessions for CHWs and Dais after exposure to these trainings.

(c) Exposure Visit for capacity building

The staff of KSK was sent on an exposure visit to three Delhi based organizations to learn from them about their methodology of reaching the adolescent girls.

Admission Strategy

An admission questionnaire was administered in the two centres, i.e. at Reetha and Kasialekh before the training commenced to understand the demographic profile of the participants their educational level, socio-economic status, relationships with members in the family, independence levels and general exposure to the outside world.

(i) Registration forms were printed and distributed from the two field centres, Reetha and Kasialekh. A registration form cost Rs. 2. The participants also had to make a financial contribution of 25 rupees a month to ensure a level of commitment, since it was intended to be a 6-8 month long intensive training covering so many components.

The KSK target group was adolescent girls between the ages of 13-19, especially those who had dropped out of the formal education system, and had studied until at least class five. Newly married girls who had married into the CHIRAG outreach villages around the two field centres were also included. Applications were invited from the girls who met the above criteria, and it was amazing to see the overwhelming response.

(ii) Participants profile

Caste

Table 6.18 : Caste profile of adolescent girls at both centres

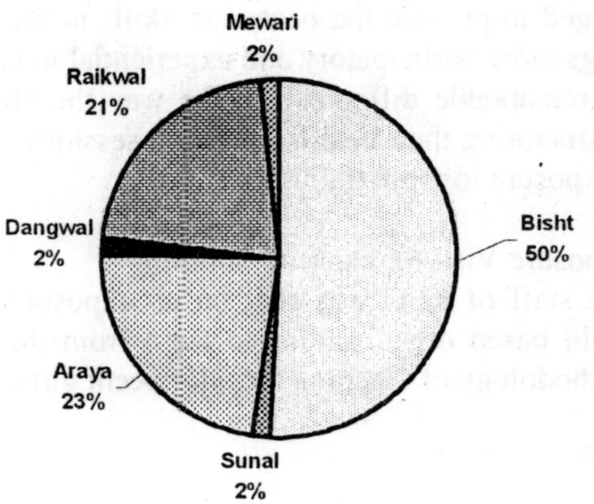

From the above table one can see that a majority of the girls who came for the training at both the centres belonged to the Thakur community, Rajputs 77 per cent (Bisht, Raikwal, Mewari, Sunal, Dangwal). 23 per cent of the girls came from Harijan families (Arya).

Education

Table 6.19 : Educational level of adolescent girls at both centres

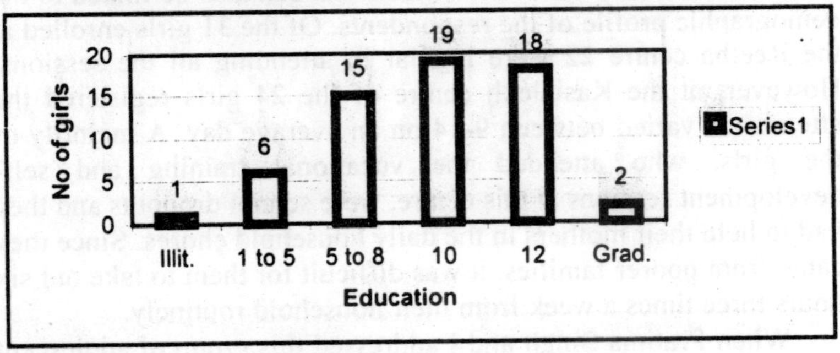

The educational level of the girls from the Reetha centre varied between class five and graduation (BA final), while the girls from the Kasialekh centre had an educational level ranging between class 8 and class 12.

Age Group

At the Reetha centre the participants were in the age group 17-20, and in Kasialekh the adolescent girls were in the age group of 15-21.

Occupation

A majority of the girls from the Reetha centre belonged to agricultural families, with a few of them coming from families with a service background. Their income was more than rupees 2,500 p.m. All the girls at the Kasialekh centre came from agricultural families with lower income levels, as low as 1500 rupees p.m. The average family size was 4-9 members. Regarding their personal profile and aspirations most of the girls from the Reetha centre stated that they would like to marry only after they were employed, whereas the girls from the Kasialekh centre were happy to marry after they were eighteen years of age. Inter-household relationships were better amongst the girls from the Reetha centre, their demographic profile also supports this, and their parents were more supportive and encouraging of the programme because of the higher education levels of the fathers and better income.

Attendance

The attendance of the girls who had finally enrolled at the two centres, 31 at Reetha and 24 at Kasialekh can also be linked to the demographic profile of the respondents. Of the 31 girls enrolled at the Reetha centre 22 were regular in attending all the sessions. However, at the Kasialekh centre of the 24 girls registered the attendance varied between 9-14 on an average day. A majority of the girls, who attended the vocational training and self-development sessions at this centre, were school dropouts and they had to help their mothers in the daily household chores. Since they came from poorer families, it was difficult for them to take out six hours three times a week from their household routinely.

When Pratima Singh and I addressed this group of adolescent girls before they finally joined the centre, there was very little participation from them during our interaction. We tried several different methods of initiating a dialogue, but perhaps it was the first time that the focus of a meeting was 'them', and not their mothers, because they were familiar with SHG and Mahila Mandal meetings. At this meeting we realized that a lot of groundwork would have to be done to mobilize the parents and enroll them into our 'dream'.

The Two Training Centres, Reetha and Kasialekh

The two Sakhis who were hired to mobilize the adolescent girls and form a group for training, had a path breaking objective before them that is to motivate the families and convince them of the significance and relevance of this integrated training for their daughters.

Keeping the views of Dr. Ravi Anand in mind about the PRERNA model of integrating vocational skills and learning, the following diagrams represent the structure at the two field centres.

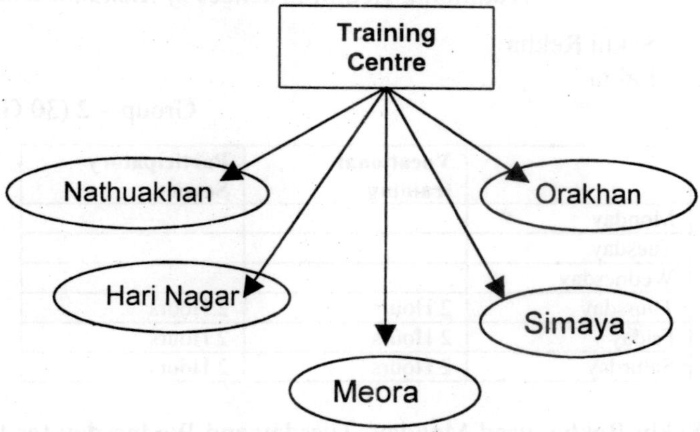

Fig. 6.4 : Details of Training centre Sitla Area (Cluster A) Reetha

1. Sakhi Radha
2. Lalita

Group – 1 (31 Girls)

	Vocational training	**Participatory Session**
Monday	2 Hours	2 Hours
Tuesday	2 Hours	2 Hours
Wednesday	2 Hours	2 Hours
Thursday		
Friday		
Saturday		

The Sakhi Radha, used Thursday, Friday and Saturday for field follow-up and meeting parents of adolescent girls attending the centre.

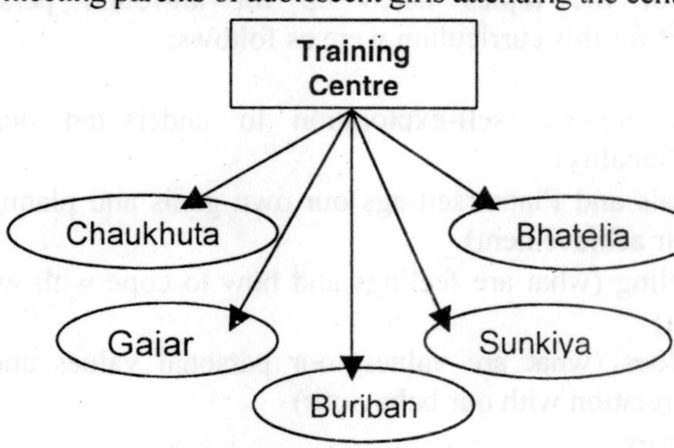

Fig. 6.5 : Kasialekh Area (Cluster B)

1. Sakhi Rekha
2. Lalita

Group – 2 (30 Girls)

	Vocational training	**Participatory Session**
Monday		
Tuesday		
Wednesday		
Thursday	2 Hours	2 Hours
Friday	2 Hours	2 Hours
Saturday	2 Hours	2 Hours

The Sakhi Rekha, used Monday, Tuesday and Wednesday for field follow-up and meeting parents.

I attended several of the sessions held at the Reetha and Kasialekh centre. Another human resource that was added to the KSK team at this point was Lalita didi who was a skilled sewing and tailoring teacher. Pratima Singh of CHIRAG had several sessions with Lalita initiating her into the methodology of using the 'self-development' sessions from the manual 'choose a future'. While Lalita took the sessions at the centres, Reetha (Monday, Tuesday, and Wednesday) and Kasialekh (Thursday, Friday, and Saturday) the Sakhis Radha and Rekha supported her and used the other days in the week to visit the community for mobilization and strengthening attendance. CHIRAG staff who had been trained at the TOTs in Dhokane also supported these sessions to make them more interesting. **(Plate 18)**

Some of the topics taken up for all-round personality development for this curriculum were as follows:

- Me, myself (self-exploration to understand our own personality)
- Goals and Plans (settings our own goals and planning for their achievement)
- Feeling (what are feelings and how to cope with what we feel)
- Values (what are values; our personal values and their correlation with our behaviour)
- Family
- Communication skills (and how to use them in handling life situations)

- Interpersonal relationships (friendship with same sex and with opposite sex)
- Community (people, mobilization and Local Self-Governance)
- Work (gender biases)

The innovative strategy followed was that along with the two hours of vocational training to integrate one aspect of personality development before proceeding for the five-day residential training on reproductive and child health.

This session continued at the field centre One, Reetha till the end of August and the first Adolescent Training in RCH was held in September 2002. At the second centre these sessions continued till November and the adolescent girls proceeded for training in RCH from November 12-17th 2002.

Strategies for strengthening attendance of adolescent girls at both field centres.

A multi-faceted strategy for enhancing participation was followed:

(i) *Home Visits :* Attendance was taken regularly at both the field centres, and at the end of every week it was easy to assess which girls were absent and from which villages. The Sakhis visited the families to find out the reasons for a girl's absence; one girl from the Kasialekh centre had not attended several sessions because she did not want to share her feelings in public. On several visits to her home, her mother shared that she loved going to school but familial constraints forced her to dropout after class 8, and she became totally silent after that. She would not interact freely with her peer group as well. Perhaps, hers is not an isolated case, as so many girls elsewhere in India also drop out after class 8. The challenge for any programme oriented to the adolescent girl must necessarily focus on bringing her into the mainstream and perhaps this initiative was a step towards that objective.

(i) Addressing mothers/women at self-help group meetings and other health meetings in the village. This strategy also helped in strengthening the attendance of the girls particularly at the Kasialekh centre.

(iii) Kendra Abhivavak *(Centre Guardians)* : In order to enhance one- to- one attention on the adolescent girls, all the staff members of Chirag who were visiting those villages to which these girls belonged, were also involved. These staff members, though not directly involved with the KSK programme, were asked to adopt two to three girls as their wards and pay individual attention to these girls. They were also supposed to interact with the families of these girls.

This helped in countering the dropout rate as attention was paid to each girl and problems discussed and solved by these guardians. The following were other members of Chirag staff who played the roles of center guardians – Neomi Pal Singh, Basanti Bisht, Lata Harbola, Kamla Bisht, Durga Bisht, Ganga Singh Bisht, Kunti Bisht, Jaswant Singh Bisht, Munni Bisht

(iv) *Meetings with role models* : Meetings were organized with persons successful in their chosen field of profession during the training sessions. The objective was to give the girls an insight into the hard work and labour that was required to get into those professions. The girls asked useful questions. The following were the persons with whom the meetings were organized:

Sl. No.	Name of the person	Profession
1	Dr. Rajesh Thadani	Manager/ Administration
2	Dr. B. K. Joshi	Professor
3	Dr. Anjali Capila	Writer/ Educationist
4	Dr. Neeta Rao	Doctor
5	Mrs. Hema Kadwal	Social worker/ Housewife
6		Auxiliary Mid Wife (ANM)
7		Gram Pradhan

(v) *Suggestion box* : There was a suggestion box placed in each training centre and the girls were asked to write whatever came to their mind on a piece of paper and drop it in the box. Writing their names was not mandatory. The messages received on these slips of paper ranged from personal questions to suggestions and problems.

This proved to be a very effective way of maintaining confidentiality and at the same time encouraging the girls to truly open up. Once a week, the box was opened and the Coordinator, Ms. Pratima Singh tried to solve the queries that arrived. There were times when she consulted subject matter experts on the questions asked before answering them. After few weeks, there came a time when most of the girls had gained enough confidence to stand up and talk about their problems in the class instead of putting them quietly in the suggestion box.

The Course Component

Keeping the objectives of the KSK programme in mind the course components focused on giving a background on personality development/understanding the self before exposing adolescent girls to individual trainings. This was followed by a detailed training on the following issues:

- Reproductive & Child health (RCH);
- Management of forest;
- Water resources, and appropriate technologies;
- Agriculture and Horticulture;
- Animal Husbandry;
- Panchayati Raj;
- Entrepreneurship skills;
- First aid;
- Legal rights;
- Self-help group.

Each module developed was field tested during the specific trainings with a group of adolescent girls. The trainings were residential and held at CHIRAG centers such as Reetha, Kasialekh and Dhokane. The duration ranging from five days to three days and groups of 20-25 adolescent girls participated in each training. The feed back received is now being used to modify the modules and keeping in mind the needs expressed by the participants during trainings, the overall curriculum of the programme is being restructured.

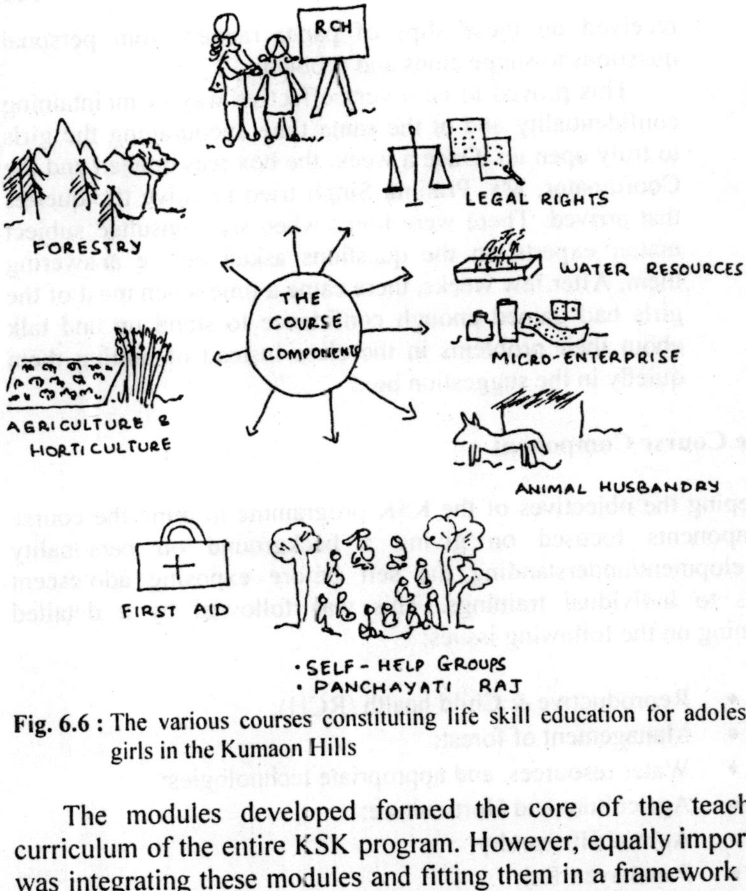

Fig. 6.6 : The various courses constituting life skill education for adolescent girls in the Kumaon Hills

The modules developed formed the core of the teaching curriculum of the entire KSK program. However, equally important was integrating these modules and fitting them in a framework that encouraged the young adolescents to think for themselves and raise their awareness levels about a variety of societal issues. The completed curriculum is therefore much more than a series of modules. It forms an integrated development package with sufficient focus given to subjects such as self-help group formation, local self-governance (Panchayati Raj) and gaining economic self-sufficiency. The fundamental guiding principle was to create a gender sensitive curriculum, which covered all the interlinked "content" areas suitable for life in the hill communities and at the same time develop a teaching methodology, which motivates attitudinal and behavioural changes. In addition, the future use of distance education was also kept in mind while developing the curriculum, which is organic in nature and will keep evolving and changing as the years go by.

Vocational Training Programmes

Vocational training such as sewing, stitching, tie-and-dye, candle making training, envelop making, book binding, food preservation, greeting card making, nursery raising and management etc. were also imparted to the girls along with the various trainings based on the course components. These trainings would enable the girls to develop entire vocational skills and start their own income generation programmes if they wanted to do so in the future.

Some Aspects of the Technical Training Modules

The entire training programme was divided into various sub-divisions, which were part of a holistic approach. A panel of expert trainers gave these trainings. Given below is the description of some major training modules.

(i) Reproductive Child Health was a 5-day residential course, which formed an essential component of the training where many key issues were highlighted for the first time. The girls were made aware of all the processes involved in the Menstrual Cycle, Child Birth, Family Planning techniques, Reproductive Health aspects related to girls and boys during adolescence and the process to womanhood and manhood. Attention was also given to the preventive measures to check the incidence of Reproductive Tract Infection (RTI) and Sexually Transmitted Diseases (STD). Community health and sanitation along with a separate session on **First Aid** also formed a part of the health training.

(ii) Forestry was an intensive 3-day residential course in the Dhokane Training centre that began by asking the young women what they would like to learn in this field. Here the focus was on trees and their properties, resources available in the different forests, direct and indirect benefits available from the forests in the area, plantation techniques, civil and reserve forest boundaries, preventive and curative measures for forest fires.

(iii) The agriculture and horticulture module was spread over 3 days but was not as intensive as the forestry course. Subject areas included soil composition, making compost, seed testing, organic-farming versus other types of farming, nursery raising and management, plant nutrition management, off season vegetable cultivation, region specific plant diseases and their bio control methods, introduction to medicinal plants and the possibilities of income generation from it and fertilizers.

(iv) Animal Husbandry was a 2-day course wherein there was a focus on certain issues including animal management, nutritional training, biodynamic composts, designing an ideal area for grazing and breeding, proper milking techniques, immunization, breed improvement, economics of animal husbandry and administration of first aid to the animals.

(v) Water Management was also a one-day course, where the young girls were trained on natural water cycle, different types of water sources, water conservation methods, filtration techniques, hand pump/water tank usage, water properties, proper sanitation practices and purification of water for drinking purposes and using water for electricity generation. Wastewater management was also an important issue that was included keeping in view the acute water shortage in the area.

(vi) Panchayati Raj was a one-day course covering issues related to Pre election voters' awareness, powers given to the panchayats by the 73rd amendment of the constitution, three tier panchayati raj system, reservation policy in the elections, *gram pradhan*, *gram sabha* and *gram panchayat*, agenda, selecting ward members, voting procedures, president and vice presidents selection. The role of women in local self-governance was the focal point of the training.

(vii) Legal Rights module was covered in one day. In this module the adolescent girls were briefed about the law, the constitution, marriage and its legal implications, the police force and bribe taking/giving. The objective of this training was to make the girls aware of the existing legal system and procedures of the country and to remove the fear of resorting to legal help in case of need. As part of the empowerment exercise the girls were made aware of the existing legal provisions that were there to protect them from the general exploitation that the women are subjected to in every sphere of life.

Training Panel

Anil Bajpai
Pratima Singh
Arvind Rana
Lata Harbola
Neomi Pal
Pranay Singh
Pan Singh Rana
Lalita
Lokendra
Chandan Chamiyal
Kishan Nayal
Rekha Rani
Radha Bisht
Munni Bisht
Ganga Anaria
Durga
Mohan Negi
Ganga Singh Bisht
Kunti Bisht

The Two Trainings on RCH

The first five-day residential training in RCH of 19 participants from the Reetha centre was held at the CHIRAG training centre at Dhokane in Almora district. The training was conducted by a two-member team from PRERNA, New Delhi, assisted by the CHIRAG staff who had been trained earlier at the TOT in June and the detailed RCH training in August 2002. A detailed profile of the NGO PRERNA is presented later in this chapter. The structure of the five-day training module developed specifically for the adolescent girls of Uttaranchal on RCH is also presented later in this chapter.

Strategy in Training : Since the RCH was going to be residential and the adolescent girls had to be away from their families for five days for the first time, a lot of ground work had to be covered to make this a possibility. One of the strategies adopted by CHIRAG was to invite the parents of the participants to the two field centres for an 'open dialogue'. The adolescent girls themselves had been instrumental in paving the way for their RCH training, as they had been sharing whatever they learnt in their sessions with siblings/aunts/mothers at home. At the meetings the KSK team representatives listened to all the apprehensions expressed by the parents, and assured them about their safety and security. The kind of issues being deliberated upon at the RCH training were also shared with them. Since this was the first training the approval and support of the parents was very important for the success of the programme. All of the parents signed letters of approval before their daughters proceeded for the training.

The trainers and training methodology : Bimila Raj and Pushpa were the two trainers from PRERNA who had travelled with me to Dhokane training centre by train from New Delhi, for the first workshop in September 2002. This training was structured in such a way that some sessions, which focused on the culture-specifics of this region, like rituals and myths related to menstruation, pregnancy and delivery were taken by the CHIRAG KSK team and the health team. This was also done to build the capacity of the CHIRAG staff to be able to conduct the five-day training independent of an outside agency.

The training methodology used was very participatory and innovative. Ice-breaking exercises, warm up games, role plays, collage making, watching a movie on a gender issue, and learning a vocational skill everyday, were interspersed with the 'learning sessions' **(Plates 19, 20, 21, 22).**

A pre-test was conducted before the workshop and the same test was administered as a post-test on the fifth day.

The second training with adolescent girls from the Kasialekh centre was held in November 2002. The CHIRAG KSK staff and the health team took the entire five-day training. Pratima Singh was the lead trainer of this workshop. The details of the workshop are presented in Apppendix I.

HIGHLIGHTS of the two trainings on RCH : I was present at both the trainings in September and November 2002. What was amazing was to see the tangible transformation of the participants. All the girls who had undergone the training were joyful, happy, full of energy and at times I noticed it was not easy for the trainers to answer their frank questions. Since the issues dealt with in the sessions were not something that are discussed so easily, it was surprising to note that from the second day the girls started 'opening up', asking questions and sharing about themselves.

Some were more articulate than the others, but as they listened to their friends I could see them opening up slowly. The exercise of writing their experiences on a piece of paper and putting it in the middle of the room, and then hearing it from another participant, seemed to demystify their experience and what they were holding on to.

The adolescent girls participated very actively in role plays, in fact the play they performed on the consequences of early marriage was so good that it generated a lot of enthusiasm in the group. The sessions on the myths and rituals related to menstruation, pregnancy and delivery in the Kumaon Hills were able to contextualize their learning, and they participated very actively in these sessions.

The skill building sessions at the end of each day like 'tie and dye' were highly appreciated by the participants **(Plate 23, 24)**. They modelled the *dupattas* they had prepared and I could sense that they were already feeling more confident. Perhaps, the unique structure of this journey (from six hours of self-development and six hours of vocational training every week for four months) to the five-day residential training was indeed special.

After five days of being together there were a lot of feelings and emotions that had got aroused. There was so much knowledge that the girls had received, they had opportunities to laugh open up, ask questions, express themselves. They had talked of issues like menstruation, sex, intercourse, masturbation, their own sexuality and all this perhaps was like a 'dam' breaking on the fifth day. Many girls were crying at the thought of going away after this '5 day camp'. They had developed a close contact with the trainers Pratima, Rekha, Radha, Lalita, Neomi who they saw as role models and in whom in a way they saw their freedom. Perhaps this long journey from 'silence' to 'openness' is a milestone in the creation of the Kishori Shikshan Kendra for the adolescent girls of Uttaranchal. For Pratima and me seeing these groups so 'opened up' was indeed a special experience, our first meeting with them on June 21st at Kasialekh was a monologue with 90 per cent of the girls just looking at the floor. What also emerged was the strong bonds that had developed between the girls of different villages – they felt like "Partners in a common destiny".

Impact of Training Analysis of Pre / Post Test Results

Reproductive and Child Health (RCH)

The Pre-test results in both centers showed limited knowledge of the adolescent girls with reference to RCH. Some attempts were made to answer questions such as: who is responsible for determining the sex of the child at birth? What is that protects one from STDs? What makes boys and girls different during adolescence? When and how does fertilization of the ova take place? About questions related to preventing conception, consequences of early childbirth, approximately half the class from both the centers wrote no answers at all. This illustrates they had no knowledge at all on certain areas. Also, as regards physiological changes during the adolescent period, 75 per cent of the class had little knowledge about this topic. With reference to questions related to boys' nightfall, menstruation and contraception the girls at Reetha had better pre-test scores with more than half the class being able to correctly answer the questions. The pre-test scores of students from the Kasialekh centre were much lower on all aspects of RCH.

The post-test results showed that the objectives of educating adolescent girls on RCH issues were clearly met. There was a great increase in the post-test scores of the participants from both the centres. However, there were a few errors made by the girls in the post-test, in issues related to the menstrual cycle, what makes boys and girls equal, and nightfall experiences. This highlights the fact that certain areas of the course could be better explained the next time or certain students be given individual attention.

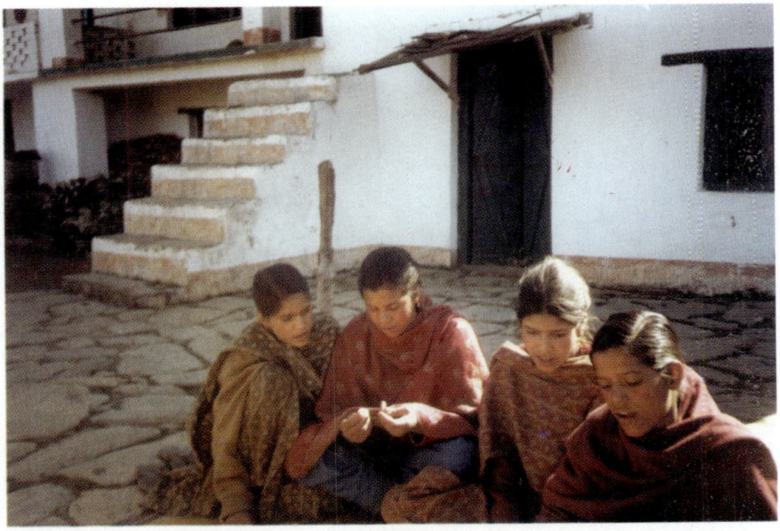

Plate 17 : Meeting adolescent girls in villages and motivating them to join the KSK.

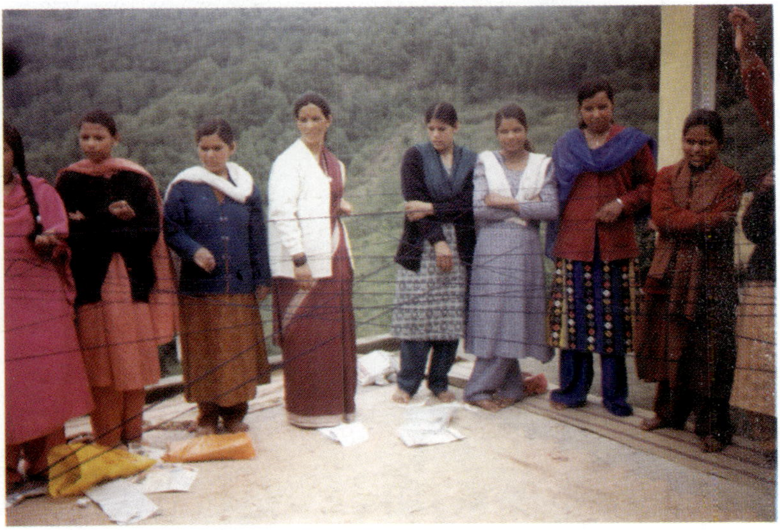

Plate 18 : Adolescent girls at the Kasialekh Centre playing an innovative game with CHIRAG staff.

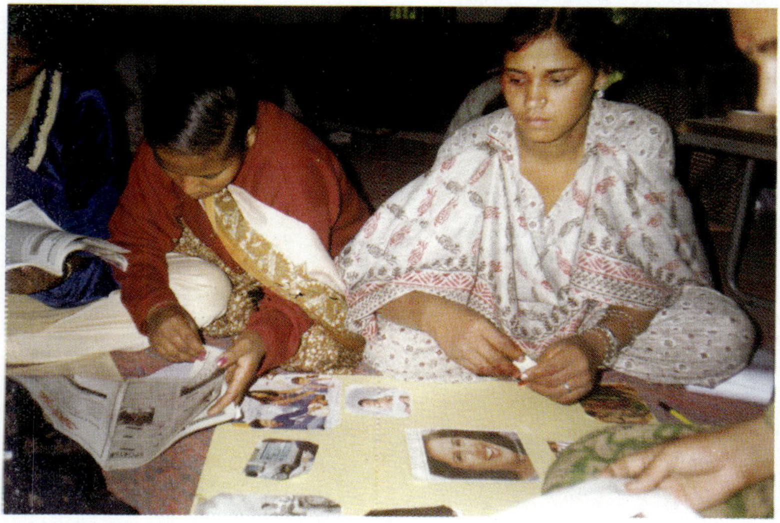

Plate 19 : Adolescent girls Reetha Centre making a collage at the first RCH Training, September, 2002

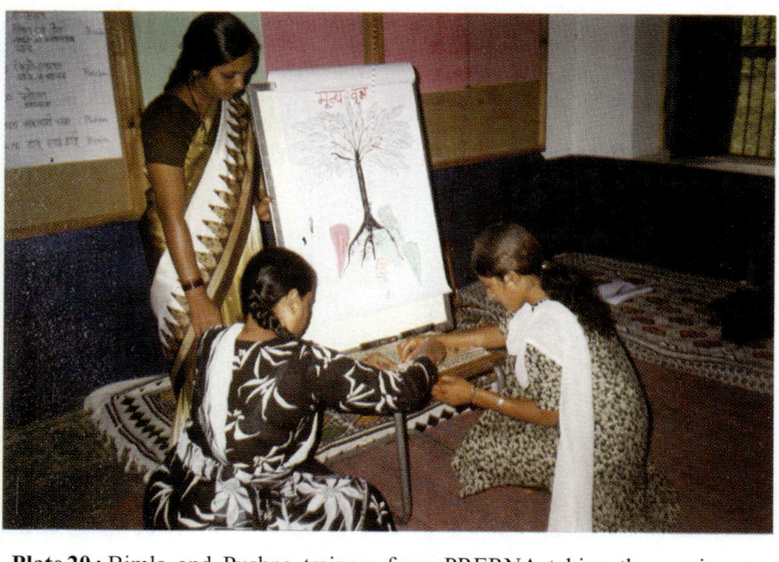

Plate 20 : Bimla and Pushpa trainers from PRERNA taking the session on Values during the first training, September, 2002.

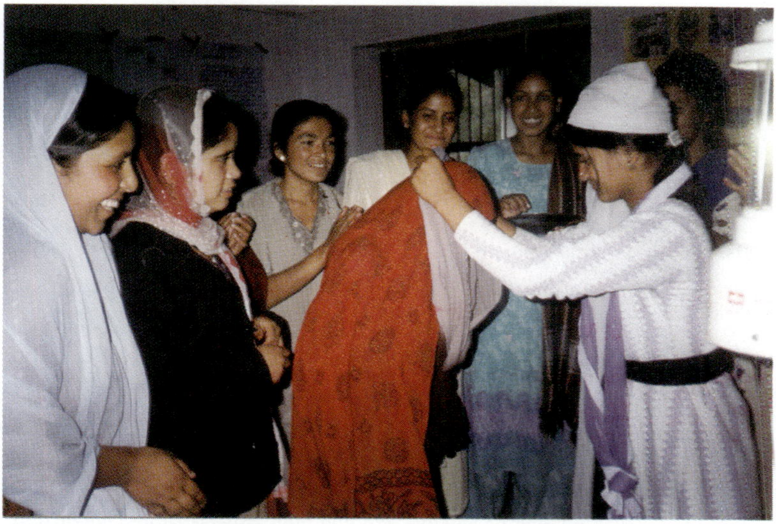

Plate 21 : Adolescent girls performing a play on 'early marriage' at the first RCH Training, September, 2002

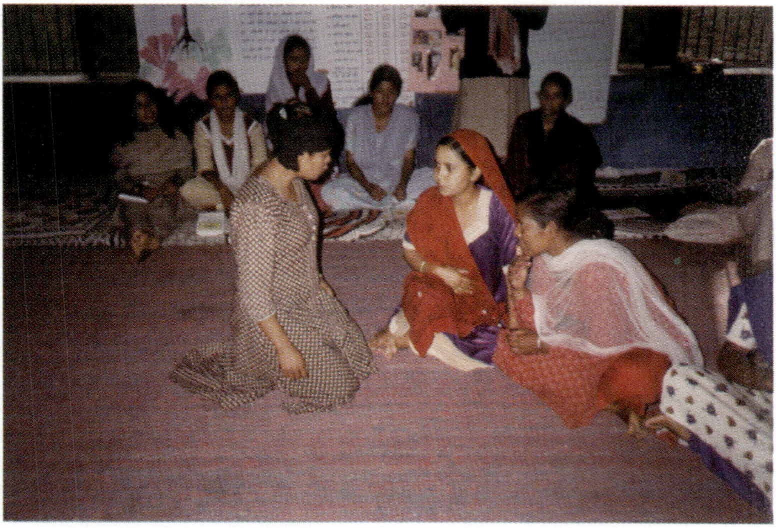

Plate 22 : Performing a role play on friendship between a boy and girl at Dhokane Training Centre

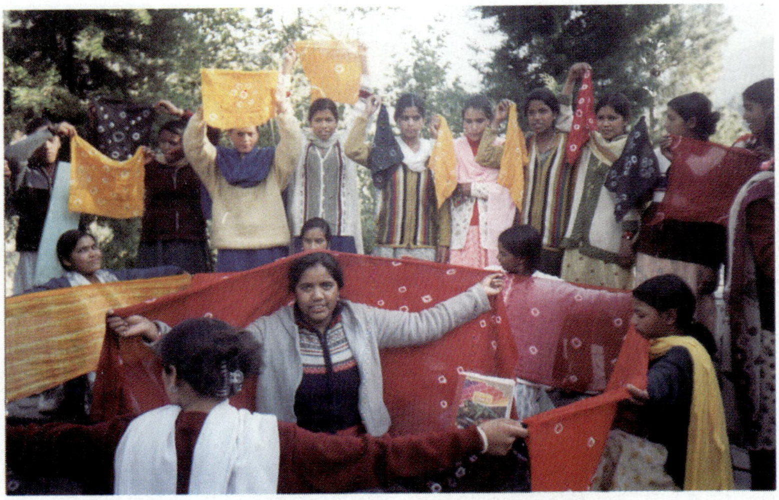

Plate 23 : Displaying their tie and dye *dupattas* with pride—Adolescent girls of Kasialekh Centre, November, 2002.

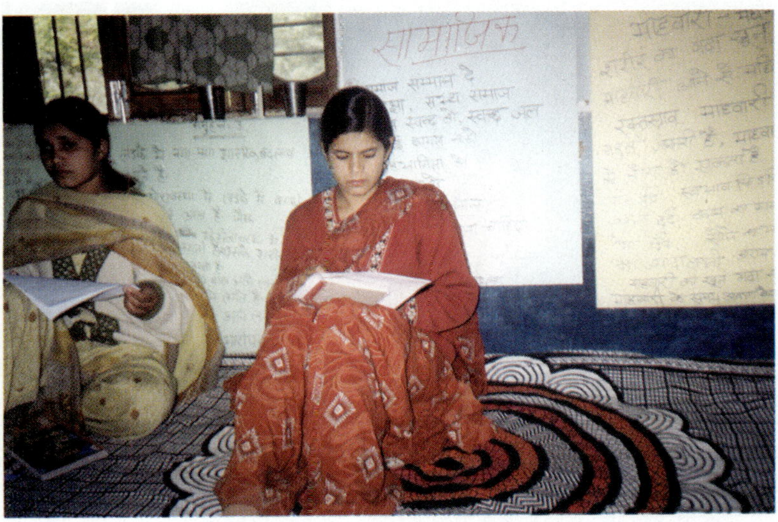

Plate 24 : Concentrating post-test —A Kumaoni girl from the Kasialekh Centre

As regards the quality of the training, the trainers and the facilities available at the training centre at Dhokane all the participants stated that they greatly appreciated the arrangements.

Innovations in the programme

Chelia Utsav

Chelia is Kumaoni word for "daughter". At the end of the first training cycle all the girls of KSK organized a festival – *Chelia Utsav* with the support from the community. The girls also participated in the bal-mela, an event organized by the women federation every year. It was a two-day affair. The women and children dedicated the first day to the cultural programmes from the community and speeches by the public representatives. The second day saw the girls of KSK presenting their cultural programmes such as a play on the problem of early marriage, a play on the concept of KSK (which was written and performed by them), a welcome song, Folk dances, classical dance, Folk songs etc. At the end of the programme Mr. Kanai Lall, Chairman of CHIRAG gave out certificates to KSK graduates.

Stalls of candles, *dupattas*, greeting cards, show pieces, games, eatables, locally made fruit/flower juice and an exhibition of posters (made by girls) were the main attractions of this function.

The objective of this *utsav* was to mobilize the community and attract those parents and adolescents who were not aware of the programme and to give importance and recognition to KSK girls in their community. In the process they also learnt the art of organizing and managing an event like this, the possibilities of generating income from the arts they had learnt and confidence building by performing in front of the community members, gram panchayat members, and their own family members. (Fig. 6.7)

General Health Check up

A commonly adopted process of monitoring the increase in level of knowledge and awareness is through pre and post-training tests. The actual impact or outcome of the training cannot be seen in a short time. However, there are some areas where the immediate impact of the trainings can be seen.

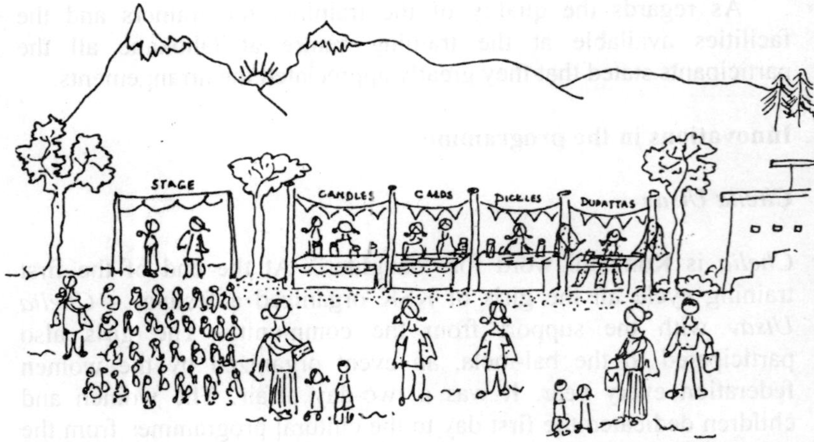

Fig. 6.7 : The 'Chelia Utsav' – Sale of Products Made by Adolescent Girls, and a Play on KSK

As anemia, urinary tract infections (UTI), reproductive tract infection (RTI), dental pain etc. are some of the general problems with the adolescents, it was decided to focus on these issues to bring about a change. A health check up was organized for the adolescent girls. Cases of anemia, RTI, UTI, dental pain and trauma/stress were diagnosed by the health team of CHIRAG. Appropriate corrective measures were taken and suggestions given in terms of personal counselling. Some cases were also referred to a qualified doctor.

Follow up : A similar checkup was done after three months where an increase was seen in the levels of haemoglobin, and there was a general improvement in the health condition of the girls. The girls had to pay a small fee for the consultation and the cost of the medicine given to them.

E. PRERANA – A PROFILE

Prerana, which means, "to inspire", was founded as a "not for profit" voluntary organization in September 1974. The founders gave expression to their vision and drive through voluntary action. Through the use of their knowledge, skills and resources, they created partnerships with people from underprivileged communities, by establishing a dialogue, generating enthusiasm, organizing and strengthening capacities of local volunteers for planning, implementing and monitoring programmes facilitating their own communities' development.

In 1983, Prerana became an associate of Centre for Development and Population Activities (CEDPA); a Washington based private voluntary organization. Supplementing its resource base with this association, Prerana forged ahead for expansion of outreach services, training and technical assistance in programme design and management to other NGO's.

Just as there had been growing concern the world over regarding the Girl Child, Prerana's experience from its programme revealed that thus far that they were mainly addressing the problems of women and children in particular and while the adolescents of the community were being left out of any development initiative that they were not addressed under any programme. A need was increasingly felt to "tap them young", with considerations that at that age adolescents were not only more eager to learn new ideas, but also were to become the future mothers.

Prerana's initiatives towards addressing the developmental concerns of the adolescent age group were formalized with the initiation of the "Better Life Option" with CEDPA in India in 1987. In 1990, Prerana further enhanced its initiatives by launching the Better Life Demonstration Project for Girls and Young Women. Keeping in view, Prerana's philosophy of integrated community development and promoting participation, Prerana took an innovative step by developing a parallel Better Life Demonstration programme for Boys and Young Men.

GOAL: To create an environment of dignity and opportunity for adolescents, enabling them to achieve their full potential of personal growth and ability to contribute to family community and societal development.

Strategies

Community Based Interventions

Better Life Options Programme: Being implemented in six urban slums along the periphery of Delhi, i.e., Aali, Lalkuan, Tajpur, Pahari, Molarband, Jaitpur and Meethapur. Their programme design includes –

- Preventive, curative and reproductive health
- Family planning

- Family Life Education (FLE)
- Literacy
- Skill Development
- Vocational Training and Income Generation
- General Training and Environmental Awareness

Learning modules include information, education and services in area of –

* Personality development
* Education
* Basic Health and Nutrition
* Reproductive health education and Family Planning Awareness
* Economic Participation
* Basic life skills training
* Social and cultural issues
* Legal rights

Prerana has adopted the peer educator approach and the module used has been developed by CEDPA.

Collaborating and Extending Partnerships with other NGOs

With the objective of extending the outreach of the programme for the adolescent girls, partnerships have been developed with other NGOs in the states of Uttar Pradesh, Bihar, Rajasthan, Madhya Pradesh and Uttaranchal. Prerana's experience has been utilized in developing proposals, designing programme and methodologies for the effective implementation, supervision, monitoring, evaluation and capacity building of partner NGOs through ongoing technical assistance.

Advocacy

Recognizing the urgency for initiating strong, sustainable and visible actions on the part of Government, Media, NGOs, Donors, Corporate sector as well as other institutions and individuals for addressing issues of adolescents, an advocacy initiative has been launched for influencing policies, resource allocation and programme directions which will aim towards familial and societal attitudes and perception about their role and life choices.

Research and Documentation

Research and documentation of innovative approaches and models of learning/sharing to strengthen future initiatives.

Prerana aims to be a professional development organization with a high emphasis on programmee innovation, learning and sharing of approaches and replicating models in integrated community development and participation. The promotion of professional volunteerism and non-charity are other strongly shared values that strengthen and provide as distinctive character to its development orientation.

F. REPRODUCTIVE AND CHILD HEALTH

Module - 5 Days

Day 1

Sl. No.	Time	Topic	Methodology
1	09:30-09:45 AM	Registration of the participants	Individual registration forms
2	09:45-10:15 AM	Introduction of the participants and facilitators Pre Test	Participatory game to introduce each other
3	10:15-10:45 AM	Aspirations and expectations from the training	Group exercise and presentation
4	10:45-11:00 AM	TEA BREAK	
5	11:00-11:30 AM	Objectives of the training Self-made Rules and Regulations for the training	Presentation Discussion
6	11:30-01:30 PM	What is Health – Forming a definition of good health. Inter-relationship of social, psychological and physical health. Factors affecting women health – in context with the hill region. Available resources at the local and administrative level.	Group exercise and presentation. Brainstorming. Lecture
7	01:30-02:30 PM	LUNCH BREAK	

Contd...

8	02:30-04:30 PM	Friendship: Identifying the qualities of a good friend Developing constructive and Healthy relationships. Friendship with the opposite sex - interpersonal communication and relationship.	Group work and presentation. Brainstorming Role Play
9	04:30-04:45 PM	TEA BREAK	
10	04:45-05:15 PM	Question Answer session	Open discussion and through question box

Day 2

Sl. No.	Time	Topic	Methodology
1	09:30-09:45 AM	Morning Prayer Recap	Presentation
2	09:45-11:15 AM	Marriage: Its social and personal significance. My mother, myself and my daughter – changing perspective Marriage in early age – its effects Roles of Husband and Wife – responsibility sharing	Group work and presentation Role play Case study Brainstorming
3	11:15-11:30 AM	TEA BREAK	
4	11:30-01:30 PM	What is Adolescence? Physical and emotional changes during adolescence Body mapping	Participatory exercise. Quiz & Lecture Group work and presentation
5	01:30-02:30 PM	LUNCH BREAK	
6	02:30-04:30 PM	Menstrual Cycle – the process Traditional and Cultural beliefs and practices Importance of cleanliness and hygiene during the menstrual cycle	Lecture Group exercise and Presentation Brainstorming
7	04:30-04:45 PM	TEA BREAK	
8	04:45-05:15 PM	Question Answer session	Open discussion and through question box

Day 3

Sl. No.	Time	Topic	Methodology
1	09:30-09:45 AM	Morning Prayer Recap	Presentation
2	09:45-11:15 AM	Male and Female Reproductive organs and their functions Reproduction – Conception and Formation of the foetus	Quiz : matching body parts with functions Lecture and presentation
3	11:15-11:30 AM	TEA BREAK	
4	11:30-01:30 PM	Conditions when conception cannot take place Who is responsible for son or daughter – X & Y chromosomes	Brainstorming and discussion Participatory game and Lecture
5	01:30-02:30 PM	LUNCH BREAK	
6	02:30-04:30 PM	Pregnancy – Ante-natal Care Dangerous signs during pregnancy Do's and Don'ts during pregnancy – region specific traditions and physical labour	Brainstorming and discussion Group exercise and Presentation Role play
7	04:30-04:45 PM	TEA BREAK	
8	04:45-05:15 PM	Question Answer session	Open discussion and through question box

Day 4

Sl. No.	Time	Topic	Methodology
1	09:30-09:45 AM	Morning Prayer Recap	Presentation
2	09:45-11:15 AM	Safe Delivery – Preparation and precautions Post-natal care Importance of colustrum	Group work and presentation Lecture and presentation Discussion
3	11:15-11:30 AM	TEA BREAK	
4	11:30-01:30 PM	Value of small family: Social and economic significance	Feature Film show Discussion
5	01:30-02:30 PM	LUNCH BREAK	

Contd....

6	02:30- 03:30 PM	Family Planning: choosing the size of the family Various methods of family planning	Brainstorming and discussion Group exercise and Presentation
7	03:30- 04:30 PM	Child care. Vaccination, malnutrition, growth chart and common ailments	Quiz and discussion Brainstorming
8	04:30- 04:45 PM	TEA BREAK	
9	04:45- 05:15 PM	Question Answer session	Open discussion and through question box

Day 5

Sl. No.	Time	Topic	Methodology
1	09:30- 09:45 AM	Morning Prayer Recap	Presentation
2	09:45- 11:15 AM	Problems related with women health – traditional and cultural practices – their significance Abortion, miscarriage, RTI, UTI, STD and HIV/AIDs	Group work and presentation Lecture and presentation Discussion
3	11:15- 11:30 AM	TEA BREAK	
4	11:30- 01:30 PM	Gender Roles. Sexual Exploitation: types and precautions. Sources of help	Group exercise and presentation Discussion
5	01:30- 02:30 PM	LUNCH BREAK	
6	02:30- 03:30 PM	Open Session Answering Questions	Discussion
7	03:30- 04:30 PM	Post-test and training evaluation.	Filling formats
8	04:30- 04:45 PM	TEA	
9	04:45- 05:15 PM	Ending the training	Group song

Case studies (programme impact)

Four adolescent girls have joined the *Balwadis* run by CHIRAG, one has become a librarian, one has become a teacher in a local school, two have started nursery raising on experimental basis, two girls have made Bio Dynamic heaps in their fields after receiving the agriculture training.

The girls are making use of the vocational trainings imparted during the training and are making candles, doing tie and dye for personal use and even selling it locally.

Case Studies Kishori Shikshan Kendra (KSK)

Adolescent girls from the two centres of Kasialekh and Reetha, shared with us their perceptions of how the training in various issues related to their life in the hills had made a difference to them, and how they would utilize this training for not only own their self-development and skill enhancement but also that of their peer groups

Case I Champa (subject) – Reetha.

Father's name – Shri Surendra Singh
Village – Simiyal
Age – 20 years
Education – Class XII

Champa is the youngest amongst the three children in the family. Her elder sister is already married and so also is the brother. Her sister-in-law (*bhabhi*) who stays at home has had no children. She suggested that both her brother and *bhabhi* should go to hospital for examination, and she would in the meantime take care of the house while they were there. Her bhabhi says that Champa treats her like a *didi*, her own elder sister, and she is fortunate to have a sister-in-law (*nanad*) like Champa. Because of this good relationship between them the family is very happy. She had also learnt at the plant nursery about carrot and radish seed plantation, which she had applied for her home also.

Champa said that she would in terms of her needs sell the seeds from what she has saved, so that this income would help in the day-to-day running of the house so that there is improvement in the family's daily life. She also thought she would give some seeds to the village and the rest to CHIRAG.

She also makes little decorative objects for the house, and says that since she joined the KSK she has learnt so many different things, and would have in its absence just stayed at home doing little else. "At KSK, she has also learnt to articulate and communicate a lot", says her mother, "unlike earlier times when she would hide whenever some guests would come at home; she speaks to them without any hesitation and offers them food." Her mother continued, "Whenever she used to come back from the KSK she would tell us about what she had learnt, and this would give us new directions also".

Case II. Saraswati (subject)	–	Kasialekh
Father's name	–	Shri Diwan Ram
Village	–	Sunkiya
Age	–	19 years.
Education	–	Class IX.

Saraswati, a member of the gram sabha of Sunkiya, has always attended the vocational classes for sewing, etc. regularity without missing a day even if there is some urgent work at home. She has unlimited potential for work and is always good in cooperation with other members. She has a family of four, her parents and brother, and here too she has worked cooperatively, specially taking care of the animals. The day she enrolled for the forest learning and van-panchayat, she at the same time sat with the women's group meetings; and is very keen to contribute to the awareness campaign for women.

After learning all this, she applied the horticultural knowledge to her home where she initiated the making of a compost-pit, so that through this means she will be able to use it for growing vegetables at home. She also encourages friends in her group to join the KSK, although these girls says that if the KSK was nearer home, it would have been possible for her to enroll many more girls to join this training centre. She herself has changed a lot after joining the KSK, because she now unhesitatingly spreads the message of its usefulness to the other women in the village.

Case III. Namita (subject)	–	Reetha.
Father's name	–	Shri Rajendra Singh
Village	–	Simiyal
Age	–	20 years
Education	–	Class XII

Namita is part of a family of five, and is eldest of the children. She belongs to a joint family where her father is the eldest of them and then her uncle (*chacha*) or father's younger brother. She says her parents do not get along well with each other and this causes a lot of tension in the family. Her father works in Nainital University and whenever he comes home there are quarrels between, and often do not speak to each other; moreover whenever her mother wants to speak, her uncle starts to scold her and everyone wants to quarrel with her. Her uncle and aunt on the other hand get along well with each other. Even when my father is not at home, she says, her uncle continues to fight with her mother. All this tension makes Namita very sad and weepy, and she wishes her parents got along well as did her uncle and aunt.

Namita says that when she learnt at the KSK about the use of manure, and knowing there was a lot of oranges (maltas) growing in her house, she could sell the juice of this fruit in the market and make money; this she would give to her mother as no one gives her any money. She said she would start this work soon, and said that earlier she did not have the capacity to think so deeply about such matter which she is now compelled to do.

It is worth mentioning here that soon after this interview Namita's hard work brought about dividends. She was selected to head the newly established library of the KSK centre. She squarely attributes her abilities for all this to the KSK centre which not only helped her to head the library but the self-confidence that she has now; in the end it has helped to support her mother.

EPILOGUE

LEARNINGS ON THE JOURNEY

All the rituals and ceremonies that mark the reproductive phase of a woman's life are a celebration or a manifestation of the sacredness of the culture of the Kumaon Hills.

Traditional beliefs give value and meaning to each phase of the woman's life. The practice of burying the placenta under a fruit-bearing tree indicates the perception of the unity of life with nature. The tree and the environment are an integral part of the nourishment cycle, which links cultural practices and practical benefit. Traditions and practices represent continuity and are a manifestation of culture, which is the embodiment of a way of life.

Culture ↔ life-cycle events ↔ health ↔ development.

This interconnectedness should form the 'basis' of the promotive, preventive and curative aspects of health care strategies. Any intervention, which is not based on the lived experiences of communities, does not become a part of a way of life. Health care is not merely a service to be delivered but it should build on people's knowledge.

Our whole model of interpreting the traditional wisdom of people, their customs, and communities needs to be re-examined. We need to understand the health practices of women in the Kumaon hills in a total context, rather than isolating them to arrive at inferences which relegates these practices as backward. The lived experiences of women related to their lifecycle events have to be viewed in the context of their world-view, and their integral relationship with the physical environment in which they live. For understanding the health practices of women one has to see their interconnectedness and inter-relatedness in a holistic manner – creating a rhythm and movement.

Culture ↔ Health ↔ Development.

What needs to be strengthened is the value behind traditional practices and perhaps a dialogue, which does not violate the values, can initiate change and take people along. It is the traditional knowledge and wisdom of women, which needs to be recognized – all this is not peripheral but integral to healthcare.

What becomes clear is the fact that village communities are governed by a set of beliefs, values and norms which individuals in that group take into account when deciding about which health practices are to be adopted and which are not to be taken up. It is not easy to go against the cultural and social norms of the majority of the members of a community. These are truisms when other studies are made but not often taken into account when health policies and planning is carried out. Outsiders coming in contact with villagers (since it is often assumed that their programme aims and means will converge with those of the people) very often forget this context.

It is important to remember that the cultural context forms a coherent system, which provides sanctions from the sacred dimension, the moral backing, which is beyond the mere empiricist or scientific comprehension of societies. For example, diets of pregnant women are said to be restricted because people believe that this will ensure a small baby and easy delivery. What is fundamental to note is that beliefs relating whether to religion, health, food or any other similar activity are all interrelated to the worldview of a community within which all explanations are given. To illustrate, the failure of folk medicine is accepted because the patient was beyond help whereas the failure of a doctor to treat and cure symptoms is not easily accepted. In short, in planning rural health programmes it would do well to keep in mind the socio-cultural context by the interventionists to eliminate the negative influences of those factors as also make use of the positive ones.

Thus, one can say that health of a society is intimately related to its value system, its philosophical and cultural traditions, and its social, economic and political organization. The health status enhancements cannot be carried out in isolation without its integration with the wider effort to bring the overall cultural social and economic and political transformation of the society.

What all this work, say as a pilot project, suggests is that all efforts of health and well being of communities is a clear goal that must become a part of developmental programmes, especially in rural areas. Thus it ensures the well being of people that deserves high priority in both research and major planned efforts at all levels.

However, the goal is not simply a functional one in terms of technologization or medicalization, since health and human behaviour is intertwined intimately with the socio-cultural milieu into which human beings are socialized. The present field study clearly points to the importance of this crucial aspect, i.e. the knowledge about the beliefs, customs, rituals, traditions, taboos and practices of village communities in the context of their health and disease status which affects them and their life.

In the absence of this overall socio-cultural approach that the public health authorities are unable to encourage the people to increasingly utilize their services since the necessary knowledge or awareness of the broad phenomenon mentioned above is either deficient or altogether lacking amongst the heath promoters. Thus there is an urgent need to understand the socio-cultural context in which health workers have to relate to the people so as to make meaningful and sustained interventions.

The problems facing the health sector today are increasingly complex, multidisciplinary in nature, and this is why new and innovative approaches are needed whereby integrated action is possible in order to operationalize concepts of environmental sustainability, economic development and community development. Decentralization and active involvement of local community in management of the system is the *sine qua non* of sustainable development in the health sector. The need for decentralization and devolution of authority might ensure that the district health authorities and block/panchyat level functionaries work in close coordination at all levels.

The work in the previous chapters and especially on adolescents shows that it is important to accept the fact that adolescence exists as a distinct and important developmental stage for all 10-19 year-old girls and boys, whether they are married or have children of their own. Only when this basic level is acknowledged then a policy on adolescents can be framed for India as a whole, recognizing it as a period of critical capability-building and heightened vulnerability for girls. It is not, as until now commonly and contrarily believed, simply a brief and inconsequential passage for girls, a time of silence, passivity, and devaluation that ends abruptly at marriage or child-bearing. Then, again, boys are considered during adolescence as threatening agents of societal destabilization. Both these images distort the fact that they are often responsible, capable and deserving of societal supports and protection. The problem is further mitigated because these young people do not constitute an organized and vocal constituency with the social and economic power to lobby on their own behalf. Their problems are generally considered as a health-centered agenda, not anything of importance in the political arena. But this is in terms of policy framing at the governmental level to which some mention has been made only in passing. In short as mentioned in Chapter 6, until recently the critical components of adolescent girls' experience has been neglected. What is required is that adolescent policies are sensitive to the different needs of girls and boys, and these, must be built virtually from the ground up. As we have seen in this pioneering work in Uttaranchal, NGOs, organizations and other private-sector initiatives can certainly catalyze and supplement governmental activity, but can there be a substitute for a public governmental commitment to adolescent girls and boys? This question needs critical attention.

In the context of the above a significant issue that needs to be addressed is that of sustainability of interventions.

Sustainability needs to be redefined in terms of social practices that enable the continuation of the 'lived experience' of societies through diverse pathways that are fluid and flexible. Sustainable development then becomes a process involving active, direct, and continuing collaboration between Government/regional institutions of Health Care, the NGOs that work with the community, and the community itself as stakeholders in the process, to ensure that all social groups, including those that were currently impoverished, transient, and politically marginalized, gain improved access to institutional Health Care Services and community networks. (Rangan, Haripriya, 2000)

The parameters of sustainability are defined by those who govern/manage/run institutions. And these are operationalized in quantitative terms. How many sterilizations, how many immunized, how many checkups !

The NGOs that work with people, while steering clear of the government or regional institutions agenda use other methodologies like 'monitoring' and 'evaluation' to assess sustainability.

Inherent in the word monitoring is a 'monitor' which means to judge or to assess performance. It does not empower, enable communities to re-examine their lived experience in a `critical manner. I am not saying that these are not important aspects of sustainability and so-called development but where do people see themselves in this agenda?

While some may argue that the processes of globalization have already underestimated the abilities of national and regional governments to strengthen the 'spaces' that are accessible to all inhabitants within their jurisdiction, it is also true that there is no better time than the 'continuing present' wherein states and civil societies in different regions of the world can re-examine and rework these concepts in enabling ways, rather than exclusiveness, to sustain regions.

APPENDIX - I

REPORT OF THE SECOND WORKSHOP FOR ADOLESCENT GIRLS OF UTTARANCHAL ON REPRODUCTIVE HEALTH ISSUES HELD AT DHOKANE TRAINING CENTRE CHIRAG, ALMORA DISTRICT

11th to 15th November 2002

List of participants at the workshop

1. Hema	village Buri Bana.
2. Leela	”
3. Jeevanti	”
4. Vimla	”
5. Prema	”
6. Hema	Sitla
7. Nandi	Garav
8. Dai	”
9. Manju	”
10. Geeta	”
11. Ganga	”
12. Saraswati	Sunhiya
13. Jeevanti	”
14. Tari	Chaukuta
15. Pratima	”
16. Vimla	”
17. Hema	Gazar
18. Radha	”
19. Rekha	”
20. Ganga	”
21. Mamta	Nathuakha.
22. Reena	Lodh
23. Meena	Sunkhiya
24. Deepa	Chaukuta

Day 1, Session I

Introduction

A game was played by Lalita , the trainer from CHIRAG, called passing the parcel, when the parcel stopped the participants had to introduce themselves by saying their name along with a skill/attribute describing themselves. After this each participant picked up a chit on which half a proverb was written. After finding their partner, they had to introduce their partner's name, describe a place the partner would like to travel to and share any incident the partner would not like to forget.

After this sharing, there was a discussion on :

1. Was it easy to enumerate one's skill?
2. Is it important to talk about one's skills.
3. Why is it important to recognize your good qualities.?
4. What is the advantage of knowing your strengths and qualities and skills in a group.?

This ice-breaking session set the tone of the workshop

Session II Working logistics. Rules of the Workshop

There was brief discussion on maintaining discipline and adhering to a time schedule.

- discipline
- Time schedule

The participants were divided into three groups ;

- Entertainment- apple
- recapitulation,-apricot
- Arrangement, logistics- mango.

The rules of the Training were determined by the participants themselves. They agreed to :

- listen carefully

- maintain discipline
- respect each other
- not make a laughing stock of each other
- be open
- participative
- answer questions if they felt like.
- ask questions without hesitation

Session III

After that the participants were asked to enlist their expectations from the workshop :

- information about health
- menstruation
- problems during menstruation
- leucorrhea, AIDS, STD, anemia
- head ache, back pain.

Other issues they raised were :

- Why is there violence against women?
- What is cancer
- Why is there burning sensation in hands and feet
- What injections should a child get
- Why do we get pimples
- Want to understand the relationship between men and women
- How are babies born
- What is white discharge

After enlisting the expectations of the workshop from the participants, the objectives of the workshop, as planned by the trainers were shared with them.

Session IV

A Pre-test comprising a set of questions to ascertain the knowledge level of the adolescent girls was administered. Most of the girls looked lost while filling up the questionnaire. They were distracted and looked around the room for support and help from each other.

Session V

Setting goals and priorities

After a brief warm up game, the trainer made the participants do an exercise of placing a nose ring on the picture of a woman. They were blindfolded. The idea behind this was to show experientially to the participants that setting a goal is important.

The objective of this game was explained to the participants. Only if we know our aim/goal can we move towards it. There was a brief discussion on the following points :-

1. What are the characteristics of a goal?
2. Why is it important to have a goal/aim?
3. Two stories were narrated about Uma and Meena.

The participants were divided into two groups and the main focal points of the stories were discussed.

1. How are these stories similar.
2. What aim did the two girls choose for themselves.?
3. How did they achieve their goals.?
4. What problems did they encounter in the accomplishment of their goals.?

Then the participants were asked to depict visually on a chart the goal/aim that they had made for their own lives . As the workshop progressed one could see the adolescent girls opening up. Four girls presented their goals as depicted on the visual. After that Rekha, the trainer from Chirag explained the importance of the five friends, five fingers in the formation of a goal. These represented why is it important, how, when , who will do it and what will be done.

Session VI

What are our values and beliefs?

The participants were given a leaf on which they were asked to write one value which was important to them, and then they were given a fruit made of paper on which they were to write an achievement that would reflect their value. The significant aspect was to see the relationship between values and achievements, and this was done by creating a

Value ....Achievement Tree

Day II

9-30 a.m. The new day began with a prayer, and a recapitulation which was presented by Prema from village Buri Bana.

Session I

The definition of good health was enlisted from the participants.

The definition that all the participants agreed upon was "Any human being who is physically and mentally healthy is a healthy person"

Taking the session forward detailed discussions were held on the following three points:

i.e., the adolescent girls were asked to share what they understood when they use the words physical, mental and emotional, and social in the context of health.

Physical Wellbeing	mental, wellbeing	emotional and social wellbeing.
1. absence of disease	• no tension	• society gives respect.
2. personal cleanliness	• rest	• education.
3. No laziness	• entertainment	• cultured society.
4. nutritious food	• information	• clean village.
5. clean water	• good environment	• equality.
6. clean air	• peace	• no discrimination.
7. clean house	• no fighting	• aware people.
8. clean clothes,	• exercise	• healthy body

After this enlisting Pratima from CHIRAG gave the participants a five minute exercise :

Think about yourself and find out what has held you back from developing yourself further. The participants were given a piece of paper on which they were to write and express their thoughts. All the chits were kept in the centre of the room and any girl read out a chit, aloud. The important issues that emerged were:

1. Tension because of discrimination.
2. No education that is why there was emotional tension and strain.
3. Lack of participation and positive of people in the village towards girls.

The girls deliberated on the social issues that were detrimental to the well being of girls and said that we are all responsible for the socio-cultural environment in which we like, this is not a blame on anyone but just a forum to get aware.

Day 2

Session II

The meaning of friendship

The participants were asked to list the expectations and qualities they want in a friend ?

Some responses were:-

1. Good behaviour towards each other.
2. No hesitation.
3. Friends in joy and sorrow.
4. Treat each other with respect.
5. Share information.

According to the adolescent girls the definition of a friend is :-
One who is there for us in pain and joy..

A story written on a card was read out by the trainer which was related tofriendship. There was a group discussion on salient points of the story to highlight the important aspects of friendship.

The next issue was what qualities do they look for in a male friend.

The qualities listed by them were :

1. Sharing joy and sorrow.
2. Good natured.
3. Keeps secrets.
4. Does not make you a laughing stock.

5. Joyful.
6. Respects your feelings.
7. Treats you as equal.
8. Respects elders.
9. Should be fair.
10. No hesitation.
11. Can ride a motorcycle.

After this the girls were divided into two groups and asked to perform a small play, one depicting a family accepting and supporting male friends; and the other depicting a situation where there was a lot of opposition to bringing male friends home. It was fascinating to see the girls perform in their local language – they were so much into the play that at moments they forgot that they were in a performance.

Main point…..Parents support and understanding is a key factor in friendship.

Session III

Communication Anil Bajpai

1. our communication skills reflect our personality
2. our communication skills motivate and inspire others.

The participants were divided into four groups and were asked to narrate:-

Group 1. One dangerous episode
Group 2. One sad episode
Group 3. One lively joke
Group 4 Description of a travel

The special skills that they were asked to observe in the narrations were :

1. Expression
2. Way of speaking.
3. Listening
4. Watching

5. Interest
6. Acting.
7. Selection of words
8. Clarity

Forms of speech, Intransitive, Transitive.

Session IV

Adolescents and body changes

Stages of life cycle.

1. Infancy
2. Childhood
3. Boy
4. Adolescence
5. Adulthood
6. Old age.

Participants discussed in detail the special characteristics of each stage and then listed the changes in a boy and girl at adolescence.

Boys	**Girls**
* Heavy voice	Onset of menstruation
* Moustache	Development of breasts
* Body growth	attracted to the opp.sex
* Broadening of shoulders	Hair in Private parts.
* Growth of private parts	Oily skin.
* Hair in private parts	Beauty conscious
* Ejaculation	Pimples.
* Hair on chest	Gets taller.

Then the session focussed on the emotional and social changes that happen in a boys and girls life.

Girls

Emotional	*Social*

1. attracted to boys	Less education
2. wants to go out	Discrimination.
3. Irritable	More responsibilities.
4. To become someone, goal oriented	Not allowed to roam freely
	Pressure to get married.
	Time constraints.
	Not allowed to speak to boys.

Boys

1. eve-teasing,	wrong behaviour
2. attracted to opposite sex	drinking/smoking,etc.
3. molestation/rape	become rowdy/rude
4. angry	irritable.

The above points were enlisted by the adolescent girls.

Pratima narrated a story to the girls about how a young girl shares her emotional feelings which she experiences during the period of pubertal changes with her friend.The participants were asked to close their eyes for five minutes and write their first experience when they experienced some emotions/feelings towards the opposite sex or when they had bodily changes at adolescence.

In order to make the five day workshop activity oriented so that girls learnt a creative skill also to enhance their self-esteem, tie and dye was taught to them by the trainees from CHIRAG. They really enjoyed this session and created beautiful "Dupattas" which they displayed the next day proudly.

The next session was body-mapping by Neaomi. One group made the internal body organs of a girl on a body-map and the other group made the anatomy of a boy. Pratima explained the functioning of these organs to the girls. The girls were totally engrossed in the body mapping exercise, one could see the fascination on their faces – what was special was the rapt attention they gave to each session.

Day 3

Prayer, recap.

The definition of health was reiterated , physical, emotional and social aspects being determinants of good health, according to the participants.

After that the experiences written about the first episode during adolescence when they experienced physical and emotional changes were read out one by one, and the participants expressed that they felt wonderful and free after their experience was read out by another participant. Such sharing is important because events which one has held on to for many years become clear and there is a sense of freedom.

Session I

Menstruation Issues

What is Menstruation ?

- A monthly occurrence where the bad blood is shed by the body
- Health of women and girls gets spoilt
- It is very important to have menstruation for women
- Get disease if there is no menstruation

Symptoms – stomach ache, back pain, irritable nature, feels more hungry, want to rest, sit separately during this period.

Menstrual Hygiene
- daily bath
- cleanliness of private parts.
- changing pads twice a day
- washing cloth and drying in sun.
- how to make home-made pads.

There was a discussion about the differences between the way women and unmarried girls are treated during this period, which is very significant in the context of Uttaranchal.

When the adolescents were asked how they would share this information with adolescent girls and women in the community they said :

- by listening to others
- Will give information to illiterate women if they elicit it.

The participants raised certain questions

- Why does menstruation stop at forty-five?
- Why does one have stomach pain during this period?

The girls were asked to share how did they feel when they first got their periods. After their sharing, it was evident that most experienced a lot of fear when they got their periods. They felt knowledge about these issues would help them in a big way.

The trainers emphasized the following points:-

1. Daily bath
2. Nutritious food.
3. Wash cloth everyday and dry in the sun.
4. Change pad frequently.
5. If pad not available use locally available materials which are clean and hygenic.
6. During pain use hot water bottle or bathe with hot water.

Question

What is irregular menstruation? The trainer explained that emotional/mental tension and overwork may cause irregular periods. However there may be other causes which need to be looked into by a doctor.

Session II

What are the traditional practices that influence women's health in this society?

Three groups were made.

1. Food intake during menstruation and what is used.
2. Food intake during pregnancy, work done and how is special care taken during period.
3. Foods forbidden after delivery, work after delivery and after how many days

Group I

Traditional practices followed during the menstrual cycle.

- No tea with milk.

- No curds.
- Some use pads/napkins/cloth.
- Some nothing at all.

Women stay in the cattle shed or in a separate room in the house, do all the outside work, do not go to temple or marriages, do not go near water sources or springs, or do extra work in fields/forests.

Group II : Pregnancy

Rice, cold water, meat, sour things, heavy food is forbidden, no checkups, keep body clean, do all work related to jungle, field, care of domestic animals, carrying heavy load, do not bath everyday, only after 4-5th day.

Group III : Post-Delivery

- Avoid fried food
- Child's lips are smeared with blood, it is believed that they will become red
- Do not give the mother water to drink, as the baby can get "Habba Dabba" (pneumonia)
- Coat walls with cow-dung.
- Plaster room with Gobar ki lipai.
- For 11 days make a small wall with cow-dung 4 inches high around the area where the post-natal woman is resting.

The girls said : Our view is that the women should eat all nutritious food, drink water, and take care of themselves and the baby. It is important to know the traditional practices so that one can adopt and practice those that are good and beneficial and avoid those that are harmful.

Session III

Marriage and Age of marriage

- Union of two souls.........................Union of two hearts
- Union of two bodies. ....new world.
- Union of two families.................. .tree laden with fruits.
- Looking for future life partner. ....clan moves on.

After this the participants were divided into three groups and asked to imagine the states and situation of "My daughter, my mother and myself :

Their projections were interesting :

My daughter

- Will marry at 25 years
- Will decide her partner herself
- Have information
- No dowry
- Small family
- Healthy body and mind

Mother

- married at 13 years
- no knowledge.
- no knowledge
- did not raise her voice
- not heard.
- not happy in married life.

Self

- Will marry at 21 years
- Will decide herself
- Will marry the person who understand man/woman relations
- Will stay wherever the husband goes
- Two children
- All decisions shared
- Equal status
- Will give no dowry.

The issues that they were asked to focus on were age of marriage, what kind of preparation for marriage, no. of children and their expectations from married life.

Regarding the issue of only the male child taking the clan forward – The girls said that if the girl child had access to education, good nutrition and care and opportunities to develop, she could also carry the name of the family forward.

Child Marriage: problems and constraints were discussed. A story was read out by Neomi about a girl called Ramia who was married a the age of 13.

Problems encountered because of early marriage: perceptions of adolescent girls

- Weakness
- Problems in uterus
- Early pregnancy
- Cannot look after child properly.
- No timely checkups
- Do not feel interested in work.
- Mental discord.
- Have to lean on parental family.
- Will have more children.

After this the participants were divided into two groups and prepared a skit on Ramia's story.

The FGD (Focus Group Discussion) after the play emphasized the following points:

- No girl should marry before the age of 18.
- Many health constraints are experienced.
- Excessive work load.
- Lack of knowledge, leads to poor health.

Next session was on the roles of husband wife in a family.
The participants were divided into three groups:

Group 1	Group 2	Group 3
Ideal husband	**Ideal wife**	**What kind of wife would you like to be**
• Self-image high	• respect elders	• friends in joy and sorrow.
• Understand wife	• good house wife	• sensible.
• Trustworthy	• takes good care of children.	• respectful
• Honest	• does not hesitate to express self	• speak sweetly and win over everyone.

• Gentle behaviour	• patient	• love all members.
• Look after elders /parents	• gives value to what her husband says	• small family
	• Honest	• Good resource manager.

When asked what they would like to do to keep their married life happy:

The adolescent girl said :

- Family planning: talk about the number of children and their education.
- Participate in decision making.
- Economically support in any way possible.

Next Session : How is a Baby Formed ?

The whole process of reproduction was explained to the girls. Neomi the trainer from CHIRAG shared with them that in Maharashtra the first menstruation of girls is celebrated a lot in the parental family.

In Uttaranchal too the first menstrual cycle after marriage is celebrated. The development of the child in the womb was explained to them with the help of cards.

4th day...After morning prayer and recapitulation

Care during pregnancy and danger signs

The trainees discussed the following issues in detail with the participants as this information was desired by them.

1. Who is at risk?
2. What should be done during pregnancy?
3. What is not to be done during pregnancy?
4. Two Tetanus injections.
5. Problems during pregnancy.
6. Preparing for delivery.
7. Dangers sign during delivery and problems.

8. Care after delivery.
9. Care of low weight babies at birth and after.
10. Immunization.

There was a discussion on nutritious diet. A reference was made to the four colors.

Brown/ yellow Green/white in a plate.

Balanced diet and its components were presented : proteins, vitamins, carbohydrates, fats, milk and milk products, green leafy vegetables, and their importance in the diet was explained to the participants.

What leads to anaemia and what are its symptoms:

1. Irritableness.
2. Weakness.
3. Giddiness.
4. Burning sensation in hand and feet.
5. Breathlessness.
6. Tired feeling
7. Mental tension.

Neomi told the girls about haemoglobin levels in the blood

Girls —12g
Boys —13g plus

Next session was a Sanitation and cleanliness.

They identified through a participatory mode , the seven aspects of cleanliness.

1. Personal hygiene.
2. Household sanitation and disposal of food waste.
3. Clean environment.
4. Waste water disposal.
5. Clean water for drinking/storage.
6. Human excreta disposal.
7. Animal waste/cow dung disposal.

Next session was on care of child and immunization

The important point discussed were :

1. Why should immunization be done.
2. Healthy child.
3. Protection against polio/T.B., etc.

The immunization schedule was explained in detail by Rekha. The rubella vaccine for adolescent girls and the Hepatitis B vaccine were also talked about. A definition on immunization was evolved from the group.

Definition : Vaccination is given for prevention of those diseases which are life threatening.

Next Session : Family Planning

The birth of a child: Fate Vs self-decision and desire.

The girls deliberated on the importance of Family Planning, lack of which would cause many problems like:

- No education for children
- Poor dietary intake.
- Economic resource crunch
- Unhappiness
- Mental tension
- Cannot attain goals and objectives.

They linked the effect this would have on society:

- no employment
- pollution
- fights
- will not have equality
- lack of fuel/energy
- will not be able to meet needs of people
- hunger
- dissatisfied society.

Going back to the five fingers discussed in the beginning for the session on goal setting. The trainees reiterated the significance of the following :

- Why — small family
- Who — husband/wife
- When — according to their wish.
- How — using contraceptive.
- What — condom, pills, copper T, operation.

Day IV : Session after lunch

Neomi gave detailed information about condoms, oral pills, copper T, Vasectomy/Tubectomy

Neomi actually showed the participants of a model of a male organ.

Neomi asked them to see the expiry date of the condom and proceeded to demonstrate how a condom is used and taken out. I noticed that the girls were hesitant to touch the condom, slowly they got over their hesitation, and started feeling comfortable about it.

It was quite amazing to see the openness of the girls as earlier in June this group was extremely shy and reticent to share any information about themselves.

Some of the characteristics of this group which attributed to their low participation, poor attendance, lack of continuity in the programme were they belonged to the economically weaker sections of society, were school drop-outs and had to help in the domestic chores with the mother.

Copper T-advantages and disadvantages

Use copper T only after one child

- Fitted into the uterus, for three years.
- One thread/cord has to be put.
- Inserted by trained Health staff
- Put this in at PHC and not at home.
- Pain in the waist – use copper T after one child, unexpected periods, going to an untrained midwife can cause injury.

Day IV. .After noon session., (14th Nov.)

Neomi —trainer, at Dhukane, session on contraceptives.

Vasectomy operation for men and women.

Reproductive health, Pratima, Rekha, Neomi.

- Growth of organs
- Are our reproductive organs healthy.
- Scrotal sacs of the male-in sound condition or not
- No pain
- No disease in private parts
- How can menstruation be regulated, regularized.

In order to get the participation of the girls the trainers asked them to share what are the problems experienced by women related to reproductive organs.

- Burning in urine
- Spots and irritation in the vaginal area
- White water discharge with bad smell
- Secretion of pus
- Irregular periods
- Pain

The aim was to show the adolescent girls what happens when the reproductive organs are not healthy. This led to the participants wanting more information on the male and female reproductive organs. A chart was put in the center of the room and the participants stood all around. Pratima explained the female organs to them and then the girls were asking to see the male organs with great enthusiasm. After that she explained how the egg formed in the ovaries moves to the fallopian tube and gets fertilized in the uterus.

Reproduction was explained in detail, about the division of the egg, about identical twins. One of the girls asked how can one tell l whether it is a girl or boy once the egg gets fertilized ? how this is determined. Does a woman determine the sex of the child ? Some other important questions asked during the sessions were :

Question : What are X and Y chromosomes?

Question : Why are women held responsible for the sex of the child?

Question : A married woman who has her period and she doesn't conceive, why?

Question : A woman repeatedly has daughters is it destiny or her fault?

Question : A menstruating woman who has repeated miscarriages, why?

Question : Why do children die after child-birth?

- poor maternal health, anaemic, repeated pregnancies, overworked, mentally tense, poor nutrition.
- low birth weight of baby.
- diarrhoea.
- any other infection.
- hole in the heart (which is rare).

Infant mortality rate in 0-1 year old is high due to diarrhoea, other causes being low birth weight, premature baby etc.

1. Mother's diet is poor and this leads to low birth weight.
2. Tetanus
3. Diarrohea
4. Delivery practices like smearing the lips with blood and other taboos of food intake post delivery make the mother who is breast feeding weak and this affects the baby also.

Next Session : RTIS, URIS, STD, AIDS

Day 5 : Prayer, recap of day 4 as well as of the whole workshop was done.

Some questions that the girls asked were read out:

- If there is bleeding from the gums , is it dangerous?
- Why is there excessive pain during menstruation ?
- Can you have sex during the periods?
- If you have small spots and itching in your vagina is it STD?
- Why is there burning in the urine?

One of the girls had a hysterical fit and kept crying. When she stopped, Pratima explained to all the girls the importance of sharing one's emotions and feelings with others or even writing it down to feel lighter! Girls are socialized to hold things and not express and sometimes all this gets too much and an individual loses control. Tears are a great reliever.

After five days of being together there are a lot of feelings and emotions that have got aroused. There is so much knowledge that the girls have received, they have had opportunities to laugh open up, ask questions, express themselves. They have talked of issues like menstruation, sex, intercourse, masturbation, their own sexuality and all this perhaps was like a 'dam' breaking on the fifth day. Many girls were crying at the thought of going away after this '5 day camp'. They had developed a close contact with the trainers Pratima, Rekha, Radha, Lalita, Neomi who they saw as role models, who share knowledge and skills, they had fascinated them, and in whom in a way they saw their freedom. Perhaps this long journey from 'silence' to 'openness' is a milestone in the creation of Yuvati Shikshan Kendra for the adolescent girls of Uttaranchal. For Pratima and me seeing this group so 'opened up' was indeed a special experience, our first meeting with them on June 21st at Kasialekh was a monologue with 90 per cent of the girls just looking at the floor. What also emerged was the strong bonds that had developed between the girls of different villages - they felt like " Partners in a common destiny".

Pratima shared her vision with the girls, that of having a newsletter of Yuvati Shikshan Kendra where in the girls can write in to the center and keep in touch by sharing what they are doing now. This batch would be the 2nd batch of 2002.

10.50 a.m. Post test difficult words, ejaculation, menstruation etc.

The participants were administered the same pre-test and given fifteen minutes to complete it. At a cursory glance it was observed that the post-test scores were good but since a number of participants in this group had low educational level, some questions were not easily understood by them. Pratima discussed each question in detail and cleared their doubts, so that they went back from the workshop with clarity about the information received.

12 noon: Towards a bright future.

Participants were divided into four groups according to their villages:

1. Gazar.
2. Sunakhiya.
3. Chaukota.
4. Bana.

They were asked to develop a plan of how they would share this information with the community and make a presentation before the group.

5th day : Last Session

Four groups made their presentations. They beautifully illustrated the arrangements of the workshop.

All the groups had given a name to their group.

The salient points that emerged during presentation were :

1. Create an environment of equality in the village.
2. Create a peaceful environment in the village.
3. Make a group of adolescent girls in which there were 10-20 girls in the age group of 13-20.
4. Choose a safe and secure place for meetings in which we can sit and talk comfortably.
5. We will talk without hesitation in the group.
6. Go door to door and collect girls.
7. Understand their problems and try to solve them with their participation.
8. We will make our future plans when all the girls have got together. It will be consensus planning.
9. While making our plan we will answer the following, why, who, how when and what.
10. We will keep time in mind while making our future plans, and decide how long we will keep our group going.
11. Our motto will be total participation of each member of the group.

12. All suggestions of each girl will be incorporated in our planning for the future.
13. We will make the future plans of our group according to the interests and needs of the adolescent girls.
14. We will give them information about health, cleanliness and share about ourselves and our failures with them.

An evaluation of the workshop was done by asking the participants to list:

- One aspect of the arrangements.
- About the content.
- About the trainees.
- Any other.
- Appreciated the nature of the trainers.
- Enjoyed themselves because of this opportunity.
- Could not sleep at night, too excited.
- Liked the content of the workshop.

One girl said she did not like the session on physical or sexual relations between man and woman. She does not understand all this, however liked the session of menstruation and found it very useful.

The more educated girls said that they were disappointed that trainees from Delhi had not come.

REFERENCES

Bannerjee, B.G. & R. Jalota, 1988, *Folk Illness and Ethnomedicine,* Northern Book Centre, New Delhi.

Bhatia, J., 1993, "Levels and Causes of Maternal Mortality in Southern India, in Studies, in *Family Planning* 25 (5): 310-318.

Bisht, L.S. 1988, "Cultural Perspective of Kumaon: Folk Songs, Dances and Literature", in *Valdiya, ibid.*

Capila, Anjali, 2002: *Images of Women in the Folk Songs of Garhwal Himalayas,* Concept, New Delhi.

Chatterjee, Meera, 1988: *Implementing Health Policy,* Manohar, New Delhi.

Das, Abhijit and Jasodhra Dasgupta, 1997: *A study of the status of women's health in Uttrakhand.*

Dumont, L., 1970, *Homo Hierarchus,* University of Chicago press, Chicago.

Farah, Francois, 2002, *Keynote address,* Third Raushni Deshpande Memorial Lecture, Lady Irwin College, New Delhi.

Gopalan, Sarla, Mira Shiva, Eds. 2000, "National Profile on Women, Health and Development", *VHAI* and *WHO* New Delhi.

Huff, Elizabeth, 2002, "Status of Mother and Child Health Management Practices in Kumaon Hills", *Internship assignment* with CHIRAG, from MSU, USA in Study Abroad Programme with Lady Irwin College.

Illich, Ivan : 1976: *Limits to Medicine,* Mario Boyars, London.

Jalal, D.S. 1988, "Kumaun: The Geographical Perspective", in *Valdiya, ibid.*

Janet Chawla : "Mythic Origins of Menstrual Taboos in Rig Veda" *EPW,* Oct.22, 1994.

Jeffery, P., and R. Jeffery and A. Lyon, 1989, *Labor Pains and Labor Power: Women and Childbearing in India,* London, Zed Books.

Joshi, Archana *et.al., Socio-Cultural Implications of Menstruation and Menstrual Problems on Rural Women's lives and Treatment Seeking Behavior* – Operation Research Group, Baroda, 1996.

Joshi, Maheshwar P. 1988 , "Kumaon: Archaeological and Historical Perspective", in *Valdiya, ibid.*

Joshi, P, 1993, "Culture, Health and Illness: Aspects of Ethnomedicine in Jausar-Bawar", in *The Central Himalayan Panorama,* S.K. Biswas, ed. The Institute of Social Research and Applied Anthropology, Calcutta.

Kakar, S. 1982, *Shamans, Mystics and Doctors,* Alfred Knopf, New York.

Kapadia, Adrian : *The Vulnerability of Power: Puberty Rituals – 'Shiv and her sisters'.*

Karkal, Malini, 1995, "Our Health: How Does it Count?- An Overview", in *Our Lives, Our Health,* ed. Karkal, Malini, Coordination Unit, World Conference on Women – Beijing 1995.

Kaur, M., G. Sisodia and S. Mehra, "Customary Practices Observed in Birth and Upbringing of Children – A study in a village of Haryana, *Indian* and Upbringing of Children – A study in a village of Haryana, *Indian Journal of Social Work*, 42(1), 75-79.

Khanka, S.S. 1988 , "Demographic Profile of Kumaun", in *Valdiya*, ibid.

Khetwal, Nirmal, 1980, *Impact of Community Development Programmes*, Unpublished thesis, Kumaun Univer. Nainital.

Kumar, Karen Trollope, 1990, "Traditional Birth Attendant Practices in Garhwal", paper presented at a seminar.

Kutumbiah, P., 1962, *Ancient Indian Medicine*, Orient Longmans, New Delhi.

Lall, Kanai, 1987, *Concept Paper* for CHIRAG and Annual Reports, Sitla, Kumaon Hills.

MATRIKA REPORT, 1999, A Celebration of Indigenous Reproductive Health Knowledge – Matrika Dai Mela, New Delhi.

Mehta, Jeejebhoy, 1996, "Aodelscent Girls in Slums", *CWDS*, New Delhi.

Mukherjee, Chowdhary, 1986, *Studies on Fertility Rates Based on the Socio-Economic Survey*, Haranand Pub. New Delhi.

Mukhopadhyay, A. 1992. *State of India's Health*. Voluntary Health Association of India.

N.K. Sethi; Ali, Almas; Kapilashrami, M.C.:2001, " Health Constraints of Uttaranchal; Population Stabilization of related Developmental Issues", *Seminar* Paper at Dehradun.

NCERT, 1999, *Adolescence Education in Schools*, New Delhi.

NIPCCD, 1999, "National Consultation Meet on Integrated Child Development Services and Reproductive and Child Health Programmes", *A Report*.

NIPCCD, 1998, "National Convention on Family Life Education: Emerging Challenges", *A Report*.

Pande, G.C. 1988 , "Role and Status of Women in Kumaun", in *Valdiya, ibid.*

Pande, G.C., 1986, "Educational Investment: Need for Change in Policy", *Southern Economist*, 24(23):13-17.

Pandey, P.C. 1978, Study of Changes in Economic Conditions of Scheduled Castes in Kumaun, *Unpublished Thesis*, *ibid.*

Pathak, Shekhar, 1988, "Kumauni Society Through the Ages", in *Valdiya, ibid.*

Pugh, Judy. 2000. *Lecture at Michigan State University.*

Rangan, Haripriya, 2001, *Of Myth and Movements – Rewriting CHIPKO Himalayan history*, OUP, New Delhi.

Sandhu, R.S., 1980, "Rites de Passage of some Scheduled Castes: Pregnancy and Birth Rites, *Eastern Anthropologist*, 24(2): 181-195.

Saxena, D.N. *Report of Family Planning and Fertility* Survey, Lucknow Univ.

Schegal, 1995, *Rural Female Adolescence: Indian Scenario*, Deep and Deep Pub. New Delhi.

Shah, I.C.V. 1988 , "Traditional Folk Art of Kumaon: Varied Expressions", in *Valdiya, ibid.*

Sharma, D.D. 1988, "Kaumaoni Language and Dialects" in *Valdiya, ibid.*

Shireen, Jeejebhoy, 1996, "Adolescent Sexual and Reproductive Behavior: A Review of the Evidence From India", *ICMR* Pûb.

Srivstava, 1979, "Incidence of Child Marriage, Widowhood, and Divorce Among Females", Occassional Papers 21, *Population Research Centre*, Lucknow.

Swain, S., 1978, "Customs and Beliefs Associated with Pregnancy and Child-birth in Rural Orissa." *Indian Journal of Social Work*, 39(1):80-84.

Thaddeus, S., and D. Maine, 1994, "Too Far to Walk: Maternal Mortality in Context." *Social Science Med.* Vol. 38(8): 1091-1110.

Tripathi, Beena, 1980, *Fertility Patterns in Kumaun*, Unpublished thesis, Kumaun Univ. Nainital.

UNFPA, 2000, " The Sexual and Reproductive Health of Adolescents: A Review of UNFPA Assistance."

UNFPA,1998, " South Asia Conference of Adolescents", *India Country Paper*.

Valdiya, K.S. ed. *Kumaun - Land and people*, 1988, Gyanodya Prakashan, Nainital, Uttaranchal.

Veena Poonacha, "Rites de passage of Matrescence and Social Construction of Motherhood Coorgs in South India – *EPW*, Jan.18, 1997.

VHAI - *State of Health in Uttar Pradesh: Health Status and Socio-Economic Development:* 1995: Lucknow.

Walsh, J., & C. Feifer, A. Measham and P. *Gertler, Disease Control Prioities in Developing Countries*, D. Jamieson et. Al., eds. Oxford University Press, London.

Werner, D & Bower, B. 1995. *Helping health workers learn: A book of methods, aids, and ideas for instructors at the village level.* Palo Alto: The Hesperian Foundation.

WHO,- 1998-99, "Reproductive Health Research at WHO: a new beginning". Biennial Report.

WHO, 2000, " Population and Reproductive Health, Facts on India", *Briefing Kit*.

WHO, 2000, " Special Bulletin on Reproductive Health", *International Journal of Public Health*, Vol.XXXIII, No.5.

Zysk, K., 1991, *Asceticism and Healing in Ancient*, Oxford University Press, Oxford.

INDEX